THE BIOHACKER'S GUIDE
TO UPGRADED ENERGY & FOCUS

An Uncommon System to Rapidly Optimize
Physical and Mental Performance

Kaizen

The Japanese have a concept called Kaizen.

It means "constant improvement."

I verbally dictated most of this book. An editor then transcribed my ramblings and did her best to make them presentable. Over the next few months, I will be reintegrating my voice.

Publishing deadlines don't always allow as much time as we'd like for these things. Typos have inevitably found their way into The Guide. I'm thankful to you, my readers, for pointing many of them out.

At this time, some mistakes remain unnoticed. If you stumble across any typos, or corrections, please email them to anthony@ thehealthblueprint.com. I welcome your suggestions to help make this book better.

Think of The Biohacker's Guide as a constantly-improving and evolving work that we are creating together. In the meantime, please forgive any unintentional typographical errors made in an effort to get this information to you as fast as possible.

THE
BIOHACKER'S
GUIDE

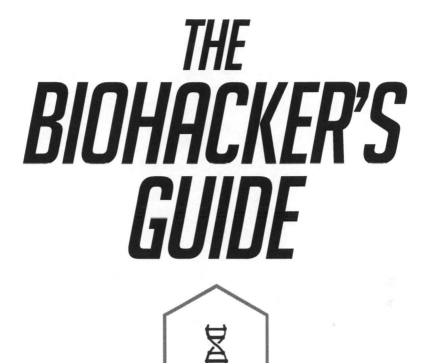

TO UPGRADED
ENERGY & FOCUS

Anthony DiClementi, CNS, NCSF-CPT
Specialist in Functional Medicine & Nutritional Neuroscience, Executive Wellness Coach

Warning & Disclaimer

The statements in this book have not been evaluated by the FDA (Food and Drug Administration). The information provided here is not intended to diagnose, treat, cure, or prevent any disease.

This book is not a substitute for a face to face consultation with your physician. It should not be construed as medical advice of any sort. I am not a doctor and I don't play one on the internet (or within the pages of this book). I am not recommending, endorsing, or supporting any of the substances or compounds (especially illegal) discussed or described in this book.

By using this information, or reading it, you're accepting responsibility for your own health, health-related decisions, and expressly release Biohacking Secrets, the Health Blueprint, and the employees of both organizations, partners, and vendors from any and all liability whatsoever, including that arising from negligence.

If you do not agree to the conditions stated above, stop reading now.

This book contains highly sensitive information and, if misinterpreted or misused, can lead to serious injury, illness, or even death. One last time, for the folks at legal:

Do not use any of the substances, products, or practices mentioned in this guide without first consulting a medical professional.

The topics discussed herein are for <u>information purposes only</u>.

Consider yourself warned.

ACKNOWLEDGMENTS

So many people make a book: the editors, the doctors, the scientists, my clients, my staff, my family, and you - the reader. Thank you.

I would also like to thank my mentors (both virtual and in real life): Russell Brunson, Richard Branson, Tony Robbins, Tim Ferriss, Elon Musk, Chris Kresser, Marc Cuban, Mark Hyman, Scth Godin, John Berardi, Bill Phillips, Eric Braverman, William Faloon, and Datis Kharrazian.

To all my clients past and present: A sincere thank you to all of you who didn't run away when I said, "Today we are going to try an experiment."

To my parents, who taught me hard work pays off, treat others the way I want to be treated and stand up for those who cannot stand up for themselves.

I also want to say thank you to Everte Farnell, the direct response copywriter that helped to make this book easier for you to read and understand. You can find more about him at www.EverteFarnell.com.

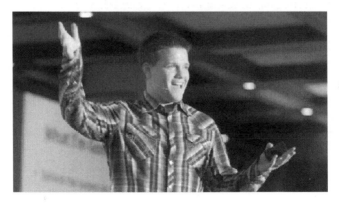

Finally, you can't expect people to read a book if they don't know it's out there. That's where my friend, business partner, and marketing savant, Russell Brunson, comes in.

Russell, to you especially, I owe my thanks and much of my success. You believed in this before anyone. I've got your back for life.

TABLE OF CONTENTS

BONUS

INTRODUCTION

CHILLIN' WITH MR. FREEZE

On a cool November Monday in Chicago I was feeling both nervous and excited as I stepped out of my 2012 Jeep Wrangler Unlimited and walked towards the entrance of Chicago Cryospa. I couldn't help but wonder if Nike sweat shorts and flip flops would appropriately fit the dress code for the occasion.

I was meeting with celebrity trainer and owner of Chicago's only cryotherapy center, Jim Karas. Jim helped get Hugh Jackman ready for his role as Wolverine in the first X-Men movie. And his true claim to fame was helping Diane Sawyer get in the best shape of her life.

The plan was for both of us to "Cryo" and then sit down for an interview.

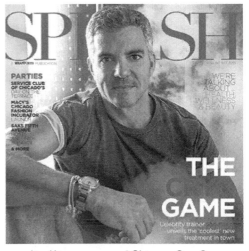

Jim Karas, owner of Chicago CryoSpa

If you're unfamiliar with cryotherapy, it's a process where you immerse the body in a liquid nitrogen chamber that chills the air to a negative 250° Fahrenheit. After a brief three minutes, the surface of your skin will sit somewhere between 20-50°(f).

Why would people subject themselves to such madness?

The reported benefits of cryotherapy include:

- Muscle and joint repair
- Restoration and faster recovery from exercise and injuries
- Weight loss
- Increased metabolic rate
- Improved mitochondrial function and biogenesis
- Anti-aging
- Ward off depression

As I entered the facility, I was greeted by a man with salt and pepper hair. He held a striking resemblance to George Clooney, but with a slightly more ethnic look.

Jim was in his mid-fifties, but didn't look a day over 40. He was wearing a tank top, workout shorts, and what looked like two sets of white tube socks underneath a pair of New Balance flip flops.

"You've got me until 1 p.m." Jim said, "and then I've got to run." He told me he had a haircut and another meeting scheduled. The next thing I knew, an attractive blonde quickly ushered us into a side room, where we were instructed to take off all of our clothes except for our boxers, and put on two pairs of socks and two pairs of white, cotton gloves. On top of the two pairs of cotton gloves, Jim added a third pair of Gore-Tex winter gloves.

A curious look must have come across my face because Jim's assistant said, "He has Raynaud's disease." Raynaud's is a circulatory condition where cold temperatures cause numbness, tingling, and achiness in the extremities, particularly the fingers and toes.

Jim went first, and he seemed entirely unfazed by the negative 250° temperatures. He carried on a conversation the entire time, never skipping a beat. He got me up to speed on the benefits of cryotherapy, his background, and the multitude of celebrities who had come through his doors. Most recently, entrepreneur, author, and peak performance strategist, Tony Robbins, stopped in. He was in Chicago for his "Unleashing the Power Within" event. In the midst of our conversation, the timer let off a loud ding, which prompted Jim's assistant, Kristen, to fire a pistol-like laser at his shin. "We take a temperature reading of the skin because it's vital that it gets down below 50 degrees to achieve the therapeutic benefits," she said. Jim's shin registered at 47°.

Now it was my turn.

I stepped into the chamber. It had a striking resemblance to a standup tanning bed with the top cut off.

Kristen then lowered the floor to ensure that my entire body was submerged with the exception of my head. "Make sure you're not touching the sides," she said, "or you can burn your skin."

I could feel cold air start to swirl around my body. An ominous mist rose from the chamber, like something from a horror movie or an early 90's rave.

Following Jim's lead, I attempted to maintain conversation throughout, but I quickly found that it required every ounce of conscious relaxation and deep breathing to keep my jaw from chattering like one of those windup toys.

Then, almost as quickly as it began, the timer sounded and Kristen opened the chamber door.

"That's it?"

"That's it," Kristen replied.

At first, there were no perceived changes in my physical or emotional state. As we sat down in Jim's office, he opened up about the strategies he uses to stay young along with the tragic events that ushered him into the health field. Both of Jim's parents passed away at a young age due to health complications. Despite this seeming genetic handicap, he believes, with a compelling certainty, that he will live to 100 and beyond.

"You can control aging, or you can let aging control you," he said. "Most people spend their lives reacting. The key to success lies in your routine. Tell me what someone does with the first 60 to 90 minutes of their day,

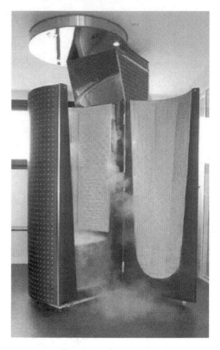

The Juka Cryosauna
(www.BiohackingSecrets.com/cryo)

and I can tell you the type of person they are."

Jim recommends planning everything, from sleep to workouts, meals, even relaxation. It's a concept that he explores in more detail in his book *"The Business Plan for the Body."* Here are just a few of the things Jim and I discussed that afternoon.

He refuses to drink water or tea without fresh-squeezed juice from an organic lemon or lime.

Many of his clients are baby boomers, and he is a big advocate of strength training. He shuns any form of cardio (this is one of the few areas where we did not see eye to eye).

Besides doing cryotherapy at least 5 days a week, other aspects of Jim's routine to which he attributes his health and vitality are an abstinence from caffeine and an uncompromising priority given to sleep.

He usually goes to bed at 9 p.m. and is up around 6 a.m., getting 8 to 8 ½ hours of sleep nightly.

In the afternoon, he naps. Usually for 20 to 30 minutes, never more. Why? Because, after 30 minutes, the body moves into a deeper, REM sleep state and you wake up feeling more tired than before you laid down in the first place.

"Most importantly," he says, "I put the right food in my body. After researching and having direct exposure to hundreds of diets over the past 27 years," he continued, "at least 50% of your diet has to come from plants. And you want those plants to be organic. If you are overweight, have high blood pressure, or have any other metabolic issue, most of those plants should be vegetables."

It was then that Jim looked down at his watch and said, "Oh shit! I've got to go. Give me a call if you have any questions or if there's anything that I can help with."

As Jim jogged up the stairs and out the front door, two things occurred to me.

The first was that I felt incredibly focused and energized.

The second was a realization that we have a lot more control over our body, health, and aging than we once thought.

It's inspiring to be around women and men who are living proof that our biological age does not have to linearly track with our chronological age. It's liberating to realize that our genes are a comparatively small part of the equation.

In life, there are things we can control, and things we have no control over. At the end of the day, we all choose what goes into our body, how we move our body, and the thoughts we allow into our mind.

THE TRUTH ABOUT BIOHACKING

"The higher your energy level, the more efficient your body. The more efficient your body, the better you feel and the more you will use your talent to produce outstanding results."

- Tony Robbins

As I write this, in my Chicago high-rise apartment, I have two, small infrared lights in my nose.

Inside the left nostril, an LED (a little smaller than a piece of candy corn) emits an infrared light with an 810 nm wavelength. These wavelength and power density parameters enable photons to reach my brain's ventral areas which are responsible for cognition, motivation, and motor control. The neurotransmitter dopamine is also produced here.

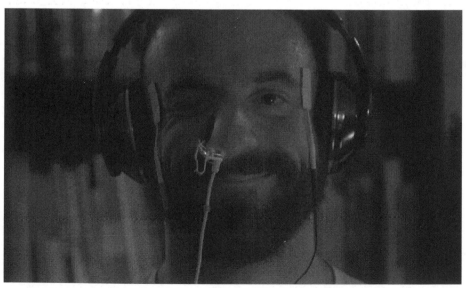

A normal day in my Chicago high-rise apartment.

INTRODUCTION

A study at the University of Texas found this type of infrared energy stimulation produces beneficial effects on frontal cortex functions such as sustained attention, working memory, and effective state. This helps us release the calming feel good chemical serotonin (the same neurotransmitter targeted by prescription antidepressants like Prozac).

This frequency is also associated with brain oscillation in the alpha state. Alpha waves help us to achieve a relaxed focus and concentration, without the jitters. Using EEG technology, scientists have found alpha brainwaves to be elevated in monks during periods of meditation.

Inside the right nostril, rests a virtually identical LED light emitting a 655 nm wavelength. This device utilizes a low level laser diode to release coherent light in the visible red spectrum. This laser is powered by a calculated dosage of energy to irradiate the capillary-rich nasal cavity.

If that all sounds like a foreign language to you, congratulations, you're normal. It will make more sense soon.

The 655 nm wavelengths are effective for circulatory and immune system enhancement.

They have been shown to improve blood flow by reducing the "stickiness" of red blood cells, decrease inflammation, cleanse the blood of viruses and bacteria, and enhance cellular energy (ATP) production.

Why stick lights up my nose? Why take supplements by the dozen?

Why not just eat right and exercise?

Really, is all this "biohacking" even necessary?

The unbridled truth is, we are moving further and further away from nature. Biohacks are designed to mimic what we should be getting naturally. The most important biohacks replicate, but are almost always

Augmentation of cognitive brain functions with transcranial lasers

F. Gonzalez-Lima* and Douglas W. Barrett

Department of Psychology and Institute for Neuroscience, University of Texas at Austin, Austin, TX, USA
*Correspondence: gonzalezlima@utexas.edu

Edited by:
Mikhail Lebedev, Duke University, USA

Reviewed by:
Julio C. Rojas, University of Texas Southwestern Medical Center, USA
John Mitrofanis, University of Sydney, Australia

Keywords: cognitive enhancement, cytochrome oxidase, low-level light therapy, brain stimulation, photoneuromodulation

Discovering that transcranial infrared laser stimulation produces beneficial effects on frontal cortex functions such as sustained attention, working memory, and affective state has been groundbreaking. Transcranial laser stimulation with low-power density (mW/cm^2) and high-energy density (J/cm^2) monochromatic light in the near-infrared wavelengths modulates brain functions and may produce neurotherapeutic effects in a nondestructive and non-thermal manner (Lampl, 2007; Hashmi et al., 2010). Barrett and Gonzalez-Lima (2013) provided the first controlled study showing that transcranial laser stimulation improves human cognitive and emotional brain functions.

different functions related to sensory and motor systems.

BRAIN BIOENERGETICS

The way that near-infrared lasers and light-emitting diodes (LEDs) interact with brain function is based on bioenergetics, a mechanism that is fundamentally different than that of other brain stimulation methods such as electric and magnetic stimulation. LLLT has been found to modulate the function of neurons in cell cultures, brain function in animals, and cognitive and emotional functions in healthy persons and clinical conditions. Photoneuromodulation involves the absorption of photons by specific

increases, the more metabolic energy that is produced via mitochondrial oxidative phosphorylation. LLLT supplies the brain with metabolic energy in a way analogous to the conversion of nutrients into metabolic energy, but with light instead of nutrients providing the source for ATP-based metabolic energy (Mochizuki-Oda et al., 2002). If an effective near-infrared light energy dose is supplied, it stimulates brain ATP production (Lapchak and De Taboada, 2010) and blood flow (Uozumi et al., 2010), thereby fueling ATP-dependent membrane ion pumps, leading to greater membrane stability and resistance to depolarization, which has been shown to transiently reduce neu-

inferior to, the benefits we would experience living a more natural, ancestral lifestyle:

– The most nutrient dense superfoods will always be local, organic plants and animals that haven't been hosed down with chemicals, genetically modified in a laboratory, or fed unnatural garbage those same animals would not eat in nature. They will never be some bar, powder, or gel.

– Movement is the best form of exercise. Master your own body weight. Get your heart rate up and sweat. You don't need a gym, or expensive fitness equipment. You do need to get off your ass and move.

Biochemical Pharmacology 86 (2013) 447–457

Contents lists available at SciVerse ScienceDirect

Biochemical Pharmacology

journal homepage: www.elsevier.com/locate/biochempharm

Neurological and psychological applications of transcranial lasers and LEDs

Julio C. Rojas [a,b], F. Gonzalez-Lima [a,*]

[a] Departments of Psychology, Pharmacology and Toxicology, University of Texas at Austin, Austin, TX 78712, USA
[b] Department of Neurology and Neurotherapeutics, University of Texas Southwestern Medical Center, Dallas, TX 75235, USA

ARTICLE INFO

Article history:
Received 8 May 2013
Accepted 15 June 2013
Available online 24 June 2013

Keywords:
Cognitive enhancement
Cytochrome oxidase
Low-level light therapy
Methylene blue
Neuroprotection
Photobiomodulation

ABSTRACT

Transcranial brain stimulation with low-level light/laser therapy (LLLT) is the use of directional low-power and high-fluency monochromatic or quasimonochromatic light from lasers or LEDs in the red-to-near-infrared wavelengths to modulate a neurobiological function or induce a neurotherapeutic effect in a nondestructive and non-thermal manner. The mechanism of action of LLLT is based on photon energy absorption by cytochrome oxidase, the terminal enzyme in the mitochondrial respiratory chain. Cytochrome oxidase has a key role in neuronal physiology, as it serves as an interface between oxidative energy metabolism and cell survival signaling pathways. Cytochrome oxidase is an ideal target for cognitive enhancement, as its expression reflects the changes in metabolic capacity underlying higher-order brain functions. This review provides an update on new findings on the neurotherapeutic applications of LLLT. The photochemical mechanisms supporting its cognitive-enhancing and brain-stimulatory effects in animal models and humans are discussed. LLLT is a potential non-invasive treatment for cognitive impairment and other deficits associated with chronic neurological conditions, such as large vessel and lacunar hypoperfusion or neurodegeneration. Brain photobiomodulation with LLLT is paralleled by pharmacological effects of low-dose USP methylene blue, a non-photic electron donor with the ability to stimulate cytochrome oxidase activity, redox and free radical processes. Both interventions provide neuroprotection and cognitive enhancement by facilitating mitochondrial respiration, with hormetic dose-response effects and brain region activational specificity. This evidence supports enhancement of mitochondrial respiratory function as a generalizable therapeutic principle relevant to highly adaptable systems that are exquisitely sensitive to energy availability such as the nervous system.

- Swimming in lakes, rivers and the ocean is the best form of grounding/earthing, reducing static electrical charge, and the subsequent inflammation that comes with our lack of contact with the Earth. That's why a good surf clears the mind. Take your shoes off. Get outside. Jump in a lake.
- Meditation is more effective than any visual, auditory, or electrical brain entrainment device you can strap to your head
- Exposing your eyes and skin to natural sunlight is better than any photobiomodulation-based technology or vitamin D supplement scientists could ever engineer.
- The best drinking water is pristine spring water from deep within the earth.

- We can't biohack or artificially outsmart the physical and cognitive degradation that takes place when we sleep for less than 7 hours. No supplement, polyphasic regimen, smartphone app or heart rate viability device can offset insufficient sleep.
- And the list goes on and on.

Look, my apartment is overflowing with a smorgasbord of biohacking tools, technologies, and devices. I love this stuff as much as you do. But before you strap on the electrodes and become an N of 1, you should have a clear understanding for why you're doing it in the first place.

For maximum results, you must see the forest for the trees.

Once you understand your desired outcomes, design an experiment. Measure. Track. That's how you'll know if it's working or if you're just some goofy douchebag with a red light up his nose ☺.

Most importantly, have fun.

This life goes by pretty fast. Enjoy the shit out of it. Tomorrow is never guaranteed. A lot of times we take ourselves too damn seriously. At the end of the day, the reason we are doing this stuff is because we want to be, do, and have more. We all want to feel good. Do more of the things that make you feel good. And do them more often.

The method of Biohacking is to strategically change your internal and external environment to rapidly enhance the body, upgrade the brain, and create an epic life. It is the art and science of optimizing human performance.

Biohacking embraces self-experimentation. It is the utilization of scientific methodology to identify the fastest, most effective strategies to create a desired end result. The essence of Biohacking is to focus on constant improvement while enjoying life where you're at right now.

Whether you're already a rockstar looking for that extra edge in your life, or your energy sucks, you're 100 pounds over weight and can barely move right now... there's something here for you.

USE IT OR LOSE IT

They say you don't know what you've got 'til it's gone.

Energy is like that. It's like air. When you have it, you don't notice it. When it's gone, you can't think about anything else.

I place great importance on energy because there was a time when I had none. I could sleep 12 hours and still wake up tired. I felt like I had early onset dementia. I would misplace my keys and forget people's names that I had just met. I would read pages in a book and not remember what I had just read.

I'll tell you more about how I found the solution in a few pages, but for now...

...I remember the first day it started. A group of my friends and I planned to go hiking. I've always been an outdoors kind of guy... hiking, biking, surfing. You name it and I love to do it.

Anyway, I woke up that morning and just didn't feel right. I was tired and a little achy. I called one of my friends in the group and told him I thought I was coming down with a cold and wasn't going to make it. I was a personal trainer and in great shape at the time, so I figured I just needed a couple days of rest.

That was Saturday. Sunday I felt the same.

I did everything you're supposed to do when you have a cold, but by Monday I was worse. A week later I was so foggy headed and tired I could barely make it through my client meeting for the week. I went to two doctors that week who said I likely had some virus. They told me to sleep and it would pass.

Two weeks later I wasn't any better. Heck, I might have been worse.

I was sleeping 12 hours a night and could barely get out of bed. And the brain fog... sometimes I felt like I might forget my own name.

After a month of this I knew something was very wrong. I went to see doctor after doctor, and they all said the same thing. They had no idea what the problem was.

Finally, desperate and disillusioned with the medical system, I started my own research. After months of scouring the internet and the library, sorting the information from the bullshit, and finding every possible cause of my problem, I had a diagnosis.

It was a self-diagnosis, but it was better than the doctors had done to that point. There was no test to con rm my diagnosis, so I had to test it for myself. I made radical dietary and lifestyle changes. Within a few days, I was starting to feel better.

Thanks to Lyme Disease, for almost two years I felt like a shadow of myself. It wasn't until I had my health stripped from me that I came to realize the irreplaceable role energy plays in our lives. If you don't have any energy:

- You're not going to have passion in your romantic relationships.
- You're not going to be able to meet, attract, and keep the quality of person that you deserve to be with.
- You're not going to be able to do a great job with your kids so that they can grow up and create happy, healthy lives for themselves. You won't be able to be the example for them that you know you're capable of being. Your kids will run circles around you and you're not going to be able to keep up.
- You're not going to be able to run your own business, or at least not at the level that you could otherwise.

ENERGY IS LIFE. ENERGY IS EVERYTHING.

This book is the result of my obsessive quest to identify which small, easy-to-implement changes produce the most powerful increases in energy and focus. Its purpose is to empower ordinary people, like you and me, to perform with superhuman stamina, strength, and focus by mastering a few extraordinary skills.

Why do the approaches within *"The Biohacker's Guide to Upgraded Energy and Focus"* work where others fail? It's because the changes I recommend in this guide are small or simple, and very often, both. I address the two biggest challenges we face today when we are trying to find effective ways to increase our energy.

The first challenge is misinformation. The explosion of the Internet has opened the door for anyone with a Wordpress website to share their two pennies. Accountability is lacking. As a result, much of the information on the web has little basis in the scientific literature or real-world "in the trenches" experience. I have made every effort to meticulously cite studies, research, and other credible sources throughout this book. On top of that, everything you read within these pages are strategies that I have personally used myself and taught to hundreds of clients in my executive coaching program.

The second problem is that generic recommendations yield generic results. Extraordinary energy, enhanced focus, and optimal performance are a product of expert customization. Your best results will always come from a custom-tailored program built based upon your:

- Age
- Gender
- Weight
- Body type

– Health status
– Genetic blueprint
– Goals
– Lifestyle
– Preferences

This is why entrepreneurs, executives, athletes, and celebrities fly around the world and pay $100,000 or more to work with me one-on-one. Working with me, they achieve that peak level of performance that only comes with a customized program.

I work with executives, entrepreneurs, world class athletes, Hollywood celebrities, and Fortune 500 corporations...

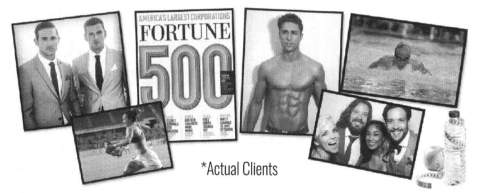

*Actual Clients

I've put everything I know into this book. The process I go through, the techniques I use, and the scientific studies I rely on.

First, I'll walk you through the foundational elements that are critical for having high levels of energy, focus, and health. Using Pareto's principle, these are the 20% that will produce 80% of your results. I always start by making sure my clients have the Foundation in place.

Next, we troubleshoot.

I help you to identify the most common, overlooked energy vampires that may be holding you back from the energy, focus, and performance you deserve. I even provide you with some of the same diagnostic tools and functional tests that I use with my clients so that you can pinpoint what may be keeping you stuck.

Then, I outline a number of the most advanced, effective, and scientifically-supported strategies for overcoming those obstacles.

BECOMING LIMITLESS

"If you crossed Tony Robbins with Dr. Oz and Rocky, you'd end up with Anthony DiClementi. His ability to help even the most frustrated clients get insane results is second to none."

- Jessica Blagaich, Los Angeles, CA

I was an NCSF Certified Personal Trainer and AASDN Certified Nutrition Specialist with a growing executive wellness coaching practice before my health declined.

Like most experts in the industry, a lot of what I was doing to help my clients was based around nutrition and exercise. And many of my clients were getting great results. However, some, despite our best efforts, never seemed to progress. I had no idea at the time that I was only working with a tiny piece of the pie.

Suddenly, in 2011, I began noticing changes in my own health. At first, I started having trouble losing weight.

Then my energy took a nosedive. I became depressed. I lost my sex drive, which is a big deal for a guy. It's a big deal for anyone. I felt more alone than I'd felt at any point in my life because I didn't think I could share what I was experiencing with anyone. Who wants to work with a health and fitness expert whose health is in the gutter, and is getting

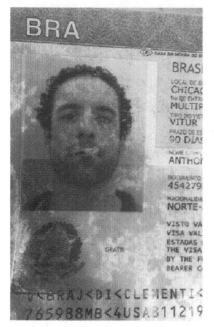

BRA

BRASI
LOCAL DE E
CHICAC
No DE ENTRA
MULTIP
TIPO DO VIST
VITUR
PRAZO DE ES
90 DIAS
NOME C
ANTHOI
DOCUMENTO
454279
NACIONALIDA
NORTE-
VISTO VA
VISA VAL
ESTADAS I
GRATIS
THE VISA
BY THE FI
BEARER O

V<BRAJ<DI<CLEMENTI<
765988MB<4USA311219

My Brazilian Visa photo in 2011. You can see my thinning, receding hairline and my dilapidated state of health.

worse, instead of better? How could I expect anyone to trust me with their health when I couldn't even fix myself? So I was keeping a lot of this close to my chest. I felt like I was on an island. Stranded and alone.

Things continued to get worse. Like I said earlier, I was seeing doctors but their efforts were no more effective than my own. The onslaught of tests kept coming back normal.

And then, I went on vacation with two of my best friends. We were in Rio De Janeiro, Brazil. My goal for the trip was to try and fake it so that my friends didn't realize what I was going through. I didn't want them to know that I was in rough shape and going through all this stuff because I didn't want to be a downer on their vacation.

After three or four days, I couldn't fake it anymore. I was in the hot tub with one of my best friends Joe when he looked at me and said, "What's going on man? Something's off."

I told him, while choking back the tears, "I know. But I don't know what to do about it. Trust me, I've been trying. This has been going on for months and it's getting worse. I'm seeing doctors. And no one's been able to help."

It was clear that I wasn't myself. Something was wrong. And Joe was the first person to say, "We gotta do something about this. We gotta get you better."

INTRODUCTION

That was my rock-bottom. I was at such a low point, that I didn't even have the energy to hide it anymore. And one of the closest people to me could see, clear as day, that I was struggling.

I felt like I'd had the curtains pulled back and the gig was up. Something had to be done.

After that, I dedicated my life to learning everything I could about Functional Medicine, nutritional neuroscience, and how to restore the body's ability to heal itself. I had no choice but to get to the root cause of what was holding me back. I read hundreds of books, research papers, and scientific journals. I consulted physicians, scientists, and experts in the world of peak performance.

A tremendous amount can be learned by studying the extremes. At one end of the spectrum, are individuals with chronic or degenerative conditions like dementia, Alzheimer's, Parkinson's, diabetes, autoimmunity, and chronic fatigue. At the other end, are people at the pinnacle of optimal performance and vitality. These are your professional athletes, top performers, and leaders in their respective fields.

If we understand what mechanisms allow us to move from one extreme to the other, the middle will take care of itself. In other words, the extremes inform the mean, but not vice versa.

This outside-in approach provided me with the tools and techniques to both heal people struggling with chronic, degenerative conditions and empower high performers to take their game to the next level.

For uncommon solutions, we have to look in uncommon places.

I worked with a number of the top functional medical practitioners in the United States. These doctors were using progressive treatment interventions to heal clients that the traditional medical system had turned its back on. In conventional medicine, one of the biggest problems is that they mostly focus on symptoms and diseases.

For example, if you go to the doctor and you have high cholesterol, you get a drug that lowers your cholesterol. If you go to the doctor and you have high blood pressure, you will normally receive a drug that lowers your blood pressure. They don't spend much time looking into why your blood pressure or cholesterol is high in the first place. The goal is just to bring the numbers down, and that's generally where things stop.

Functional medicine works in the opposite way. Rather than simply treating the symptoms, functional medicine seeks to uncover the root cause of the problem. Symptoms are important, of course. They give us clues that help us figure out what underlying mechanisms may be contributing to the problem. However, when you look at the root cause and fix that, the symptoms tend to resolve themselves.

Imagine someone has a thorn in their foot. There are a number of ways to ease their pain. For instance, you could apply a numbing agent, like novocaine, to the area surrounding the thorn. This would provide the patient with some degree of relief. However, in functional medicine, the goal is not to relieve the symptoms. The goal is to remove the thorn.

"Pain is temporary, It may last a minute, or an hour, or a day, or a year, but eventually it will subside and something else will take its place. If I quit, however, it lasts forever."

- Lance Armstrong

Case in point, I was diagnosed with chronic Lyme disease, which is known as "the great imitator" because it mimics the symptoms of over 200 other diseases. I had body aches, low energy, brain fog, and a laundry list of other health issues. I even had pre-diabetic blood sugar levels despite eating what I thought was a healthy diet.

It felt like I was operating at 10% capacity. A symptom-based treatment plan would have been like playing a game of Whack-A-Mole.

One of the doctors I worked with jokingly referred to me as Humpty Dumpty. He said, "You're so broke, we've got to put you back together piece by piece." That's kind of what happened. Every system in my body had started shutting down, and, one by one, we had to put them back together. Piece by piece, we had to rebuild my Foundation.

Here are the 7 areas I refer to as The Foundation to upgrading your energy and focus:

- Nutrition
- Movement
- Stress Management
- Sleep
- Supplements
- Hydration, Oxygenation, and Light
- Habits and Mindset

Once all of those pieces were in place, I then had to identify and eliminate those conditions that can suck the energy right out of us and destroy our ability to focus.

We do that in the Troubleshooting phase, where we strategically address any relevant limiting factors including:

- Gut dysfunction (digestive issues)
- Nutrient imbalances
- Toxic overload
- Low testosterone & HGH (Human Growth Hormone)
- Adrenal fatigue (HPA Access Dysregulation)
- Hypothyroidism
- Blood sugar and metabolic issues

- Neurotransmitter imbalances
- Chronic infections
- Brain inflammation
- Immune dysregulation (Inflammatory imbalance)
- Impaired methylation (and genetic mutations)
- Mitochondrial dysfunction
- Circulation and oxygen deliverability issues
- Poor posture, movement patterns, and bio-mechanics
- Estrogen dominance, elevated androgens, and PCOS (in women)

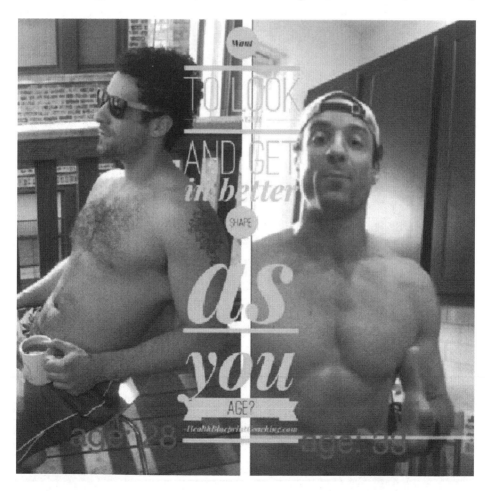

INTRODUCTION

By applying these uncommon strategies that I learned with the help of some of the top functional medicine practitioners in the world, I was able to start improving my situation. I began to feel my energy levels rise with each passing day.

As I continued to build and work through this unorthodox system, I was able to lose weight faster and easier than I had ever lost it before. I was never the guy who walked around with six-pack abs, even when I played soccer in college.

Once I started healing my body and addressed those compounding factors, I naturally ended up in the best shape of my life. I had a six-pack for the first time; I was leaner than I had ever been. At that point, I realized that a lot of the stuff that I was doing before, that I thought was right, was actually holding me back.

I learned to identify the underlying mechanisms and fix the root cause of my fatigue, poor focus, and suboptimal health. In doing so, I learned how to help other people, I also learned that many of the energy-related challenges we face go far beyond diet and exercise. A lot of the foods that we are led to believe are healthy are the very foods that are zapping our energy, causing brain fog, and actually keeping us from having the body we want.

I learned the hard way that a lot of the workouts and exercises that I was doing were running my hormones into the gutter and killing my ability to build fat-burning muscle.

Before I had my health crisis, when I wasn't getting the type of results I wanted, my solution was to get more strict with my diet, push harder at the gym, or both. What I should have focused on was restoring balance in the body.

The results of my journey back to life became the framework I use with my executive coaching clients today. And, when we started applying this system in their lives, the results were nothing short of amazing.

Just recently I had a client, name Everte Farnell, who was 100 pounds overweight. For 15 years he had steadily gained weight no matter what he did. When I did my initial consultation with Everte I wasn't sure I was going to be able to help him. He was incredibly knowledgeable about food and exercise. He had a good diet, he exercised and he kept getting fatter.

Finally, during our conversation he mentioned that he always felt bloated when he eats wheat/gluten. That was the answer, he had food allergies. Once he started on the foundational program, and cut out food allergens, he dropped *20lbs in one week*. His weight loss slowed after the first week, but has continued at a steady rate.

And he's not the only client who quickly and easily drops weight. Many clients lose weight faster and easier than ever before. Even men and women who've tried for decades without success. They have more energy and feel better than they have in years - sometimes ever.

And many high level business professionals report hours of additional productivity every day.

Today, I teach these uncommon biohacks to world-class athletes, corporations, traders, executives, and entrepreneurs. The strategies I teach succeed where others fail *because they're based on science*. They've been tested in the real world by hundreds (in some cases thousands) of clients, and proven to work. Anyone can do them.

Perhaps most importantly, they work quickly. These rapid results inspire you so that you stay motivated to move forward. My system doesn't require that you have superhuman levels of discipline, willpower, and motivation. The only real requirement is consistent application of the techniques and principles.

Having said that, it's important to make it clear that I am not a doctor. I want to be completely transparent about that. And the folks at legal insist I remind you that the recommendations in this book are not to be considered medical advice or a substitute for a face-to-face consultation with a medical professional.

I'm a researcher, biohacker, and executive wellness coach specializing in nutritional neuroscience, functional medicine, and peak performance. I have faced and conquered extreme adversity with my own health, and this has afforded me a unique perspective, position, and skill set.

Today, I teach executives and high-level entrepreneurs how to build a lifestyle that rapidly enhances the body and mind, and helps them

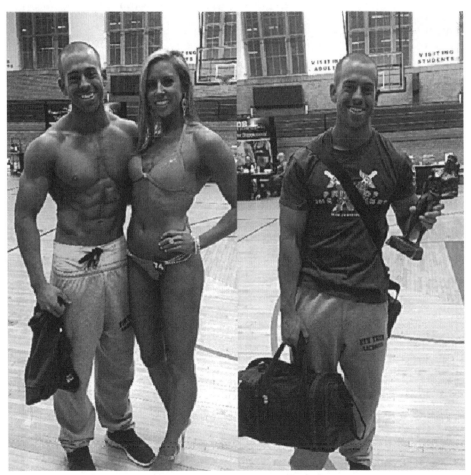

One of my clients, Sean, after his first fitness competition.

gain an edge in every area of their lives. My mission is to give *you* unique tools that will help you to change your mind, change your body, and change your life.

During the course of my journey, I have had a lot of time to reflect on the question of what health is and what it really means to me. Even though today I'm in the best shape of my life and feel better than I felt even before I was sick, I still experience symptoms of Lyme disease from time to time.

I no longer desire a life without pain because pain makes us stronger and *it shapes who we become.*

- We are all warriors.
- We fight for change.
- We fight for progress.
- We fight for a better life.
- We fight to understand who we are and what we believe in.
- We all fight wars in our work, in our bodies, in our minds, and for each other.
- We are all warriors, and only by confronting our fears, overcoming adversity, and pushing through the pain do we earn the privilege of living out our dreams.

LIFE MOVES PRETTY FAST

The world wants to neuter you. They want you to let go of your "unrealistic" hopes and dreams.

They want you to be mediocre. But mediocrity is for losers.

People will always try to bring you "back down to Earth" because when you burn bright it shines a painful light on their own compromises, insecurities, and abandoned dreams. A need for the acceptance of others will make you invisible in this world. Life is too short not to live up to your full potential and be the best version of yourself.

Nearly 70% of Americans are overweight or obese (American Heart Association, 2014), and over 67% of Americans are unhappy (Harris Poll, 2013). In fact, according to a Harvard study, the number of people diagnosed with depression is increasing by a staggering 20% each year.

If that's normal, I say f*#k being normal.

To change your body, change your mind, and change your life, you need a different skill set than the normal crowd. You need more effective strategies and new behavior patterns. I'm going to hand those to you right here in this book. You'll be able to rewire yourself and have the epic life you want and deserve.

My #1 professional responsibility is to my clients. Whether that's a client who has invested seven figures to work together, or someone who has ordered this book for free, my mission is to always give you 100% of my energy, attention, and focus, and never take for granted all that you are investing in me.

People once plagued by obesity, alcoholism, and life-threatening degenerative diseases have used this information, as well as my personal guidance, to regain control of their bodies and their lives.

Successful executives and entrepreneurs have used these strategies to produce the energy and focus required to build multi-million dollar businesses and achieve their physical and genetic potential.

And I am the secret weapon for many professional, world-class athletes, allowing them to gain an unfair advantage over their competition.

I can help you do, be and accomplish more than you dream about right now. It all starts with one simple decision, which is to never again accept a life that is less than you are capable of living.

And remember, Rome wasn't built in a day. Be patient. Trust the system. Focus on change, and the results will come.

There are going to be days where you don't feel like doing the things you know you need to do to accomplish your goals... *do them anyway.*

There's a pernicious misconception that fit, healthy people have these superhuman levels of motivation and discipline. They don't. What they do have is habits, and they intentionally create habits that empower rather than dis-empower them.

Until now you've likely never had accurate information about your health. You deserve better information than a lot of what's out there polluting the internet. You deserve the life you want and can have.

RESEARCHING ROADBLOCKS

One of the biggest traps I see clients fall into is the over-accumulation of information. With the entire collective knowledge of human history available with a Google search from your smart phone, too many people get caught in analysis paralysis. And it's keeping many people from actually getting shit done. To avoid that problem, I've chosen not to include dozens of lower-impact biohacks to minimize option overload. And, for each section in The Foundation, I have provided "The One Thing" that will produce the highest return on investment. Hopefully that helps keep decision fatigue in check.

Timothy Noakes, PhD, co-authored over 400 research papers. He once stated, "Fifty percent of what we know is wrong. The problem is that we don't know which 50%."

Listen to your body and trust your instincts. How you feel in response to a hack is the most accurate data point for determining whether it is having a positive or negative impact on your well-being.

Trust your intrinsic biofeedback mechanisms over laboratory studies, which can be biased and rarely take into account your unique genetic blueprint. And remember, if you find the science boring, too dense, or you're overwhelmed by a certain portion of this book, please feel free to skip it. I include it for those who are interested in corroboration of the claims and methods I'm showing you. You don't need to know any of it. The methods will work without knowing the scientific details.

MASTER THE FOUNDATION

The Foundation represents your most important inputs for energy, vitality and focus. These are the things we would be getting naturally were it not for our modern genetic-environmental mismatch.

Trying to enhance performance, or restore imbalances in the body, exclusively through the use of biohacks, nutraceuticals, or technology when we are missing these foundational elements is like putting the cart before the horse.

Ideally, we want each of these seven categories represented in some form as you go through your day. To reiterate, the seven categories I consider The Foundation of upgraded energy and mental clarity are as follows:

- Nutrition
- Movement
- Stress Management
- Sleep
- Supplements
- Hydration, Oxygenation, and Light
- Habits and Mindset

These are the highest-leverage areas when it comes to looking, performing, and feeling your best. Quantum shifts occur when we close the gap between what our bodies need for optimal gene expression and the stark contrast of what we actually get in our modern lifestyles.

Most of my executive coaching clients come to me frustrated by one, or more, of the following:

- Diet resistant, hard-to-lose unwanted weight
- Frequent stomach and digestive trouble
- Feeling bloated or swollen
- Body aches, pains, tightness, and stiffness (especially in the lower back and/or knees)
- Poor sleep, insomnia, and low energy
- Brain fog, mood swings, anxiety, and stress
- Acne, rashes, and other skin problems

The more symptoms an individual has, the more important it is to take immediate action to correct the underlying issue. To be considered as consistent with the principles of Functional Medicine all of my treatment methods must fulfill four key criteria. They are:

- Do no harm (Hippocratic Oath)
- Improve symptoms as well as overall function and quality of life
- Help to reverse the underlying causes of the imbalance
- Improve the long-term prognosis for the client

The human body is a survival machine. By strategically exposing it to calculated amounts of good stress, we are able to create a healing effect. These good stressors and eustress can be physically and emotionally unpleasant in the short term, but therapeutic in the long term.

Distress (bad stress), however, when left unchecked, interferes with physical and psychological growth, energy production, and desirable metabolic adaptations. Examples of distress include:

- Over-training
- Inefficient sleep (quantity or quality)

- Carbohydrate restriction combined with glycolyticly-demanding, high-intensity training
- Chronic stress
- Chronic infections
- Exposure to toxins at a rate that exceeds our body's capacity to eliminate them (i.e. alcohol, mercury, food allergens, hormones in commercial meat and dairy, chemicals, antibiotics, vaccines, genetically modified foods, etc.)

Good stress (eustress) facilitates physical, emotional, and biological growth. Examples of good stress include:

- Caloric restriction (when strategically done short term)
- Exercise (resistance training, steady state cardio, high intensity intervals, etc.)
- Fasting (intermittent fasting and longer term fasts)
- Dry saunas (hyperthermic conditioning)
- Ketogenic diet
- Cold exposure (and Contrast Hydrotherapy)
- Learning new skills (i.e. juggling, mountain climbing, unicycling)
- Oxygen deprivation (hypoxic training)
- Resisted breathing
- Acupuncture
- Stretching, myofascial release, trigger point work, and deep tissue massage (the kind that "hurts so good")

And, lastly, here are some principles and truths you'll want to put to work for you as you take steps to upgrade your energy, focus, and performance:

- The more you move, the more energy you will have. Electricity is vital to life and we are bioelectric beings. Movement charges your internal battery in much the same way generators convert mechanical energy into electrical energy.

- The fastest way to change your emotional state and feel more energetic is to change your physiology (i.e. Change the way you breathe and move your body).
- The more you sleep (up to 9 hours), the more energy you will have.
- The more organic green vegetables that you eat, the more energy you will have and the more effectively you will eliminate toxins.
- The more clean, structured water you drink, the more energy you will have.

Meditation is one of the most powerful biohacks to upgrade your focus and manage your stress. After hundreds of interviews with top-performers across dozens of industries, three-time bestselling author Tim Ferriss found meditation to be the one commonality among most of them. Your mind is your most powerful ally. Use it to visualize your life as it will be in the future. Play pretend. Imagine. Think thoughts that make you *feel good*.

Use your emotions to guide your decisions and actions. Be the hero in your life's story. Imagine your life like a Hollywood movie. What would the hero of your story do?

Now, do that.

Your energy is a direct reflection of your daily habits and routine. Do the most important thing first. What separates high performers is their ability to commit, plan ahead, stay focused.

Move with purpose. A man who moves with purpose doesn't have to chase people or opportunities. His light causes other people and opportunities to pursue him.

There's always room for us to evolve and upgrade ourselves. Be happy and content with where you are now, knowing that room for improvement will always exist. Cultivate independent thinking. Design your test. Measure and track. The biohacking experiment never ends.

If you find this book helpful, please share it with friends, family members, and co-workers. Tell them how they can get a copy for free (for a limited time) at www.BiohackingSecrets.com.

Pay it forward.

Your friend,

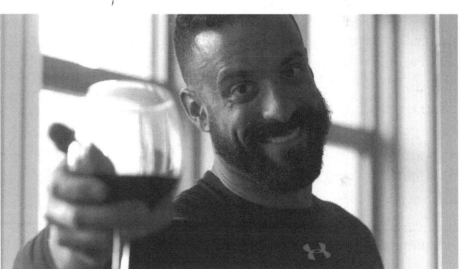

P.S. We thought it would be fun to include some pictures of clients I've helped over the years. So if you come across a picture that seems a bit random, that's probably why. Enjoy!

Nutrition

- 80% organic plants, mostly vegetables, and most vegetables should be green
- 20% protein, mostly wild-caught fish & oysters
- Lots of healthy plant based fats (extra virgin olive oil, c8 mct oil, coconut oil, avocado, nuts, seeds

THE FOUNDATION
OF UPGRADED ENERGY & FOCUS

Stress Management

- Meditate 5 minutes daily
- Get out in nature
- Cold thermogenesis
- Hyperthermic conditioning
- Audio visual entrainment
- Pulsed-electromagnetic fields (PEMFs)
- Neuro-linguistic programming
- NuCalm

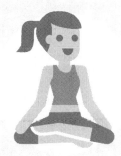

Movement

- 80% aerobic and mobility/flexibility-based, build a bigger aerobic engine first
- 20% strength and resistance training, sprints and high-intensity interval training
- Aim for 20 to 30 minutes of fasted steady-state training in your aerobic training zone at least three days a week.

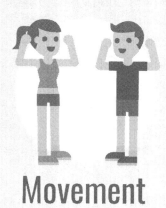

Sleep

- Set aside at least 7 ½ hours per night for time in bed
- Manipulate temperature to optimize sleep onset and offset
- Earthpulse and SR1 Deltasleeper
- "Bridge the Gap" segment intending exercise
- Binaural Beats

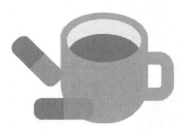

Supplements

- Magnesium Glycinate
- Methylcobalamin B12 sublingual lozenge
- Docosahexaenoic acid (DHA)
- CoQ10 as Ubiquinol
- D-Ribose
- Bioactive B vitamin complex with: Methylfolate, Vitamin B6 as P5P, Riboflavin as R5P, Vitamin B12 as methylcobalamin, Betaine anhydrous
- Take nutrients in their natural form and avoid synthetic versions

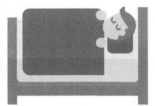

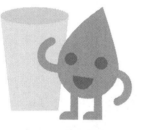

Hydration, Oxygenation, & Light

- Mountain Valley Spring Water
- Hydration: Use a reverse osmosis water filtration system & drink structured water
- Oxygenation: Wim Hof method and deep, diaphragmatic breathing
- Light: 20 minutes of full spectrum sunlight per day to the retina and exposed skin

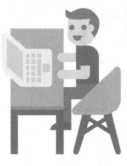

Habits &Mindset

- The 5 Minute Journal
- Create and execute a Daily Action Plan (DAP)
- Segment Intending, Visualization, Play Pretend, Imagine Your Desired Future As Present Reality

NUTRITION

It is possible for you to get all the nutrition you need strictly from food, without any supplements. It's also very unlikely to happen. For someone to get everything they need from food, while also triggering desirable gene expression, one would have to:

- Follow a whole food, plant-based diet
- Have constant access to toxin-free, nutrient-dense foods
- Eat local, seasonal produce close to the time it was picked, or pulled, from the Earth
- Drink and bathe in clean water that hasn't been adulterated, destabilized, or clustered because of the addition of toxic chemicals - like chlorine and fluoride - or exposure to copper pipes. Copper pipes cause the water to lose electrons which changes its energetic properties and makes it more difficult for our bodies to utilize.
- Get at least 20 minutes of direct sunlight daily to their retina and exposed skin
- Sweat everyday for at least 20 minutes
- Spend more time each day moving and standing than sitting.

- Get at least 7 hours of quality sleep per night. This requires no less than 7.5 hours in bed.
- Live a low-stress life or manage stress with daily meditation, relaxation, or deep breathing practices.
- Have strong social bonds and relationships that provide feelings of love and connection.

That's not very likely in our modern world. And I'm assuming there are no underlying health issues which may require additional interventions.

The truth is that there's an inverse relationship between the integration of new, healthier habits and the enjoyment that we get from food and social activities.

Why? Because most of the best tasting foods are loaded with chemicals that have the same effect on our brain as street drugs like heroin, cocaine, and opium. You take away that high and suddenly life can be a lot less enjoyable.

Beyond that, most social events involve alcohol and late nights that throw off our hormonal balance and circadian rhythms. So, in our effort to be healthier, we pass on many social activities. This cuts us off from our most valued human need - love, connection, and social bonds.

Do you now understand why many people aren't willing to change their behavior patterns long enough to create the necessary shifts in their health? The sacrifices are too great. That's why optimizing our physical and genetic potential almost always requires the utilization of tools, technologies, and biohacks that transcend a nutrition-only approach.

IT STARTS WITH YOUR NUTRITION

There is no area that will have a greater impact on your energy and focus than your nutrition.

Four hundred years before the birth of Christ, the Greek physician Hippocrates, considered to be the father of modern medicine, said "Let food be thy medicine, and thy medicine be thy food."

Today we have corporations engineering pseudo-foods (think Cheetos, soda, Twinkies), that trick our brains into interpreting them as evolutionarily beneficial. Thousands of years ago, foods high in fat and sugar equated to high caloric density which, in turn, meant sustained energy. These companies employ teams of scientists, referred to as "food engineers," to create products (let's not call them foods) that are addicting and, most importantly, sell. These chemical engineers manipulate them to entice us to overeat.

Once they've landed on a product that sells, they find the cheapest ingredients they can to make it profitable. Lunchables, for example, lost money until Phillip Morris did away with real meat and cheese and

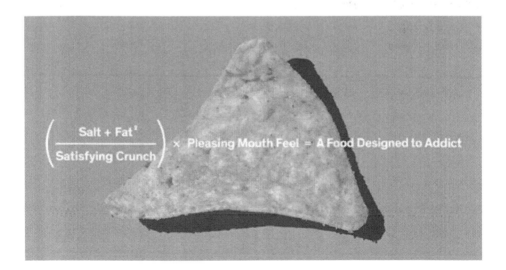

$$\left(\frac{\text{Salt} + \text{Fat}}{\text{Satisfying Crunch}} \right) \times \text{Pleasing Mouth Feel} = \text{A Food Designed to Addict}$$

started loading them up with various forms of genetically engineered corn and soy.

After working one-on-one with hundreds of clients of different genders, ages, ethnicities, and backgrounds, I'll be the first to admit that there is no one-size-fits-all diet. The right diet for you will depend on a number of different factors, such as your:

- Age
- Weight
- Gender
- Goals
- Health status
- Genetic blueprint
- Lifestyle
- Preferences

To simplify what can be a complex topic, let's eliminate body re-composition (burning fat, building muscle) as a motivating variable. Because how I would design a customized nutrition program for someone looking to get lean and toned would differ from one intended to maximize energy and cognitive function.

So, what should we eat to feel good and maximize energy?

LeBron James eats Paleo.

Novak Djokovic cut gluten and dairy from his diet. In less than a year, he went from winning sporadically to winning every grand slam in the game.

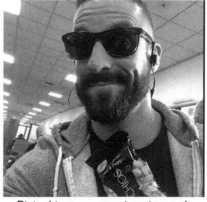

Pistachios are a great go-to snack

Rich Roll, athlete and advocate of plant-powered wellness, completed five Iron Man marathons in seven days, while on a vegan diet.

After analyzing hundreds of studies on nutrition, I can see how someone could get very confused thanks to all of the contradicting results, so let's start with the things experts agree on.

Most experts worth their salt, can pretty much agree that a healthy diet should:

- Keep blood sugar stable and be low in sugar, flour, and processed foods
- Include mostly plants, predominantly a wide variety of green vegetables. But also include others, by eating across the color spectrum (orange, yellow, red, purple) to ensure a diverse intake of free radical scavenging anxtioxidants, phytochemicals, and to produce synergistic nutritional benefits.
- Be low in toxicity by eliminating chemicals, pesticides, antibiotics, vaccines, hormones, GMOs, preservatives, additives, and artificial sweeteners as much as possible
- Contain good, quality plant-based fats[1] and Omega-3's

---

[1] Most people do well with higher quantities of quality plant-based fats. These types of fats can be found in extra virgin olive oil, avocados, coconut oil, MCT oil, seeds, and nuts. There are, however, some exceptions for individuals with sensitivities to various types of nuts, fat malabsorption, low stomach acid, gut dysbiosis, and a number of other conditions.

If animal products are consumed, it is best that they are organic, free range, pastured, or grass-fed. These meats have been shown to have a superior fatty acid composition, higher contents of antioxidants, vitamins, and minerals, as well as fewer chemicals and hormones than their conventional counterparts. Grass-fed beef can be ordered on line and delivered to your doorstep through many companies like Butcher Box (www.getbutcherbox.com), Massa Meats (www.massanautralmeats.com), and U.S. Wellness Meats (www.grasslandbeef.com).

- Provide sufficient Protein[2] - what constitutes sufficient protein varies greatly, depending on your weight, age, gender, underlying health issues (adrenal fatigue, blood sugar issues), goals, and who you ask.
- Be based around local, seasonal, fresh foods - these are required for maximizing the amount of nutrients you get from a food

We live in an accumulation-oriented society. When something is missing from our lives, we look first to what we can add to remedy our situation. What we usually need to do is eliminate and simplify.

While you get this stuff figured out, simplify your nutrition. In extreme cases, I've had clients on detoxes where they ate nothing but salads for weeks at a time. And you know what, they felt better than they'd felt in years afterwards. Of course I helped them build back up after, but I share this example to illustrate a point.

Eliminate foods that can elicit an immunogenic and allergenic response in the body. Like we saw with tennis pro Novak Djokovic, when we remove the energy vampires lurking on our plate, we unlock our ability to tap into our physical and genetic potential.

---

[2] Omega-3 fats should come from fish, caught in the wild, preferably, or krill, which have a higher bio-availability. When eating wild-caught fish, you should focus on smaller species such as sardines, anchovies, and herring. These have been shown to contain lower amounts of mercury when compared to predatory fish like swordfish and tuna. Wild Planet Sardines in Extra Virgin Olive Oil are one of my staples when traveling or in need of a quick snack on the go.

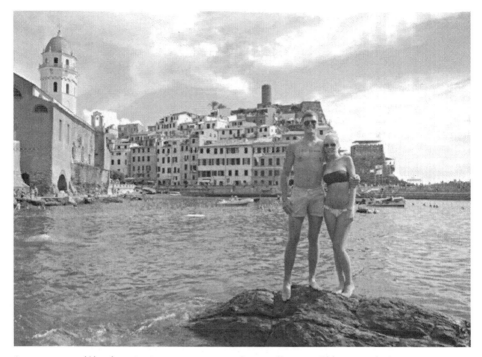

Woody enjoying some sun on the small town of Vernazza Italy.

DITCH THE DIETARY TOXINS: ADDITION BY SUBTRACTION

We've got an epidemic on our hands, really. So many people are facing autoimmune conditions and low-level food sensitivities. The problem is that they haven't yet made the connection that the adverse health effects that they are experiencing are caused by the foods that they are putting in their body.

Most people imagine if they had food sensitivities or low-level food allergies, they'd eat shellfish (or insert your cliche food allergen of choice) and their face would explode into a swollen mess of rashes and histamine. In reality, this is the exception rather than the rule.

The research illustrates that these allergies are much more subtle. They trigger multiple inflammatory pathways in the body, and they can manifest themselves in a number of different ways.

There are also food sensitivities, like gluten for example, that don't always exhibit physical symptoms or show up on blood tests. Why?

Well, for one, many of the testing methods are imperfect. The most accurate and reliable way to assess a potential gluten sensitivity is through a 28-day elimination/provocation-diet. You eliminate gluten 100% for a full 28 days. Then, after four weeks, have a meal with a moderate to high amount of gluten. Let's say pizza, in this case. Observe how your body responds to the pizza over the next 72 hours. Any changes in energy, mood, bloating, brain function, or your ability to make a fist can be indicative that there are more pronounced consequences of ingesting those gluten-containing foods occurring on a cellular level.

Nutrients. 2015 Feb 27;7(3):1565-76. doi: 10.3390/nu7031565.

Effect of gliadin on permeability of intestinal biopsy explants from celiac disease patients and patients with non-celiac gluten sensitivity.

Hollon J[1], Puppa EL[2], Greenwald B[3], Goldberg E[4], Guerrerio A[5], Fasano A[6].

⊕ Author information

Abstract

BACKGROUND: Intestinal exposure to gliadin leads to zonulin upregulation and consequent disassembly of intercellular tight junctions and increased intestinal permeability. We aimed to study response to gliadin exposure, in terms of barrier function and cytokine secretion, using intestinal biopsies obtained from four groups: celiac patients with active disease (ACD), celiac patients in remission (RCD), non-celiac patients with gluten sensitivity (GS) and non-celiac controls (NC).

METHODS: Ex-vivo human duodenal biopsies were mounted in microsnapwells and luminally incubated with either gliadin or media alone. Changes in transepithelial electrical resistance were monitored over 120 min. Media was subsequently collected and cytokines quantified.

RESULTS: Intestinal explants from all groups (ACD (n = 6), RCD (n = 6), GS (n = 6), and NC (n = 5)) demonstrated a greater increase in permeability when exposed to gliadin vs. media alone. The increase in permeability in the ACD group was greater than in the RCD and NC groups. There was a greater increase in permeability in the GS group compared to the RCD group. There was no difference in permeability between the ACD and GS groups, between the RCD and NC groups, or between the NC and GS groups. IL-10 was significantly greater in the media of the NC group compared to the RCD and GS groups.

CONCLUSIONS: Increased intestinal permeability after gliadin exposure occurs in all individuals. Following gliadin exposure, both patients with gluten sensitivity and those with active celiac disease demonstrate a greater increase in intestinal permeability than celiacs in disease remission. A higher concentration of IL-10 was measured in the media exposed to control explants compared to celiac disease in remission or gluten sensitivity.

This study shows that wheat consumption causes intestinal permeability in all individuals, not just those who are sensitive to grains and gluten.

The other reason many gluten sensitivities don't show up on blood tests is because they're not gluten sensitivities at all. They're glyphosate sensitivities.

This toxic herbicide is heavily sprayed on all non-organic wheat crops and subsequently ends up in your breads, cereals, pastas, crackers, and other flour-based foods. That's why some people are fine when they make the switch to organic wheat products which are not sprayed with glyphosate.

It's another reason that organic does matter.

The Detox Project (www.detoxproject.com) tests for glyphosate residues in your water and body. If glyphosate levels in your body are high, they recommend a 3-week detox. I add additional customizations for my clients to further improve detoxification and remove accumulated glyphosate from the pineal gland and brain. This may include liposomal melatonin along with a number of other natural detoxifying compounds based on the client's genetics and health status.

Other foods containing this toxic herbicide are: soy (including all non-organic soy derivatives), corn (including high fructose corn syrup and all other non-organic corn derivatives), canola oil, cotton, and sugar beets.

In March 2014, The International Agency for Research on Cancer (IARC) classified glyphosate as a "probable carcinogen." Rats fed

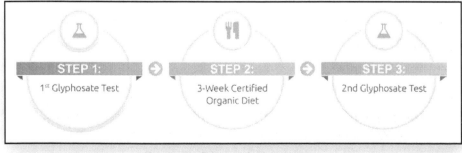

STEP 1: 1st Glyphosate Test

STEP 2: 3-Week Certified Organic Diet

STEP 3: 2nd Glyphosate Test

The Detox Project glyphosate test.

genetically modified foods containing glyphosate developed massive cancerous tumors, birth defects, reproductive disorders, and increased mortality.

Many people who have sensitivities to gluten or glyphosate develop intestinal permeability, a condition that opens the doorway for autoimmunity. However, these clients don't always experience the digestive symptoms indicative of compromised intestinal integrity.

Many of the modern illnesses that continue to soar, year over year, are autoimmune in nature. These include:

- Rheumatoid arthritis
- Lupus
- Multiple sclerosis
- Thyroid disorders
- Celiac disease
- Psoriasis

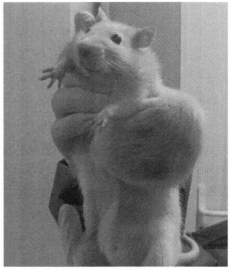

So how can you tell if you are experiencing immunogenic or allergenic reactions to certain foods without being poked and prodded with needles or forced to endure a gauntlet of expensive laboratory testing?

Rats fed genetically modified foods containing glyphosate developed cancerous tumors.

You can start by paying attention to whether you experience any of the common symptoms on a monthly basis:

- Joint pain
- Muscle pain
- Aches

- Diet-resistance, hard-to-lose weight
- Difficulty making a tight fist (swollen hands)
- Brain fog
- Difficulty concentrating or focusing
- Fatigue or low energy
- Cold intolerance
- Psoriasis, eczema, or other skin conditions
- Hair loss
- Gas, bloating, constipation, diarrhea, or other digestive symptoms
- Dry eyes, skin, or mouth
- Numbness and tingling in the hands and feet (peripheral neuropathy[3])
- Multiple miscarriages
- Blood clots
- Irritability and low mood
- Depression
- Anxiety
- Schizophrenia and bipolar disorders[4]
- Unwanted cravings, excessive hunger, and binge eating
- Sinusitis (sinus congestion)
- Stuffy nose
- Post-nasal drainage (a runny nose may be a sign you're eating something potentially problematic)
- Watery eyes

---

[3] A common cause of peripheral neuropathy is a vitamin B12 deficiency. This is something worth investigating if you experience numbness or tingling in your hands and/or feet.

[4] There are many case studies of physicians who have been able to induce schizophrenic and bipolar characteristics in clients by exposing them to high levels of immunogenic and allergenic foods--particularly grains and dairy.

The worst part about food sensitivities is that it's usually the foods we love that are the most problematic. For me, it's peanuts, peanut butter, chocolate, and dairy (cheese in particular). I used to take down an entire brick of cheese in one sitting without skipping a beat.

If there's a food that you find yourself frequently craving, that you have a really hard time not eating in excess, there's a good chance a low-level food sensitivity or autoimmune aspect may be at play.

The idea is to bring more conscious awareness to how the foods we put into our bodies affect our energy, health, cognitive functioning, and even weight. To truly assess the impact of these foods, we have to first know what it feels like to be in our healthy, natural state. Often we've been eating this stuff for so long, we don't know what normal is anymore.

That's why I require many of my clients start their program with a 3-4 week, customized detoxification protocol. There are always slight modifications based on the individual, but the overall objective is to get that person back to baseline so they can feel what it's like to not be inflamed and bogged down with toxins.

In terms of nutrition, the most important thing for optimizing your energy and focus is to minimize or eliminate these food allergies and runaway immune responses (systemic inflammation). Most importantly, you want to minimize the *big four* toxins, which are:

- Grains (breads, cereals, pizza, pasta, flour, wheat, crackers, chips, etc.). The most problematic grains are wheat, barley, rye, and their derivatives.
- Dairy
- Alcohol
- GMOs (genetically modified organisms) including corn, soy, canola oil, cotton, sugar beets, and derivatives of these crops)

The first three are self-explanatory. Avoiding GMOs, however, can be a little trickier. I recommend you:

- Eat organic as much as possible
- Check your labels for derivatives of the most commonly genetically modified crops (corn, soy, canola)
- Avoid products made by companies on the "Monsanto Companies" list on the next page. Many clients are surprised when I reveal that V8, Green Giant, Healthy Choice, Power Bar, and a number of other "healthy" brands may be the very reason they're overweight, sick, and tired.

There are many healthy and allowable forms of the foods you enjoy in these categories if you know where to look.

Take yogurt, for example. Stonyfield has a dairy-free organic soy yogurt that's delicious. Organic means no GMOs, pesticides, herbicides, chemicals, or artificial sweeteners. You won't want to go nuts and eat 15 of these yogurts a day or you'll be taking in a lot of xenoestrogens, which may impact hormonal health in some individuals. However, when responsibly consumed, soy constituents like genistein and other soy isoflavones have been shown to help maintain healthy cellular biological function and proliferation.

There a countless examples of healthy alternatives to the foods you love. You just need to know where to look, and what to look for. Integrating these types of toxin-free substitutes is one of the ways my clients are able to keep their sanity, still experience pleasure from food, and simultaneously make choices that are good for their bodies.

I recommend my clients avoid GMO's because most GMO's are modified so farmers can indiscriminately use glyphosate. There are

MONSANTO COMPANIES
DO NOT BUY

Aunt Jemima
Aurora Foods
Banquet
Best Foods
Betty Crocker
Bisquick
Cadbury
Campbells
Capri Sun
Carnation
Chef Boyardee
Coca Cola
ConAgra
Delicious Brand Cookies
Duncan Hines
Famous Amos
Frito Lay
General Mills
Green Giant
Healthy Choice
Heinz
Hellmans
Hershey's Nestle
Holsum
Hormel
Hungry Jack
Hunts
Interstate Bakeries
Jiffy
KC Masterpiece
Keebler/Flowers Industries
Kelloggs
Kid Cuisine
Knorr
Kool-Aid
Kraft/Phillip Morris

Lean Cuisine
Lipton
Loma Linda
Marie Callenders
Minute Made
Morningstar
Ms. Butterworths
Nabisco
Nature Valley
Ocean Spray
Ore-Ida
Orville Redenbacher
Pasta-Roni
Pepperidge Farms
Pepsi
Pillsbury
Pop Secret
Post Cereals
Power Bar Brand
Prego Pasta Sauce
Pringles
Procter and Gamble
Quaker
Ragu Sauce
Rice-A-Roni
Smart Ones
Stouffers
Sweppes
Tombstone Pizza
Totinos
Uncle Ben's
Unilever
V8

several studies that suggest GMO's are safe, and many that say they are not. Some suggest GMO crops can even lead to cancer. I don't know the answer, but I do know glyphosate causes many people problems, and so we avoid it.

Seems simple enough, right? I thought so too. Until I realized how many ingredients that may be derived from GMO corn don't have the word "corn" anywhere in their name. LiveCornFree.com publishes an eye-opening list of over 50 ingredients derived from corn.

To help you make better choices, here's a more in depth list of common food allergens and sensitivities:

- Dairy
- Grains
- Soy
- Eggs
- Peanuts
- Tree Nuts (including nut butters)
- Alcohol
- Coffee
- Tea
- Chocolate
- Shellfish
- Yeast
- Stoned fruits (peaches, plums, cherries, apricots)
- Canola oil
- Corn
- Wheat
- Gelatin
- Meat (beef, chicken, mutton, pork)

- Seeds (sesame, sunflower, poppy are most common)
- Nightshades (potatoes, tomatoes, eggplants, peppers)
- Mushrooms
- Legumes
- Caffeine
- Processed foods
- Canned foods
- Highly glycemic fruits (watermelon, mango, pineapple, grapes, raisins, dried fruits, etc.)
- Sugars and sweeteners (honey, agave, maple syrup, coconut sugar)

Also, pay close attention to:

- Gluten cross-reactants (coffee, chocolate, whey protein, corn, quinoa, oats, hemp seeds, rice, sesame, soy, yeast)
- Hidden sources of gluten (modified food starch, food emulsifiers, food stabilizers, artificial food coloring, malt extract, the clarifying agents in some red wines)
- Overlooked sources of gluten (processed condiments: ketchup, mustard, salad dressings, deli meats, beer, soy sauce, imitation crab meat)
- Health products (proteins, especially whey, branched-chain amino acids, pre-workout formulas)
- Any products that contain artificial sweeteners (Sucralose, which can cause brain inflammation, migraines, fatigue, disrupted gut microbiome)

Ninety-five percent of healthy people don't have to worry about cutting out these foods, especially if they don't want to.

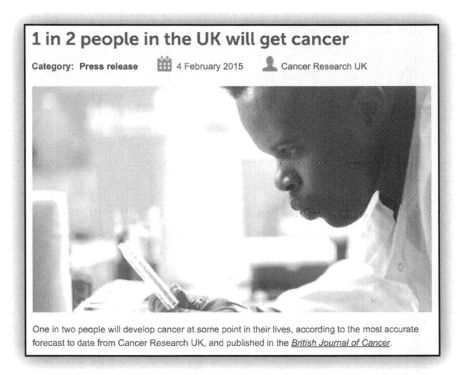

1 in 2 people in the UK will get cancer

Category: **Press release**   📅 4 February 2015   👤 Cancer Research UK

One in two people will develop cancer at some point in their lives, according to the most accurate forecast to date from Cancer Research UK, and published in the _British Journal of Cancer_.

If your objective is to take your performance to a higher level, I encourage you to review the list above, noting the foods that you eat the most frequently. Once you identify them, experiment by cutting or eliminating those foods for 28 days to see how you feel.

Studies have shown that a single serving of gluten can cause an inflammatory response that can last upwards of 21 days in sensitive individuals. This is why I recommend that clients remove these foods for at least 28 days. This helps them to get a more accurate assessment of their response and sensitivity levels.

If you're dealing with a chronic health issue, my recommendation would be a little more stringent. I would encourage you to cut out all of these foods, or as many as you can, for 28 days. This would be an all-out elimination diet. During this time, you would focus on small amounts of wild-caught fish, some organic chicken and turkey, and a variety of organic plants. Most of those plants should be vegetables, and most of those vegetables should be green. I would also recommend some organic berries (1/2 to 1 cup per day) and some sweet potatoes, yams, or squash.

For beverages, focus on mostly water from a clean source. You can also include almond milk. Just make sure it doesn't contain carrageenan. Carrageenan is a thickening agent which has been implicated in a number of cancers and shown to exacerbate digestive issues. It's also injected into participants in studies on anti-inflammatory drugs because it initiates a rapid inflammatory response in the body.

Other allowed beverages include herbal teas, organic green tea, yerba mate, guayusa, and coconut milk (as long as you know you aren't sensitive to coconut).

I recommend including a vegan protein powder, too. This will allow you to make one of your daily meals a shake. There are a number of good options out there, many of which I use with clients. The important thing is to make sure you check the ingredients and there aren't any of the foods that you're trying to avoid. Whey and casein, for example, are both dairy. My current favorite can be found at www.biohackerprotein.com.

This 28-day elimination diet is ultra-simple. While restrictive, it does come with many benefits.

Most people will spend, on average, 28,000 days on Earth in their lifetime. If you had the opportunity to invest just 28 of those 28,000 days, to exponentially upgrade your energy and focus, health, mood, body composition, and quality of life, would you do it?

When you face challenges, and you decide to push forward in spite of them, that is strength. That is the process that leads to high performance. High performers are willing to do the things other people aren't.

If you don't want to dive into a 28-day elimination diet right away, you don't have to. There are some other things that you can try first.

THE 28-DAY ELIMINATION DIET
EAT THIS:

FIRST 28 DAYS:

- Vegetables
- Organic Berries
- Starchy Tubers
- Wild Caught Fish and Seafood
- Whole Food Probiotics
- Healthy Plant-Based Fats
- Bone Broth
- Fresh Green Vegetable Juice
- Organ Meats
- Vegan Protein Powder
- Seeds

Do not eat dairy or yogurt of any kind

THEREAFTER TEST/ADD:

- All Healthy Meat (grass-fed beef, pastured eggs)
- Organic Fruit
- Organic Sprouted Lentils/Beans
- Nuts and Nut Butters
- Grass-fed Ghee & Butter
- Lard, Tallow, and Fat
- Hydrolyzed Beef & Collagen Protein Powder
- Raw, Organic Dairy from Pastured Cows
- Organic Grains
- Nightshades

In the next section, you'll learn about some the most important principles to follow when it comes to your nutrition. You'll discover which superfoods will provide you with the greatest levels of energy and mental clarity.

CASE STUDY: JIM – YOUR DIET EXISTS TO SERVE YOUR LIFESTYLE

For obvious reasons, I can't give someone's personal information in this book, so when I present a case study, I want to assure you they are based on a real person and the data is accurate, but the names and personal details have been changed to protect the client's privacy.

Jim was a 33-year-old investment banker. He had never really worked out or given much thought to his diet or health. Once he turned 30, he started noticing less energy and more stiffness throughout his body. He also had some difficulty concentrating, especially in the afternoons after lunch. He knew he needed to make some changes, but he wasn't sure how.

Jim hadn't played sports growing up and had never exercised. Like many of us, the idea of him going to the gym and working out - without what he felt to be adequate knowledge or experience, was intimidating.

The first time Jim and I met in person, I couldn't believe my eyes. Most of the guys I work with are between 30 to 60 years old. Jim's chronological age was on the lower end of that range, but he looked like he was in his late 40's, or even early 50's.

He was probably about 50 pounds overweight. Most of that weight had set up camp around his midsection. His hairline was thinning and receding. He was somewhat shy, lower energy, with a quiet demeanor, and he didn't keep eye contact for long. While standing and sitting, he was hunched over.

His body screamed to me, "I need help!" Not just with physicality, but with his mental game as well.

I knew Jim would be one of the toughest cases I had ever taken on.

I still remember that first session vividly. Within three minutes of a very low-intensity warm up, he looked like he had just finished the Boston Marathon breathing through a snorkel. He was gasping for air.

We moved on to the chest press machine. We started at around 40 pounds per side. Jim did a few reps and then looked at me and said, "Less weight. This is too heavy." So I reduced the weight. This continued, until there was nowhere left to put the pin in the machine.

Despite the shaky beginning, we eventually got Jim stronger and making some serious progress.

Nonetheless, I started noticing a pattern. Each week, by the time we got to Friday, Jim was a machine. But by the time Monday rolled around, it was like we had lost three weeks of progress. Exercises and rest periods that he could have breezed through just days earlier, left him gasping for air.

Jim also exhibited symptoms of circulatory issues, often manifesting themselves as tightness or burning in his calves and feet. It was like I was training a completely different person.

I had seen this before, but never to this degree. When we talked about it, we were able to identify the culprit. Five days a week, Monday through Friday in Jim's case, he ate pretty well. But, then, starting around 5 p.m. on Friday through the weekend, it was a free for all. This extended cheat day included egregious amounts of cocktails, beer, breads, pizzas, pastas, and cheese.

His weekly slump suddenly started to make a little more sense.

What we were experiencing every Monday was the result of an acute, inflammatory response that was precipitated by the cascade of toxins Jim was bombarding his body with every weekend.

I sat down with Jim and asked him what he wanted to achieve. Essentially, he told me that he wanted to get in better shape, he wanted to have more energy, and he wanted to do both of these things to the highest degree possible without having to sacrifice all of the foods that he loves. Now that we were clear about the desired end result, I could design our roadmap.

I put together a plan for Jim that involved what I referred to as "strategic feasting." This would allow him to maximize his results without deprivation or even the frustration that can sometimes come with eliminating many of the foods we enjoy. Where is Jim today?

By simply making a few small shifts, compounded by consistent daily action, Jim got his weight down to 212 pounds. His performance at work took off and he was courted by a competing firm who offered a substantial pay raise. His mood, energy, marriage, bank account, and body are all in better shape. And it's not because he made any radical lifestyle changes. All it took were a few intelligent shifts that built momentum with practice. Jim is probably never going to rock six pack abs or bang out 30 floor-to-overhead 135-pound clean and presses sub-3-minutes. Those things aren't important to him. The perfect diet for each of us is one that takes into account our goals, health status, genetic blueprint, preferences, age, and gender. Your diet exists to serve your lifestyle, not the other way around.

HOW TO EAT TO WIN

You've learned that there is no perfect, one-size-fits-all diet for everyone and why the perfect diet for you is one that takes into account everything that makes you unique.

There are a number of principles and practices you can implement today, that will pay dividends in increased energy and focus.

Nothing will directly affect how you feel, how you think, how you look, and your overall quality of life more than your nutrition. Most people are sabotaging themselves with foods that make them feel like crap. I recommend that you start out strict and focus on the foods that most humans respond well to. Then, you can begin to experiment by incorporating additional foods back into your diet. As you do, you'll want to assess the response that your body has to the foods you reintroduce and weigh out the benefits versus the costs of keeping each one in your diet.

For most people, I believe that if you are dialing into these principles five days a week, you can give yourself two days with more latitude. Any days you plan to deviate from the program, I recommend you postpone the first cheat meal for the day as long as possible. For instance, you may want to hold off and save that cheat meal for dinnertime. Overeating is much more likely to take place when we consume immunogenic and allergenic foods early in the day. Why?

Because it initiates a roller coaster effect, characterized by spikes and dips in blood sugar that make us even hungrier. Here's how it usually goes down:

- You eat some processed food containing carbohydrates.
- Blood sugar goes up.
- Your body releases insulin to shuttle that glucose (sugar) into your cells where it can be utilized.

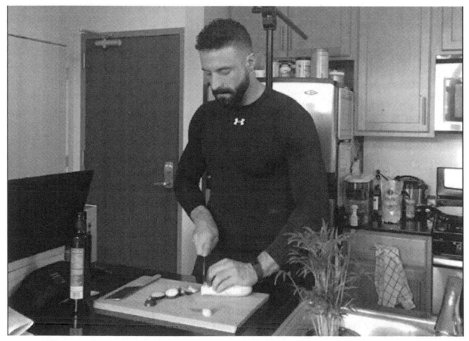

Diversify your antioxidants and polyphenols by eating different types of leafy greens and a wide variety of vegetables across the color spectrum.

- Sometimes the body can release too much insulin, causing a drop in blood sugar that exceeds normal baseline levels (this is a condition known as reactive hypoglycemia). It's more common in folks with energy- and weight-related issues.
- Our body is an intelligent system consisting of many feedback loops. In order to bring blood sugar back within the healthy range, we experience feelings of hunger.
- So, we eat more.
- But do we eat kale or broccoli? Not a chance. We grab more of those manufactured pseudo-foods because they give our brain a warm and fuzzy shot of feel good neurotransmitters as soon as they hit the tongue.

This viscous cycle has a tendency to continue until we either: (a) eat ourselves into a food coma or (b) go to bed for the night. And that, my friend, is why it's better to delay that first cheat meal as long as you can.

When you postpone those cheat meals and dietary deviations, it shortens the window available for us to make bad decisions and allows us to start the next day with a clean slate.

FROM SUPERMODELS TO SUPER BOWLS

At age 38, New England Patriots quarterback, Tom Brady is on top of his game with no signs of slowing down. He's publicly expressed his intent to continue playing into his 40s and, the way it's going, things look promising.

So, with 28 being the average retirement age in the NFL, what's Brady's secret to staying on top? Well, it may have something to do with his ridiculously healthy diet.

In a 2016 interview, Brady's personal chef, Allen Campbell, reveals how Tom fuels himself for peak performance: "Eighty percent of what they eat is vegetables," Campbell said. "[I buy] the freshest vegetables. If it's not organic. I don't use it. And whole grains: brown rice, quinoa, millet, beans. The other 20 percent is lean meats: grass-fed steak, duck every now and then, and chicken. As for fish, I mostly cook wild salmon."

You're probably aware that Tom Brady is married to Victoria's Secret Angel and "The World's Richest Supermodel" Gisele Bundchen. She eats the same way. Their children eat this way.

These principles apply whether you're a supermodel or competing in the Super Bowl. Your nutrition is, without exception, the foundation of looking, feeling, and performing at a world class level. Is it more expensive to eat this way? Yes.

It doesn't have to be though. If I can teach you how to cut you monthly food expenses by 30% to 50%, while eating organic, would that be something that interests you? I do exactly this for many of my coaching clients (www.BiohackingSecrets.com/coaching).

Let's break down how I recommend you eat to maximize energy and focus. First, make 80% of the food that you consume plants. This includes mostly vegetables, with the exception of tomatoes, potatoes, and mushrooms (only at the beginning). Focus on organic, fresh green vegetables with their natural water content (structured water) and life force. Include lots of different types of leafy greens and a wide variety of vegetables across the color spectrum (purple, red, orange, yellow, and deep blue). A few examples are: Asparagus, Spinach, Lettuce, Broccoli, Cauliflower, Artichokes, Garlic, Onions, Zucchinis, Squash, Cucumbers, Turnips, Watercress, Herb Salad Mix, Romaine, Kale, Charred Collards and Arugula.

Your healthy fats will also come from plant-based sources (again, just to start). Use extra virgin olive oil or MCT oil on your salads (along with

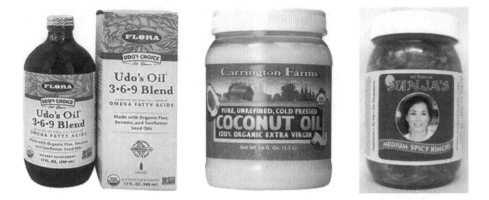

Bragg organic apple cider vinegar as a dressing and organic seasonings for variety and flavor). Healthy fats can also come from: Coconut oil, MCT oil, Pure Caprylic acid (C-8 MCT oil), Udo's oil blend, Flax, Chia seeds, Pumpkin seeds and Sunflower seeds.

You'll want about half of your vegetables to be raw and the other half lightly cooked in some healthy fats in order to enhance nutrient absorption. There's an inverse relationship when it comes to nutrient content and nutrient absorption in raw versus cooked veggies. Raw veggies have more nutrients, but they're not as easy for the body to absorb. Lightly cooked vegetables have slightly fewer nutrients but those nutrients are more easily absorbed.

Be sure to include some whole food probiotics like: Sauerkraut, Kimchi (Sunja's is my personal favorite), Pickled ginger, Fermented cucumbers, Coconut yogurt, Kombucha, and Bubbie's brand pickles.

If you struggle with any digestive symptoms like gas, bloating, constipation, or diarrhea, you'll probably respond better to lightly cooking your vegetables and minimizing their intake in the raw form.

Limit animal proteins as well, unless you have adrenal fatigue or blood sugar issues.

When it comes to fruits, your focus should be on those that are nutrient dense, low-glycemic, and organic. Individuals who want to lean out should stick to a maximum of 1 cup of the following organic berries per day: Raspberries, Blackberries, and Blueberries.

To a lesser degree, folks maintaining their body weight or focusing on recomposition can include organic: Apples, Pears, Apricots, Peaches, Plums, and Cherries.

Avoid dried fruit. It's a form of concentrated sugar, and it no longer contains its natural water content, which plays many important roles ranging from hydration to digestion, bioelectric conductivity, absorption, and the assimilation of nutrients. Plus, dried fruit is much lower in the antioxidant glutathione, which we find in raw, organic vegetables and fruits.

Individuals who are healthy, close to their ideal body weight, and who engage in glycolytically-demanding workouts (like high intensity interval training) can also include: Sweet potatoes, Yams, Squash, and Plantains.

If you don't consume adequate carbohydrates proportionate to your energy expenditure it can downregulate thyroid hormones, create a catabolic (muscle wasting) internal environment, kill sex drive, make you moody, and screw up your digestion.

Many people who start eating healthier mistakenly avoid all impact carbs and, in doing so, deprive the good bacteria in their gut of the beneficial fiber it needs to thrive. Getting this fiber from acellular, plant foods is beneficial whereas getting it from fiber added to processed "health foods" can have unwanted ramifications like diverticulosis (a digestive disease characterized by inflammation of the colon).

UFC Heavyweight Champion and WWE superstar Brock Lesnar was forced to end his rising MMA (mixed martial arts) carrier prematurely because of this debilitating condition. I would have been honored to have the opportunity to work with an athlete like Brock, to help him heal, and see if we could get him a few more years on top.

That covers 80% of your nutrition program. Simple and effective.

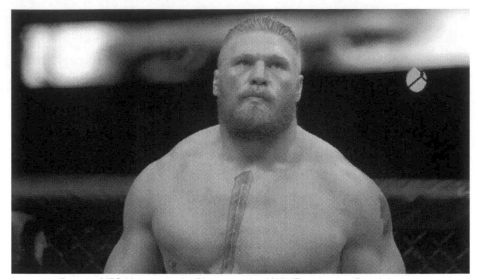

Former UFC Heavyweight Champion and WWE superstar Brock Lesnar

The other 20% of your foods come from mostly wild-caught fish. You'll want to focus on smaller, non-predatory fish because they have lower mercury and environmental toxin content.

There's often concern from my personal clients about protein, so I'll address it here too. If you are healthy, and getting adequate calories in your diet, you don't have to worry about not getting enough protein. The healthiest countries in the world eat far less protein than we do. And yet we are the nation force-feeding ourselves protein while getting fatter and sicker by the day.

This doesn't mean that going strict vegan or vegetarian is the answer. The problem with strict vegetarian diets is that they are missing many of the critical nutrients we need for optimal biological functions. A lot of studies have shown that vegans and vegetarians are susceptible to deficiencies in fat-soluble vitamins like vitamin A and vitamin D, long-chain fatty acids like DHA and EPA, calcium, zinc, iron, and B12.

Should you choose to focus on a vegetarian diet with the inclusion of wild-caught fish, the risk of these deficiencies can be mitigated with an intelligently-designed supplement protocol.

After the 28-day detoxification/elimination/provocation period, many clients find that compliance and sustainability increase with the inclusion of certain other healthy meats. A few recommendations are: Free-range chicken, Free-range turkey, Grass-fed beef, Grass-fed lamb, and Organ Meats.

These foods help to address some of the potential deficiencies that are probable with a meat-free, plant-based diet.

Your best choices are organic, grass-fed beef and pastured meats from a local farm. This meat is ideally consumed as close to the time of slaughter as possible. Not only does this ensure the highest level of nutrient content is consumed, but it also minimizes the proliferation of certain bacteria which multiply as time passes. High levels of these bacteria can aggravate histamine intolerance and digestive issues in some individuals, the consequences of which may include brain fog, fatigue, skin problems, and respiratory problems.

The second best option, when you can't get local and fresh meat is organic meats. Be sure to avoid factory-farmed meats (these are the kind used in almost all restaurants and grocery stores).

Many people thrive on plant-based fats while keeping animal fats to a minimum. This can be attributed to gut issues, fat malabsorption, hypochloridia (low stomach acid), and chronic infections. Later on, I'll explain how the biofilms (groups of microorganisms in our systems) use fats as one of the key components of their structures.

Organic free-range eggs are also an excellent source of healthy fats like choline, B vitamins, and nutrients. If you experience joint pain, back pain, aches, stiffness, or nagging injuries, I advise that you first rule out any sensitivity to eggs (even organic, free-range sort) before

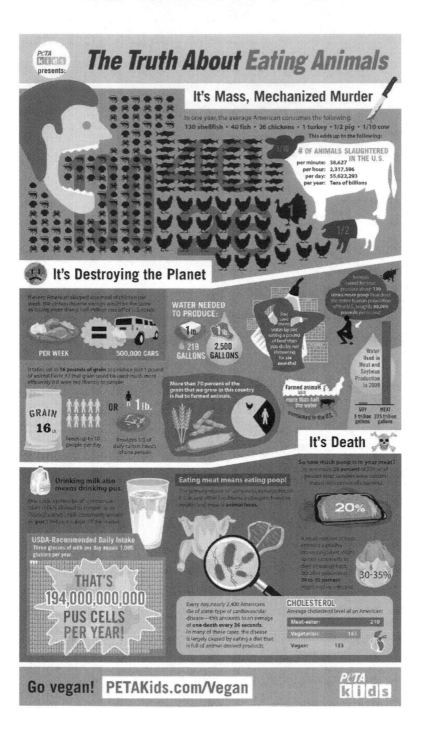

The Truth About Factory Farms
(Confined Animal Feeding Operations or CAFOs)

CAFOs or "factory farms" raise large numbers of animals – typically 1,000 or more – in a small area, and feed them grain-based, genetically modified food that includes antibiotics and hormones to maximize their growth in a short period of time.

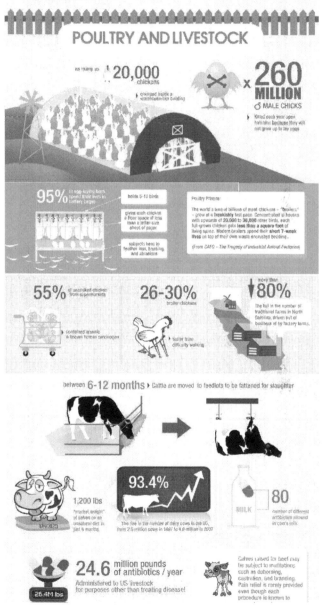

POULTRY AND LIVESTOCK

as many as **20,000** chicks

crammed inside a warehouse-like building

x **260 MILLION** ♂ MALE CHICKS

Killed each year upon hatching because they will not grow up to lay eggs

95% of egg-laying hens spend their lives in factory cages

holds 5-10 birds

gives each chicken a floor space of less than a letter-size sheet of paper

subjects hens to feather loss, bruising, and abrasions

Poultry Prisons:

The world's tens of billions of meat chickens – "broilers" – grow at a breakishly fast pace. Concentrated in houses with upwards of 20,000 to 30,000 other birds, each full-grown chicken gets less than a square foot of living space. Modern broilers spend their short 7-week lives on top of their own waste-encrusted bedding...

(from CAFO – The Tragedy of Industrial Animal Factories)

55% of uncooked chicken from supermarkets

contained arsenic a known human carcinogen

26-30% broiler chickens

suffer from difficulty walking

more than ↓**80%**

The fall in the number of traditional farms in North Carolina, driven out of business of by factory farms.

between **6-12 months** ▸ Cattle are moved to feedlots to be fattened for slaughter

1,200 lbs
"market weight" of calves on an unnatural diet in just 6 months.

93.4%
The rise in the number of dairy cows in the US, from 2.5 million cows in 1987 to 4.8 million in 2007

MILK **80**
number of different antibiotics allowed in cow's milk

24.6 million pounds of antibiotics / year
Administered to US livestock for purposes other than treating disease!

26.4M lbs

Calves raised for beef may be subject to mutilations such as dehorning, castration, and branding. Pain relief is rarely provided even though each procedure is known to...

reintroducing them to your diet. Some of the most nutrient-dense foods include: Organ Meats, Wild game and poultry, Fish and shellfish, Eggs, Meats, Fruits, Vegetables, Nuts and seeds, and Herbs and spices.

HOW MUCH FOOD TO EAT

In short, you want to eat enough to maintain energy levels and hormonal health, but no more.

Numerous studies have found a 20% to 40% calorie restriction causes favorable gene expression, improved biomarkers of health, and increased longevity. Eating less can also improve mitochondrial function (these are the small energy powerhouses of our cells), and improve the body's ability to detoxify.

Eat light throughout the day. Take in enough to maintain energy levels and focus, without postprandial (after meal) grogginess. Intermittent fasting is one strategy that works well for many people. I will explain some implementation strategies for this momentarily.

Make dinner your largest meal of the day. This is where you would include a larger portion of wild-caught fish, organic, free-range poultry, or some of the other options that have been discussed.

In terms of specific quantities, here are my recommendations:

- Unlimited organic, non-starchy vegetables (the green stuff).
- Some organic berries (depends on activity levels, age, muscle mass, carbohydrate tolerance, underlying health issues). Most clients do best limiting to one cup per day.
- Small portions of healthy animal protein once or twice per day. Make wild caught fish and oysters your primary source. If there are health issues at work, more protein may be required short term.
- Lots of plant-based fats. Limit if you're trying to lose weight as they are calorically-dense.

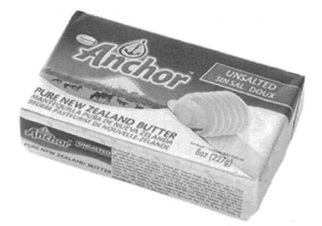

For healthy clients, after the 28-day elimination diet, we test the following one at a time: Butter from grass-fed cows (Kerrygold brand, Anchor), Organic ghee (a clarified butter from grass-fed cows), Animal fat from healthy, pastured animals, Nuts and seeds (raw, organic, sprouted; Go Raw is a good brand), Chia, Flax, Pumpkin, Sunflower, Nuts, and Nut butters[5].

When you are first starting out, you should avoid or minimize: sugar, dairy, grains, potatoes, soy, corn, rice, canola oil, alcohol, and derivatives of these foods.

For physically active individuals with healthy insulin sensitivity, or people trying to add muscle, we test: Organic white rice, Organic sprouted brown rice, Organic potatoes, Organic corn, Organic grains, and Organic, raw, full-fat dairy from grass-fed cows (occasionally).

Insulin is anabolic (muscle-building). To prevent unwanted weight gain or inflammation that can result from elevated insulin levels, we determine the minimum effective carbohydrate load for each individual and try to limit any spikes in blood sugar to once or twice a day.

---

[5] You can test nuts and nut butters as long as you don't experience any pain or inflammation. Soaking nuts increases their digestibility and absorbability.

QUALITY OVER QUANTITY

For five of the past six years, my mom and I watched helplessly as my father's physical and mental capacities deteriorated. I say helplessly because, for those first five years, he refused to let us take him to a doctor for help.

When his situation was too pronounced to ignore, and numerous friends and family members had spoken up, we finally convinced him to see a specialist.

I put together a nutrition and lifestyle-based protocol, and a progressive supplement program to counteract the observable neurodegeneration. At the Parkinson's screening, one of the first questions the doctors asked him was whether he had grown up on a farm. My father responded, "No."

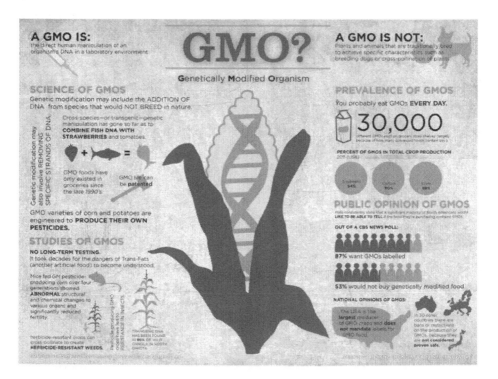

Fortunately, my mom was by his side. She politely interjected, "Gene, you spent every summer on your parent's farm."

Curious now, my mother asked the doctor why.

He explained that, in recent years, a strong correlation between pesticide and herbicide exposure and the onset of Parkinson's later in life has been observed.

Let's circle back real quick to the Monsanto herbicide glyphosate that's used on genetically modified foods. We already know it is a probable carcinogen, in addition to being linked with obesity and early death. Well, now we can add Parkinson's and neurodegenerative brain disorders to the list.

Over the past 20 years, we have witnessed a meteoric rise in modern degenerative diseases like dementia, Alzheimer's, Parkinson's, and cancers. Is it any coincidence that GMOs first hit the shelves of our grocery stores in 1994? Then, in 1996, the first glyphosate-resistant weeds were detected. This meant farmers had to use higher and higher quantities of this carcinogenic herbicide to produce the same result.

In the field of epigenetics - which studies the turning on and off of genes based on environmental triggers - there's a saying that goes, "Our genes load the gun, but it's our environment that pulls the trigger." Experts now estimate that as much as 60% of our genetic expression is determined by environmental factors, as opposed to our genes.

What environmental factor, do you suppose, influences our genes more than any other? It's impossible to say for sure, because we are all different. But food is right up there with the top contenders.

What we are realizing is that certain individuals, my dad being one of them, aren't able to eliminate environmental toxins as well as some other people (i.e. "the loading of the gun").

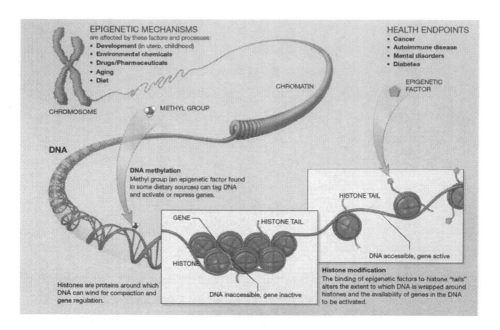

EPIGENETIC MECHANISMS
are affected by these factors and processes:
• Development (in utero, childhood)
• Environmental chemicals
• Drugs/Pharmaceuticals
• Aging
• Diet

CHROMOSOME

METHYL GROUP

CHROMATIN

HEALTH ENDPOINTS
• Cancer
• Autoimmune disease
• Mental disorders
• Diabetes

EPIGENETIC FACTOR

DNA

DNA methylation
Methyl group (an epigenetic factor found in some dietary sources) can tag DNA and activate or repress genes.

GENE

HISTONE TAIL

HISTONE TAIL

DNA accessible, gene active

HISTONE

DNA inaccessible, gene inactive

Histones are proteins around which DNA can wind for compaction and gene regulation.

Histone modification
The binding of epigenetic factors to histone "tails" alters the extent to which DNA is wrapped around histones and the availability of genes in the DNA to be activated.

When exposed to toxins like herbicides and pesticides ("the pulling of the trigger"), conditions like Parkinson's can result.

Does anyone still believe organic doesn't matter?

A 2014 study in the British Journal of Nutrition found higher anti-oxidant and lower cadmium concentrations as well as lower incidents of pesticide residues in organically-grown crops. Another recent study confirmed organic produce to have higher levels of beneficial flavonoids (flavanols, isoflavones, flavones, catchins, flavanones) because these anti-oxidants protect plants, too. Plants not sprayed with pesticides and chemicals have to increase the levels of anti-oxidants that they produce in order to protect themselves from insects and other environmental threats.

Similar benefits and principles are found when we investigate wild-caught fish and organically-raised animal products. These foods have been found to have a healthier fatty acid composition, a higher Omega-3 to Omega-6 ratio, and higher levels of CLA (conjugated linoleic acid).

CLA is a healthy fat that helps to build lean muscle, burn fat, and increase energy levels.

Organic food provides the body with more anti-oxidants, vitamins, and minerals, and possesses less harmful elements such as chemicals, hormones, antibiotics, vaccines, and genetically-modified organisms.

Conventional meat comes from animals that are frequently fed a diet which largely includes genetically-modified corn and grains. This, of course, is absorbed into the meat, which we then consume.

A study done by researchers at the University of Zurich found an association between processed meats and the increased risk of dying from cancer and heart disease.

Another study, conducted at Columbia University, found a direct correlation between the consumption of cured meats (salami, ham, bacon, jerky, sausage) and the development of cardiovascular disease. Conventional factory-farmed and CAFO meat has also been implicated in cases of Alzheimer's, dementia, obesity, fatigue, and early death. A report from *"The Week"* found Methicillin-resistant Staphylococcus Aureus (MRSA), a dangerous bacteria that are extremely resistant to antibiotics, in many pig farms in Canada. Canada sells many of its live pigs to the US each year.

Here's where it gets kind of nasty, in addition to genetically-modified grains, many cows are also fed chicken excrement (poop), dead chickens, and feathers.

Until recently, these cows were also being fed other dead and rotting cow carcasses. That's what led to the outbreaks of Mad Cow Disease (bovine spongiform encephalopathy), the human form of which results in dementia and death within 13 months. Consequently it was made illegal to continue feeding cows other decaying, dead cows due to these risks. It is still legal, however, to feed cows chicken feces and dead, decaying chickens.

These unnatural practices are not without consequence. Emerging research suggests that Alzheimer's, dementia, and these other shrinking brain disorders may be linked to two diet-related problems:

- The first is the consumption of excess sugar.
- The other is the creation of neurodegenerative proteins that comes from feeding cows (a natural herbivore) infected animal meat (i.e. chickens).

Researchers identified proteins tagged TDP-43, in an estimated 97 percent of people with amyotrophic lateral sclerosis (ALS) and 45 percent of those with one form of dementia.

According to research published in 2011, the TDP-43 protein was found in 25% to 50% of Alzheimer's patients where it was clumped inside brain and nerve cells rendering them dysfunctional. It has been suggested that Alzheimer's may be a slow-moving version of Mad Cow Disease.

The only way to avoid these potential threats, and keep your brain healthy and sharp, is to eat organic and know where your food is coming from.

THE 80/20 RULE: EAT 80% PLANTS

Many people, especially people who have a solid nutritional knowledge-base, are eating way too much meat. This includes the grass-fed, free-range, organic varieties.

There was one particular infographic that went viral years ago. Essentially, there was an image of a plate and a glass. The plate was divided down the middle. Half of the plate was filled with green plants, the other half consisted of meat, and the glass contained water. Underneath the picture it said, "It's not that hard people!" At the time,

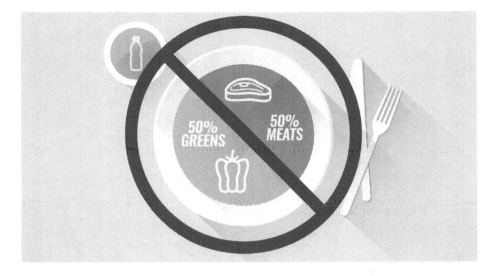

this visual helped a lot of people realize that they needed to eat less processed stuff and more real food. That knowledge is now mainstream.

What ended up happening was many people were misled to believe that calories don't matter, as long as you're eating the right kinds of foods. While this may be true, in the short term, for someone coming off a Standard American Diet (SAD), it is not the truth.

That's why many of my clients come to me after experiencing initial improvements in health, fat loss, and energy, despite eating copious amounts of calorie-dense foods (i.e. coconut oil, nuts, and grass-fed beef). Once their hormones have normalized, the rate of their progress slows substantially or reaches a stalemate.

Calories matter. Especially when it comes to energy and focus.

One of the *only* proven ways to increase human life expectancy is caloric restriction. It is hypothesized that this is because we expend large quantities of energy to digest food. Furthermore, digestion and the associated metabolic processes produce free radicals and increase oxidative stress. If our antioxidant status is strong enough to neutralize these free radicals, no ill effects are observed.

N Engl J Med. Author manuscript; available in PMC 2010 Apr 8.

Published in final edited form as:

N Engl J Med. 1997 Oct 2; 337(14): 986–994.

doi: 10.1056/NEJM199710023371407

PMCID: PMC2851235

NIHMSID: NIHMS182771

Caloric Intake and Aging

Richard Weindruch, Ph.D. and Rajindar S. Sohal, Ph.D.

Author information ▶ Copyright and License information ▶

In postindustrial societies, overeating, inactivity, and obesity have emerged as new challenges in public health.[1,2] Considerable effort is now being devoted to determining the pathophysiologic consequences of overeating. Several lines of evidence suggest that caloric intake influences the rate of aging and the onset of associated diseases in animals and, possibly, humans.[3-5]

The observation that laboratory rats not only live longer but also have fewer age-associated diseases when their food intake is restricted dates back to the 1930s.[2-7] Numerous subsequent studies have found that when the ad libitum food intake of mice and rats was reduced by 30 to 60 percent, the average life span and the maximal life span (the mean survival of the longest-lived decile) increased by similar amounts.[3] In contrast, rats with nearly unrestricted caloric intake (92 percent of the average unrestricted intake) that were kept lean with exercise and weighed about 40 percent less than sedentary control rats with the same caloric intake had an increase in the average life span but not in the maximal life span.[8] In all these studies, the life-extending benefits of caloric restriction depended on the prevention of malnutrition and a reduction in overall caloric intake rather than any particular nutrient.[3-5]

Because caloric restriction can markedly prolong the life span, it is being widely studied to determine the mechanisms of aging. An increasing body of evidence suggests that cumulative oxidative damage to macromolecules such as protein, lipids, and DNA has a major role in aging. Caloric restriction attenuates both the degree of oxidative damage and the associated decline in function.[7] We will review evidence that caloric restriction prolongs life in laboratory animals, evokes an array of responses, including a decrease in oxidative stress and damage, and may retard the aging process in humans.

Link between caloric intake and aging.

Unfortunately, many of us are living in a nutritionally dilapidated state with poor antioxidant status. To get our body back to homeostasis, we must:

– Improve our antioxidant status
– Decrease oxidative stress or
– Both

The recommended course of action is to eat smaller portions, and consume more foods that are naturally high in nutrients and

HIGH	MEDIUM	LOW
Organ meat	Whole grains*	Refined grains (i.e.bread, pasta, crackers, etc.)
Meat, wild game and poultry	Legumes*	Sugar
Fish and shellfish	Plant fats and oils**	Industrial seed oils
Eggs	Animal fats and oils**	Processed food and snacks
Fruits	Dairy products	Sugar-sweetened beverages
Vegetables		Artificial ingredients
Nuts and seeds*		Alcohol
Herbs and spices		Natural sweeteners

Whole grains, legumes, and nuts and seeds contain substances called "nutrient inhibitors" that impair the absorption of some of the nutrients they contain.

**Plant and animal fats are relatively low in nutrients, but they play other crucial roles, including helping us to absorb the nutrients in other foods.*

Foods ranked by nutrient density and bioavailability.

antioxidants, like raw organic plants. When we decrease our digestive burden by eating less, or by choosing foods that are easier to digest, the outcome is lower levels of oxidative stress.

For most people, plants are easier for the body to digest than animal protein. This is even more true for individuals with low levels of stomach acid, a condition known as hypochloridia. The exception is when clients are dealing with gut dysfunction. It can be hard for these folks to break down raw veggies. In these cases, I suggest starting out by lightly cooking your veggies in healthy, plant-based fats like extra virgin olive oil, coconut oil, or MCT oil.

Less energy required to break down food means more energy for other things. It also means lower inflammatory markers and a decreased rate of aging on a cellular level.

If you have a plate in front of you, about 80% of that plate should consist of plants, and the remaining 20% should be:

- *Most Frequently:* Wild-caught fish and oysters
- *Less Frequently:* Organic, free-range chicken and turkey
- *Least Frequently:* Organic grass-fed beef, Wild game, Duck, or Bison

Again, these suggestions are provided in the context of optimizing energy and brain power. They are not necessarily as relevant when it comes to improving body composition or nutrient status. To accomplish these desired outcomes simultaneously would likely necessitate a customized program.

Wild caught fish and these recommended animal proteins provide the body with bioavailable forms of essential nutrients like vitamin A, vitamin D, iron, vitamin B12, and animal-based Omega 3 fats. Many of these essential nutrients can be difficult to obtain in a strict vegan or vegetarian diet.

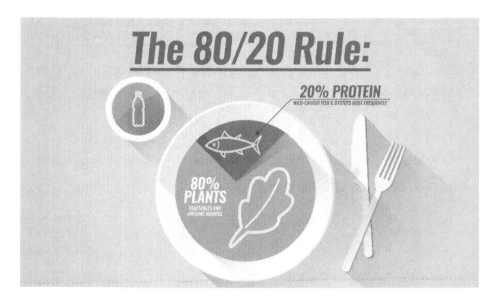

By basing 80% of your food volume around plants, mostly vegetables and some organic berries (fruits if you're within a healthy weight range), we lower our exposure to systemic inflammation, metabolic diseases (insulin resistance, high blood sugar, leptin resistance), heart disease, cancer, and diabetes.

SUCCESS LEAVES CLUES

The following is a short list of some historical figures you may not have known were vegetarians and vegans:

- Albert Einstein (He believed that "nothing will benefit human health and increase chances for survival of life on earth as the evolution to a vegetarian diet.")
- Leonardo Da Vinci
- Mark Twain
- The Beatles
  - Paul McCartney
  - John Lennon
  - George Harrison
  - Ringo Star
- Elen DeGeneres
- Madonna
- Nikola Tesla
- Plato
- Abraham Lincoln
- Justin Timberlake
- Charlie Chaplin
- Steve Jobs
- Benjamin Franklin

- Ariana Huffington
- Sir Isaac Newton
- Thomas Edison
- Ralph Waldo Emerson
- Deepak Chopra
- Bill Clinton
- Hank Aaron
- Henry David Thoreau
- John Harvey Kellogg
- Carl Lewis
- Vincent Van Gogh
- Henry Ford
- Charles Darwin

It's not just about morals, ethics or, even, health...

Today 18% of worldwide greenhouse gasses are produced by livestock and meat production.

That's more than cars, buses, planes, boats, and trains combined.

Perhaps more important than driving less or switching to electric cars, the greatest decision we can make to preserve our planet is eating less meat. This is especially true for red meat.

I recommend red meat be consumed no more than once a week to optimize your own health and that of our one and only planet.

Look back at the list above.

It includes some of the most successful and brilliant minds in human history.

Success leaves clues.

THE SECRET TO A HAPPY BELLY

The human gut microbiome has been the subject of extensive research in recent years. Our knowledge of the resident species and its capacity to impact energy production, cognition, hormonal health, and body composition is rapidly growing. Your gut is home to a complex community of over 100 trillion microbial cells.

The gut microbiome impacts energy and cognition through various mechanisms, including:

- *The Immune System:* Approximately 70-80% of your immune system is located in your gut.
- *Neurotransmitters and Mood:* Around the same percentage (70%) of the body's feel good neurotransmitter serotonin is produced in the gut. Serotonin boosts your resistance to stress and elevates your mood.
- *Digestion, Absorption, and the Simulation of Nutrients:* When gut health or intestinal integrity (leaky gut, inflammation) are compromised, it prevents us from properly digesting, absorbing, and transporting nutrients throughout the body which handicaps energy production.

A key aspect of maintaining high levels of energy is making a conscious effort to consume foods that support the growth and replication of good bacteria while avoiding substances that can disrupt this delicate balance, damage the intestinal lining, and cause systemic inflammation.

Our gut contains both good and bad (pathogenic) bacteria. When we consume dietary toxins (the immunogenic and allergenic foods we discussed earlier), this can allow the pathogenic bacteria to gain a foothold and disrupt the delicate microbial ecosystem in our gut.

This imbalance, referred to as gut dysbiosis, can lead to hard-to-lose body fat, inflammation, depression, skin conditions, brain fog, bowel disorders, and chronic fatigue.

Here are two strategies to keep your belly happy and healthy:

- *Avoid the Bad Stuff (acellular carbohydrates and toxins):* Refined carbohydrates, sugar, processed foods, antibiotics, birth control, non-steroidal anti-inflammatory drugs, commercial dairy, artificial sweeteners, industrial seed oils (corn oil, canola oil, soybean oil, and vegetable oil), wheat, grains, and alcohol. For female clients interested in more information on hormonal birth control and how it impacts our biology long term, I recommend picking up the book Sexy by Nature: The Whole Foods Solution to Radiant Health, Life-Long Sex Appeal, and Soaring Confidence by Stefani Ruper.

- *Consume a Diet High in Cellular Carbohydrates:* This includes vegetables, tubers, and fruits. These carbohydrates are cellular in nature, meaning they are surrounded by fibrous cell walls. This fiber feeds good bacteria in the digestive tract.

These cellular carbohydrates serve to:
- Lower inflammation
- Strengthen your immune system
- Increase the production of serotonin
- Help to maintain a healthy body weight

All of these are integral components to energy production, focus, and high performance.

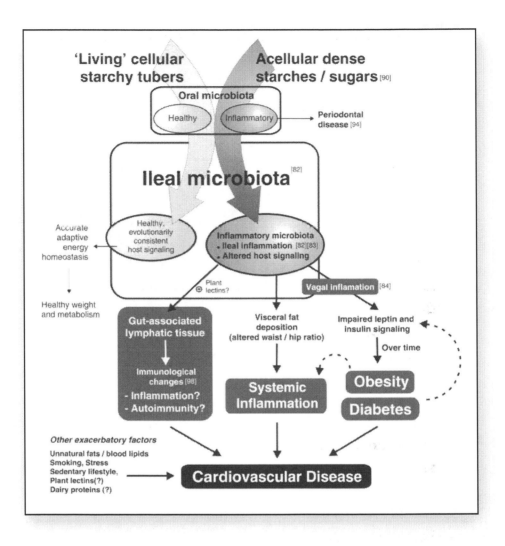

Now let's contrast an ancestral diet, rich in plant-based cellular carbohydrates, with a modern man-made diet that's been overrun with acellular carbohydrates.

Acellular carbohydrates are much higher in carbohydrate density than anything we would have encountered on an ancestral diet. They lack the fiber necessary to slow the subsequent spike in blood sugar and insulin release that takes place whenever we eat carbs.

Again, this comes down to an issue of quality over quantity.

A harmful misconception is that carbohydrates make us fat, sick, and tired. For people who are overweight, insulin resistant, or dealing with other metabolic issues, there is some truth to this. There are many examples of traditional, indigenous cultures, such as the Tukisenta in Papua New Guinea, who get 95% of their calories from cellular carbohydrates. Yet, the Tukisenta are lean, energetic, and have excellent biomarkers of health.

The reason why industrialized diets are so harmful is not because of the quantity of carbohydrates they contain. It's because those carbohydrates lack living cells and have a completely different impact on the gut microbiome compared to plant-based cellular carbohydrates.

The Lesson: Eat real food. Mostly plants. Make most of those plants vegetables. And make most of those vegetables green. Focus on quality over quantity. Here's a helpful rule of thumb when making food choices. Ask yourself:

- *Question #1:* Did this food exist somewhere on Earth 10,000 years ago? If the answer is yes, move on to question two.
- *Question #2:* Did this food exist in, or close to, the form I'm about to eat it somewhere on Earth 10,000 years ago?

If you get a "yes" to both questions, you're probably good to go. Dig in.

CASE STUDY: VITA

In a past life, I was a trainer and yoga instructor at David Barton Gym (DBG) in Chicago. David Barton was known for having some of the best personal trainers and fitness professionals in the world.

I am not here today because of talent. I am here because of an obsession. I am obsessed with constantly learning, growing, and evolving to help my clients get results faster and easier.

We are all created equal. And you can be anyone you want to be if you are willing to put in the time and hard work. I am not talented. I am obsessed. Teaching yoga and training clients at David Barton was an opportunity to "sharpen the ax" and learn from some of the greatest fitness professionals on the planet.

A world class mixed martial artist will seek out the best teachers in each of his fighting disciplines in order to become a more well-rounded, lethal fighter. The difference was that my disciplines were not Jiu Jitszu, boxing, Muay Thai, or wrestling. They were nutritional neuroscience, exercise physiology, functional medicine, and executive coaching.

To grasp what it was like at David Barton Gym, imagine a New York-style-nightclub meets cutting-edge fitness training facility. There

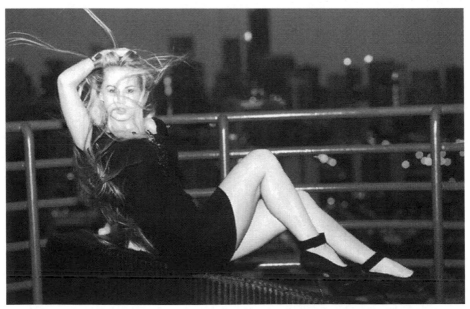

Vita's story illustrates the damage that conventional meats and farming can cause.

was minimal lighting. Deep house music blasted from the speakers and reverberated off the gym walls. And the clientele were young professionals in their late 20's, 30's, and 40's. DBG members were there just as much to be seen as they went there to train.

Vita was a 23-year-old Ukrainian bombshell who started at the front desk before she was taken under the wing of the gym manager, Lauren, and groomed to be a trainer.

Vita had the type of body most women would kill for. It was well known that many wives of Vita's male clients were not thrilled about the idea of their husband spending hours every week with another woman, especially a woman like Vita.

Vita moved to the US from the Ukraine when she was just 21 years old. Even in the Ukraine, she was very healthy. She avoided processed and refined foods. She cooked almost all of her meals at home, and knew exactly what was going into her body. She maintained these same habits after moving to the US.

This is where things get a little weird.

Even though Vita was eating the exact same foods, in the same quantities, and doing the same workouts she had done in the Ukraine, she gained over 20 pounds in the first three months she was living here.

She was frustrated and confused. How could it be possible for someone to gain more than 20 pounds of fat, that quickly, without changing a single aspect of her lifestyle aside from geographic location.

Things didn't stop there.

Partly because she felt helpless and partly due to other chemical influencers, Vita became depressed. Her energy was lower than it had ever been. She quickly found herself in a challenging position many of us have been in ourselves. She knew she had to workout to improve her situation, but she was tired all the time.

Completely bewildered, Vita started looking for answers. In her search, she stumbled upon a movie called Food Inc. which blows the whistle on our nation's food industry, exposing how the US food supply is controlled and manipulated by a handful of corporations that put financial profit ahead of consumer health.

In Food Inc., the filmmaker takes his camera into slaughterhouses and factory farms where chickens grow too fast to walk properly, cows eat feed pumped with toxic chemicals, and illegal immigrants risk life and limb to bring these products to market at the cheapest possible costs. It wasn't until Vita became aware of the radical differences in how food is produced in the US compared to the rest of the world that these changes started making sense. Many people who immigrate to the US have similar experiences.

Since Vita was on a budget, buying everything organic wasn't really a viable option for her. So what she ended up doing was cutting back on a lot the meat that she was consuming.

Most of the chemicals, hormones, and antibiotics in meat are stored in the fat. When Vita consumed animal protein, it was almost exclusively lean fish and poultry, to minimize exposure to these toxins. She eliminated commercial dairy entirely. To compensate for less meat and dairy, she ate more vegetables.

In less than two months, Vita's weight was back to normal. Her energy as high as it had ever been, and she dropped the 20 pounds without even trying.

I mention Vita because she is a perfect, isolated case study about the damage that conventional meats and farming can cause our bodies. The exact same types of foods and portions in the Ukraine and in the US, and a completely different result. The only difference was how the animals were raised and harvested. Factory farming and non-organic food have severe ramifications to our body.

THERAPEUTIC KETOSIS

Mitochondria are bacteria-like organelles inside our cells. They take nutrients and convert them into ATP (adenosine triphosphate), which is the primary energy unit in our body.

Impaired cellular energy production, also known as mitochondrial dysfunction, was once thought to be a rare condition that affected only one in every 4,000 people. However, recent research has shown that there are varying levels of this disorder, and its prevalence is much more common than we once suspected. Now it is believed that mitochondrial problems affect as many as 1 in every 50 people.

Mitochondrial dysfunction has been implicated in a wide range of modern degenerative conditions, ranging from chronic fatigue, pain, fibromyalgia, depression, anxiety, chronic stress, autism, cancer, diabetes, and mental disorders like bipolar disease and schizophrenia.

There are two types of mitochondrial dysfunction: primary and secondary. Primary mitochondrial dysfunction is a result of a genetic mutation that's inherited from our mothers. Secondary mitochondrial dysfunction is a result of environmental factors like exposure to toxins, poor diet, lack of sunlight, inadequate sleep, and a sedentary lifestyle.

Studies show that patients with chronic fatigue syndrome (CFS) are much more likely to have mitochondrial dysfunction than true CFS. Additionally, mitochondrial dysfunction is suspected to be related to a number of other conditions, including Lyme disease.

A study conducted in 2012 showed bactericidal antibiotics, like those used in the treatment of Lyme disease, induced mitochondrial dysfunction, and oxidative damage in mammalian cells. This means that many Lyme patients, who are already starting out with suboptimal cellular ATP production, may find their energy levels further compromised after the administration of the antibiotics.

When I was undergoing treatment for Lyme disease, I was on oral antibiotics of various types for almost an entire year. There were days I could sleep 12 or even 14 hours and still wake up exhausted. A key aspect of my recovery was addressing and improving mitochondrial function and cellular energy production.

Therapeutic ketosis of the most effective interventions for improving mitochondrial function. This can be achieved through a ketogenic diet or intermittent fasting.

Therapeutic ketosis is a natural state that can be induced by prolonged periods of decreased glucose. Additional benefits of therapeutic ketosis, courtesy of www.ketogenic-diet-resource.com, include: Freedom from hypoglycemia, food fixations, and sugar cravings, Lack of hunger, Lower blood pressure, Drop in Cholesterol, Increase in HDL Cholesterol, Drop in triglycerides, Drop in fasting blood sugar and fasting insulin levels, Decreased levels of C Reactive Protein (CRP) and HbA1c proteins, More energy, Decrease in stiffness and joint pain, Clearer thinking, Changes in your sleep patterns and an improvement in sleep apnea symptoms, Weight loss, Heartburn relief, Decreased gum disease and tooth decay, Improved digestion and gut health, and Mood stabilization.

Sci Transl Med. 2013 Jul 3;5(192):192ra85. doi: 10.1126/scitranslmed.3006055.

Bactericidal antibiotics induce mitochondrial dysfunction and oxidative damage in Mammalian cells.

Kalghatgi S[1], Spina CS, Costello JC, Liesa M, Morones-Ramirez JR, Slomovic S, Molina A, Shirihai OS, Collins JJ.

⊛ Author information

Abstract

Prolonged antibiotic treatment can lead to detrimental side effects in patients, including ototoxicity, nephrotoxicity, and tendinopathy, yet the mechanisms underlying the effects of antibiotics in mammalian systems remain unclear. It has been suggested that bactericidal antibiotics induce the formation of toxic reactive oxygen species (ROS) in bacteria. We show that clinically relevant doses of bactericidal antibiotics-quinolones, aminoglycosides, and β-lactams-cause mitochondrial dysfunction and ROS overproduction in mammalian cells. We demonstrate that these bactericidal antibiotic-induced effects lead to oxidative damage to DNA, proteins, and membrane lipids. Mice treated with bactericidal antibiotics exhibited elevated oxidative stress markers in the blood, oxidative tissue damage, and up-regulated expression of key genes involved in antioxidant defense mechanisms, which points to the potential physiological relevance of these antibiotic effects. The deleterious effects of bactericidal antibiotics were alleviated in cell culture and in mice by the administration of the antioxidant N-acetyl-l-cysteine or prevented by preferential use of bacteriostatic antibiotics. This work highlights the role of antibiotics in the production of oxidative tissue damage in mammalian cells and presents strategies to mitigate or prevent the resulting damage, with the goal of improving the safety of antibiotic treatment in people.

Therapeutic ketosis via carbohydrate restriction, fasting, and exogenous ketones were instrumental in my recovery from Lyme disease. This is also one of the most effective strategies for improving energy levels and cognition.

You may have heard from your physician that ketosis is a life-threatening condition. If so, then your doctor may be confusing diabetic ketoacidosis (DKA) with nutritional ketosis (keto-adaptation).

Diabetic ketoacidosis occurs when a diabetic (usually a Type 1 diabetic) fails to receive adequate insulin and effectively starves. Insulin is the transport of protein that shuttles sugar from our blood into our cells, where it can be used to produce energy.

Therapeutic ketosis, on the other hand is also a powerful performance-enhancing tool for healthy members of the general population.

As we age, we lose the ability to process carbohydrates. This is a condition called decreased carbohydrate tolerance. Consequently, our bodies becomes less sensitive to insulin.

Long-chain fatty acids (LCFAs) do not cross the blood-brain barrier. Through the process of beta oxidation in the liver, Coenzyme A then begins to break down these fatty acids. The byproducts of beta oxidation form water-soluble ketone bodies.

Ketones can readily cross the blood-brain barrier and get inside the cells and into the mitochondria. The two main types of ketone bodies are Acetoacetate (AcAc) and Beta-hydroxybutyrate (β-HB). It usually takes 24-28 hours for someone to get to levels that are considered mild ketosis (above 0.5 millimolar). Many people mistakenly assume they are in ketosis. Anyone who has tried to verify a ketogenic state, using ketone levels in the blood, has probably found it to be more difficult than anticipated. You can't just skip breakfast, drink a cup of Bulletproof Coffee, and go ketogenic.

Fasting is, however, the quickest way to get into ketosis.

This may explain why most of the studies on intermittent fasting show the greatest benefit occurring right around the 24-hour mark. Less time may prevent ketosis from taking place.

Therapeutic ketosis has been shown to have numerous beneficial effects on gene expression and results in desirable epigenetic changes, both on an acute and long-term basis.

The ideal ketogenic diet is around 20% to 30% protein and 70% to 80% fat. Carbohydrates sources consumed come exclusively from non-starchy vegetables, with a focus on the green variety.

When we restrict carbohydrates, blood sugar stabilizes and insulin levels decrease. The body, and particularly the liver, will then start to mobilize fatty acids for fuel.

I recommend that you aim for mild to moderate ketosis, which is between 1 to 3 millimolars. This will provide the energy, cognitive health, longevity, performance and real-world benefits without potential adverse effects. When you get into higher millimolar ranges, mild metabolic acidosis may result, and this will need to be compensated for by the kidneys and liver. The most effective nutritional practices for inducing therapeutic ketosis are:

- Intermittent fasting
- The Ketogenic Diet
- Caloric restriction
- Exogenous ketones

Some of the tools that I recommend for increasing ketone levels are:

- Pure Caprylic acid (Bulletproof Brain Octane, Parrillo CapTri)
- MCT oil
- Raw, organic, extra virgin coconut oil

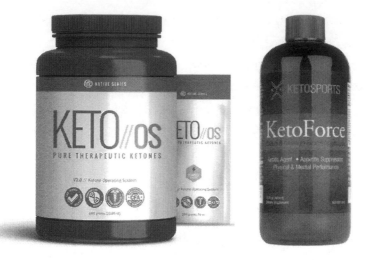

- Keto-OS exogenous ketones by Pruvit (http://biohacks.pruvitnow.com)
- Keto Sports KetoCaNa exogenous ketones
- KetoSports KetoForce
- Scivation Xtend Raw branch chain amino acids (no color, no sweeteners, no flavor)

Exogenous ketones supplements are particularly helpful in easing the transition into ketosis and making fasting more enjoyable and sustainable. There are products that contain beta-hydroxybutyrate salts and offer the following benefits:

- They raise blood ketone levels
- They increase endurance
- They decrease oxygen utilization
- They accelerate ketosis, and this eases the metabolic transition into ketosis
- They also provide caloric energy that cannot be stored as fat

For bodybuilders and athletes, it's important to have a calorie surplus to push insulin levels up and to drive metabolic processes. Twenty to thirty percent of your diet is protein coming from wild-caught fish, free-range poultry, and pastured (grass-fed) organic meats.

Healthy fats come from: Pastured egg yokes, Extra virgin olive oil, Raw, organic coconut oil, MCT oil, Pure Caprylic acid (C8-MCT as found in Bulletproof Brain Octane and Parrillo CaprTri), Butter from grass-fed cows (less frequently than plant sources), Organic ghee from grass-fed cows (less frequently than plant sources), Nuts, Seeds (flax, Chia seeds, pumpkin seeds), Avocado, and Udo's Choice oil blend.

When it comes to carbohydrates, you should aim for 35 or more grams of fiber from: Organic, non-starchy vegetables, Leafy greens, Herb salad mix, Spinach, Kale, Charred collards, Romaine Spring Mix, Arugula, Lettuce, Mustard greens, Turnip greens, Broccoli, Asparagus, Green beans, Celery, Artichokes, Cabbage, Cauliflower, Mushrooms, Brussels sprouts, Bean sprouts, Broccoli sprouts, Bok Choy, Cucumber, Okra, Onions, Peppers, and Snow peas.

Each meal should have lots of fiber from green vegetables to help keep you in ketosis, and always eat your vegetables with a source of fat.

Big salads will be a staple of your diet. Be sure to add many different types of organic, non-starchy vegetables. You should also include avocado and base your dressings around extra virgin olive oil, MCT oil, pure Caprylic acid, and apple cider vinegar.

The most important fat to include as part of your therapeutic ketosis is C-8 Caprylic acid MCTs as found in Brain Octane and Parrillo CapTri. These medium-chain triglycerides are the fastest to metabolize in the brain because your liver does not have to process them. It takes the body 26 steps to convert sugar into ATP. It takes only three steps for your body to convert C-8 Caprylic acid MCTs into the ATP required to fuel cellular energy.

You would need almost 20 tablespoons of coconut oil to get the equivalent effects of one tablespoon of C-8 Caprylic acid MCTs.

I have provided a detailed breakdown for measuring your state of ketosis using blood tests, urine, and breath tests in the "Keeping Track: Self-Monitoring" section of this guide.

The easiest, most accurate way to monitor your ketone levels at home, that I've found...and the one I use, is the Precision Xtra by Abbot. Blood ketones are best tested in a fasted state, so it's recommended to do this in the morning prior to breakfast. Again, you'll want to aim for 1-3 millimolars.

Potential contraindications and adverse effects of the ketogenic diet include:

- Increased cholesterol
- Kidney stones
- Gastroesophageal reflux
- Risk of ketoacidosis in Type 1 diabetics

Not all people do well on ketogenic and high-fat diets. We occasionally see this in individuals who are dealing with digestive issues, especially when the ketogenic diet is high in animal fats.

It can also be problematic for individuals with chronic infections since many pathogens used dietary fat to build protective biofilms, which prevent our body's immune system from doing its job.

Lastly, individuals with fat malabsorption or body aches may do better limiting excessive dietary fats and supplementing with a quality digestive enzyme that includes lipase.

For a more in-depth exploration of therapeutic ketosis or the ketogenic diet, I recommend checking out:

- www.Ketogenic-diet-resource.com
- www.KetoNutrition.org
- Anything by Dom D'Agostino (start with his podcast episode of The Tim Ferriss Show)
- www.EatingAcademy.com and anything else by Peter Attia (The Tim Ferriss Show podcast is a good intro to Peter's work as well)

THE CYCLICAL LOW CARB DIET

Let's say that you've tried a ketogenic diet or fasting, and decided they are not a good fit. The good news is that you can still experience many of the same benefits simply by moderately restricting your carbohydrate intake. A cyclical, low carbohydrate diet may:

- Increase energy production
- Increase mitochondrial efficiency
- Increase fat utilization during exercise and physical activity
- Increase the efficiency of glycogen utilization
- Increase health and longevity
- Activate biological pathways responsible for building and repairing lean muscle tissue

Simply by making plants, particularly non-starchy vegetables, your primary carbohydrate source, you will lower your body's carbohydrate load. These cellular carbohydrates, wherein the carbs are surrounded by fibrous cell walls, have lower carbohydrate densities when compared to grains and processed foods.

They also feed the good bacteria in the gut, which has been shown to lower inflammation, strengthen the immune system, boost energy, elevate mood, and improve hormonal health.

Raw, organic vegetables and fruits are also highest in the antioxidant glutathione, which we need to neutralize free radicals, protect our mitochondria, and eliminate toxic heavy metals from the body.

Finding your optimal carbohydrate intake requires a little experimentation.

The goal is to consume enough carbohydrates to support energy expenditure and hormonal health, without overburdening the digestive system or triggering the storage of excess body fat.

You'll also want to vary higher carb days with lower carb days. Most people do best with high carb days on heavy training days and lower carb days on days they are less physically active. Of course, high and low are relative terms based on each individual's carbohydrate tolerance, health status, and goals.

As a general rule of thumb, a good place to start is 65-100 grams of carbohydrates per day for men and 50-75 grams of carbohydrates per day for women.

CASE STUDY: MIKE – TRAIN LESS, EAT SMARTER, FEEL BETTER

Mike was a 26-year-old professional model living in Chicago. He was tall, with a naturally lean build. He had been a swimmer his entire life, and he had a solid knowledge base of health, nutrition, and fitness.

Armed with this knowledge, Mike was one of the few men out there able to maintain sub-10% body fat year-round.

Mike ended up coming to me because he was stuck. Many of the strategies that he successfully used in his early 20's to stay lean were no longer working.

He was frustrated and concerned about how these changes would effect his livelihood. His career is centered around his physical appearance, and he was finding himself having to spend hours a day at the gym and getting so strict with his diet that it was having a negative impact on his social life.

While Mike looked great on the surface, he was exhausted. His interest in sex had decreased, making him wonder if he had low testosterone. The situation was only made worse when he tried to compensate by adding more high-intensity CrossFit-style workouts and essentially eating chicken breasts and broccoli for most of his meals.

This combination of glycolytically-demanding workouts and extremely low-carb dieting had brought about a symptomatic pattern that I've seen more and more with my male clients as of late. I helped him order some necessary blood tests, which confirmed my suspicions.

Mike's laboratory results confirmed that he had the testosterone levels of a 70 year old man.

He also had compromised thyroid hormone function, confirmed by T4, T3, reverse T3, and TSH (thyroid stimulating hormone) blood work.

Part of the problem was a mismatch between Mike's energy outlay, from his demanding workouts, and his carbohydrate intake. I reintroduced a variety of organic fruits and starchy tubers into his nutrition program. They included: Raspberries, Blackberries, Blueberries, Apples, Pears, Sweet potatoes, Yams, Squash, Plantains, Cassava, Organic wholegrain germinated brown rice, White potatoes and organic jasmine rice (occasionally).

I instructed him to consume these insulin-spiking carbohydrates post-workout, or with dinner, and always alongside a healthy, low fat protein source and plenty of fiber.

Since Mike needed to maintain extremely low levels of body fat, we made sure that meals which spiked blood sugar were low in dietary fat. His meals were either high-fat and low-carb, or high-carb and low-fat.

I recommended that Mike consume around 0.7 grams of protein per pound of lean body mass. And the protein he consumed should come from wild-caught fish and organic poultry. I calculated Mike's lean body mass using the Boer, James, Hume formulas. Then, I removed the outlier and averaged the remaining two results. He was required to get at least 35 or more grams of fiber per day, and if he chose to eat nuts, grains, or legumes, I advised that he soak them prior to cooking in order to maximize nutrient bio-availability and minimize potential digestive complications.

In less than a week, Mike's energy was higher than it had been in months. His mood had elevated, he was less stressed, and he was sleeping much better at night.

You see, carbs trigger the release of serotonin. By consuming most of his carbohydrates with dinner, Mike was able to feel more relaxed, and this induced a deeper, more restful night's sleep. It is a fallacy that eating carbs at night will make you fat. If anything, the opposite is true. Eating carbs for breakfast spikes blood sugar and insulin levels, which adversely impact lipolysis (fat burning).

I ran into Mike a couple of months later. His sex drive had returned, and he was dating again. He looked great and, best of all, his nutrition program was actually sustainable. He didn't have to carry tupperware with him everywhere he went. He trained less, ate smarter, and felt better.

In the next section, we are going to discuss a biohack that, if it were a pharmaceutical drug, would be worth billions of dollars every year. This biohack is good old fashioned exercise. The really great news is, thanks to modern advancements in sports medicine and scientific studies, we are able to get much more out of exercise programs with much less work. Here are a few of its benefits:

- Patients with knee arthritis who exercised for one hour, three times a week, reduced their pain and disability by 47%.
- In older patients, it reduced incidence of Alzheimer's and dementia by 50%.
- In patients that were at a high risk of developing Diabetes, exercise coupled with other lifestyle interventions reduced progression to clinical Diabetes by 58%.
- Post menopausal women who exercised for just four hours a week had a 41% reduction in their risk for hip fractures.
- Anxiety and stress were reduced by 48%, according to the meta-analysis.
- Patients with depression[6] were able to reduce their symptoms by 47%.

One study followed over 10,000 Harvard alumni for over 12 years, and those who exercised regularly ended up with a 27% lower risk of death than those that did not get the treatment. It is also the #1 treatment intervention for fatigue and increasing natural energy levels, and perhaps most importantly, exercise has been shown, in study after study, to improve quality of life.

In the next section, you are going to learn some of the most effective exercise strategies for increasing energy, cognitive function, and performance, along with some breakthrough tools and technologies for accelerating your results.

---

[6] Patients who had depression did just as well with this intervention as they would have if they had been taking prescription antidepressants. In many cases, they even did better than they would have if they were taking prescription meds.

NUTRITION BIOHACKS

This is not an all-inclusive summary from this section but will help you get started until you are able to explore in more detail.

The One Thing: Make 80% of your nutrition organic plants. Most of those plants are vegetables, and most of those vegetables should be green. Wild-caught fish is your primary source of protein. Think of vegetables as the main dish. Wild caught fish and starchy tubers (sweet potatoes, yams, squash) or organic berries are your sides. Include liberal plant-based fats like avocado, raw organic chia seeds (in shakes), extra virgin olive oil, raw organic extra virgin coconut oil, MCT oil, and C8 pure caprylic acid MCT oil.

Biohack #1: To understand your body better, pay special attention to what makes you feel good and what makes you feel bad.

In this chapter, I have advised that you do so by eliminating common immunogenic and allergenic foods from your diet for 28 days, and then strategically reintroduce them one at a time to observe their impact.

As you reintroduce these foods, pay close attention to what effects they may have on your energy, mood, pain and stiffness, and cognitive function over the next 72 hours.

Biohack #2: Minimize the *big four* toxins, which are: Grains (especially wheat, barely, rye, and their derivatives), Dairy, GMOs (i.e. Corn, soy, canola oil, and their derivatives), and Alcohol. Remember, what you *don't* eat is far more important than what you do eat.

Biohack #3: One of the most effective interventions for improving mitochondrial function is therapeutic ketosis, which can be achieved through a ketogenic diet or intermittent fasting.

Biohack #4: If not a ketogenic diet, I recommend a cyclical, low-carb diet to:

- Increase energy production
- Increase mitochondrial efficiency
- Increase fat utilization during exercise and physical activity
- Increase the efficiency of glycogen utilization
- Increase health and longevity
- Activate biological pathways responsible for building and repairing lean muscle tissue

Biohack #5: Drink nutrient-dense shakes and juice organic green vegetables. Best results are experienced having one shake for a meal daily. This should be made in a blender, not a NutriBullet or other device which do not provide enough room for blended greens and whole foods. I recommend:

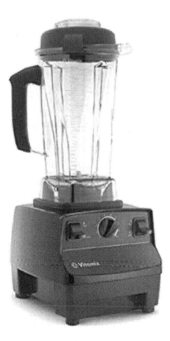

- *Blender:* Vitamix 5200 Blender and Blendtec Total Blender
- *Vegan Protein Powder:* Sunwarrior Warrior Blend Protein and Vegan Shakeology (best tasting vegan protein I've found; www.biohackerprotein. com)
- *Juicer:* Champion Commercial Juicer and Breville 800JEXL Juice Fountain Elite 1000-Watt Juice Extractor

Biohack #6: Make it convenient to eat healthy. Some of my favorite go to foods include: Wild Planet Wild Sardines in Extra Virgin Olive Oil, Wild Planet Wild Alaska Pink Salmon, Wild Planet Wild Albacore Tuna, Crown Prince Oysters in Olive Oil, Nick's Sticks Free Range Turkey Sticks, Raw veggies and guacamole available at any grocery store, and Go Raw Sprouted Organic Pumpkin Seeds.

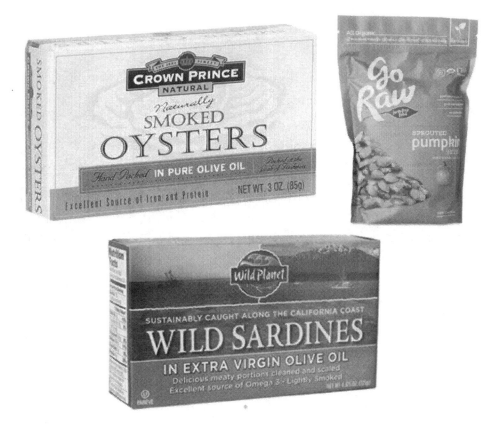

Health bar manufacturers require the use of syrup (such as sugar, honey, maple, corn, rice, tapioca, agave, or sugar alcohol), which increases the glycemic load of the product, can send you running for the bathroom, and may be toxic. Using a proprietary technology, WarriorBar is made with no added sugar, sugar alcohol, or syrups and uses non-denatured bioactive whey protein from grass-fed cows.

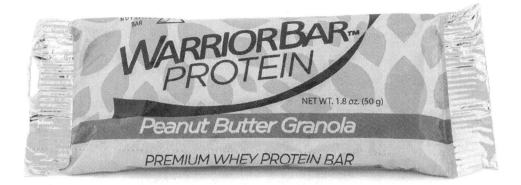

These services also make eating healthy more convenient:

- *Instacart (www.instacart.com):* Get groceries delivered to your door in 1 hour. Shop online from stores like Whole Foods and Costco. Your first delivery over $10 is free. This is a game changer for my busy clients.
- *Peapod (www.peapod.com):* Another online grocery shopping and delivery service.
- *Door to Door Organics (www.doortodoororganics.com):* Farm fresh food delivered to your front door.
- *Luvo Inc (www.LuvoInc.com):* Local, organic, preservative-free meals, products and ingredients. Great for people who work and travel a lot. Many options do contain grains, so not recommended for individuals with autoimmune issues.
- *Green Chef (www.greenchef.com):* Fresh, organic meals delivered to your doorstep.
- *Factor 75 (www.Factor75.com):* Factor 75 delivers healthy prepared meals to your home. Their organic meal plans are designed for a variety of diets including paleo.
- *Thrive Market (www.ThriveMarket.com):* Buy healthy food from top-selling, organic brands at wholesale prices. Shop for

gluten-free, non-gmo, non-toxic products for a wide range of diets. While their unique selling point is wholesale pricing. I've heard mixed things. But nothing a little ethical bribe can't smooth over. They are offering a free 15-ounce Nutiva organic coconut oil to our readers at BiohackingSecrets.com/Nutiva.

- *U.S. Wellness Meats (www.grasslandbeef.com):* Healthy meat and other organic products delivered to your doorstep.
- *Massa Meats (www.massanaturalmeats.com):* Healthy meat, delivered.
- *Arizona Grass Raised Beef Company (www.azgrassraisedbeef. com):* Another healthy meat delivery option.
- *Amazon.com:* Where I buy most of my supplements and biohacking gear.
- *Eat Purely (www.EatPurely.com):* Chef-made, organic meals delivered in 20 minutes (this is a lifesaver when I'm working late and the fridge is bare; currently Chicago-only). Save $20 on your first order with promo code "ANTHONYD2".
- *Hi-Vibe Organic Juice Bar (www.hi-vibe.com):* My favorite organic superfood juicery in Chicago. My go-to is the G-8 green

detox juice. It's all power greens, low sugar, no fruit. Ask for Nick.

- *Radish (www.goradish.com):* Healthy meals delivered hot and ready to eat in under 20 minutes. Whenever possible they use organic and locally farmed produce. The menu changes every day, which keeps it from getting boring. You build your meal starting with 7 healthy items for you to mix and match. Meals start at just $10. Another lifesaver when I'm bunkered down working on big projects. Save $10 on your first order with the promo code "BIRMET".

- *Sprig (www.sprig.com):* If you're really pressed for time, Sprig offers healthy, organic meals delivered in 15 minutes. Sprig is geared towards the folks who wondered why nobody ever came out with 7-Minute Abs. I just had a Jerk Chicken Salad with Fruit & Pepper Relish and one of the best dark chocolate chip cookies I've ever tasted (okay, maybe two, don't judge). Get $10 off your first order with promo code "DICLEME360".

Biohack #7: Make healthy food taste good. Many recipes that are Pescetarian, Paleo, vegan, vegetarian, and Mediterranean Diet fit the criteria recommended in this guide. Some ingredients that will add great flavor to your food include:

- *Salad Dressings:* Extra virgin olive oil, Bragg apple cider vinegar
- *Herbs and Spices (ideally fresh):* Garlic, Ginger, Cinnamon, Cumin, Turmeric, Sage, Rosemary, Chile Pepper, Saffron, Parsley, Basil, Curry, Thyme, Cayenne Pepper, Oregano, Cilantro, Fennel
- *Seasonings:* Himalayan sea salt, Bragg Sea Kelp Delight, Bragg Sprinkle, Bragg Nutritional Yeast, Borsari Seasoned Salt, Dorot frozen garlic cubes, Dorot frozen basil cubes, Bragg Liquid

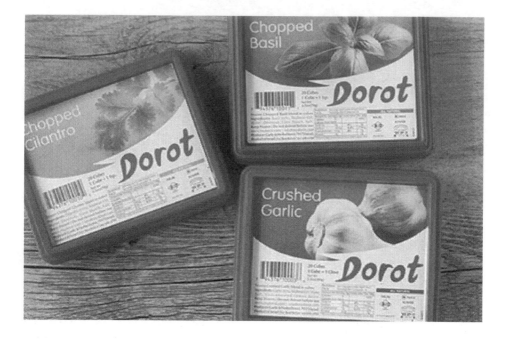

Aminos, and Nori Komi Furikake (this dried mix made of sesame seeds, seaweed flakes, salt, and a little sugar kicks up vegetables, soups, rice, and salads. Plus, no MSG which is an excitotoxin, a class of chemicals that overstimulate neuron receptors and can trigger migraines in some individuals).

- *Hot Sauces:* Cholula Hot Sauce, Sriracha Hot Sauce

Order a few highly-rated, organic seasonings on Amazon and see which you like.

MOVEMENT

English businessman and investor, Sir Richard Branson, is best known as the founder of the Virgin Group, which is comprised of over 400 companies. In his 65 years on this planet, he has accrued over $5 billion in net worth. Branson has an infectious personality, a seemingly endless supply of energy, and the kind of unmatched productivity you'd expect from someone running over 400 companies.

A few years ago, a group of entrepreneurs was visiting Branson at his home on Necker Island. They had all gathered to learn from the man himself and to share ideas on how to grow and improve one another's business.

During the meeting, one of the attendees asked Branson the question every business owner wants to know, "How do you become more productive?"

Branson sat back and thought for a minute, and the attendees waited, eagerly anticipating his response. After a long pause, Branson responded with just two words, "Work out."

Working out (and, specifically, building a bigger aerobic engine) is the answer to many of the most challenging questions I get asked by executives, entrepreneurs, athletes, traders, and high-level business professionals today:

Q: How do I increase my energy?

A: Work out.

Q: How do I get more confidence?

A: Work out.

Q: How do I strengthen my immune system?

A: Work out.

Q: How do I minimize down time?

A: Work out.

Q: How get a deeper, more restful night's sleep?

A: Work out.

Q: How do I increase my attention to detail and stay focused for longer periods of time?

A: Work out.

Q: How do I get a better body and elevate my mood?

A: Work out.

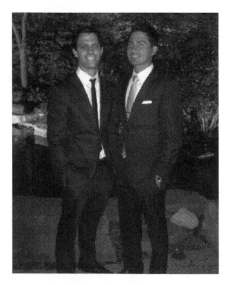

The solution to so many modern challenges is a simple one. Perhaps that's why so many of us ignore it.

Or, perhaps it's because so many of us are doing it wrong.

There are some key differences between a workout program for improving body composition versus one designed to increase energy, focus, and productivity.

Many people, especially men, think that they want a lean, ripped body and washboard six-pack abs. Looking good is important, and it does play a role in confidence and how we feel about ourselves. But I believe that what most of us really want is to feel good. The reason why we pursue a better body and outward displays of strength and fitness, like six-pack abs, is because we believe that these physical characteristics will bring about the good feelings that we desire.

In recent years, steady-state cardiovascular exercise has gotten an undeserved bad rap. Although resistance training, cross-fit, power lifting, and other high intensity exercise programs are very effective for burning fat and building muscle, they pale in comparison to cardiovascular exercise when it comes to increasing energy, focus, and productivity.

Sir Richard Branson loves to start his day with a swim or a game of tennis on Necker Island. He estimates that by investing one hour into exercise, he adds four additional hours of productivity to his day.

There's plenty of scientific literature that confirms Branson's assessments. Dozens of scientific studies have found that steady-state endurance exercise produces many metabolic and cardiovascular benefits, including:

- An increase in oxidative capacity of skeletal muscle (greater number and size of mitochondria)
- An increase in skeletal muscle myoglobin concentration (myoglobin is the primary oxygen-carrying protein in muscle tissues)
- A greater ability to oxidize fatty acids for energy
- An increase in stored glycogen
- A decrease in resting heart rate
- An increase in resting and exercise stroke volume
- An increase in maximum cardio output
- An increase in VO2 max (which is one of the only things that has been scientifically proven to correlate with an increased lifespan in humans)

Regular exercise also protects us from disease in several ways. One of the main ways that it does so is by preventing oxidative damage and lowering inflammation, which are the primary mechanisms behind most modern degenerative conditions. This likely explains why people who are sedentary have up to 2.5 times the risk of developing heart disease.

Academy Award winner Matthew McConaughey is known for always being in great shape and rarely one to wear a shirt when he can get away with it. McConaughey was voted "Sexiest Man Alive" by People Magazine. He has one simple rule when it comes to exercise. He says, "My rule is to break a sweat a day... whether that's going for a run, whether that's dancing, whether that's loving, just break a sweat a day."

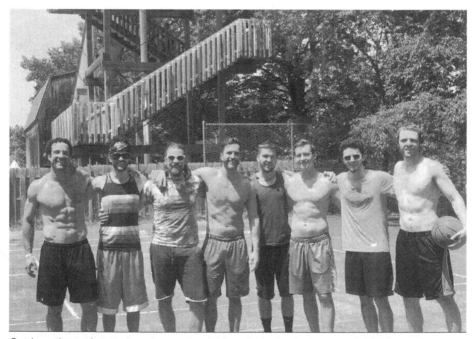

Outdoor play isn't just about having fun (although that's a big part of it). It's also an engaging way to workout, boost endogenous Vitamin D production & strengthen social bonds.

One 2006 study, published in Psychological Bulletin, analyzed over 70 studies on exercise and fatigue involving more than 6,800 people. What they found was that people who completed a regular exercise program reported far more energy and less fatigue than those groups that did not exercise. In fact, the average effect of exercise was greater than the improvements seen from the use of stimulant medications, including those used for attention deficit hyperactivity disorder (ADHD) and narcolepsy.

Every group studied, from healthy adults to cancer patients to diabetics, as well as to those with heart disease, all benefited from consistent exercise.

There are two mistakes that most of us make when it comes to aerobic conditioning:

1. Exercising at the wrong intensity (either too high or too low)
2. Exercising for the wrong duration (either not long enough to trigger physiological benefits, or so long that the workout exceeds the body's ability to recover)

I've hated running my entire life. Even 18 years of competitive soccer couldn't convert me to a fan of running. It wasn't until the past couple years that things finally took a shift. After studying scores of scientific studies, it is clear to me that an optimally, a well-rounded training program should address all three major energy systems:

- *The Phosphagen System* (also known as the Creatine Phosphate System, 3 to 30 seconds, This includes power lifting, bursting, and sprinting)
- *The Anaerobic System* (also known as the Glycolytic System, 30 seconds to 2 minutes, resistance and interval training)

- *The Oxidative System* (also known as the Aerobic System, greater than 2 minutes)

I spent the first 30 years of my life training only two of the three energy systems. I avoided cardio like the plague.

Performing exercise that targets the phosphagen and anaerobic systems will improve your body's capacity to do work and your physical ability to perform athletic activity. They are also the most effective energy systems to target when your primary objective is body re-composition and building muscle.

The oxidative system, which we target by performing lower-intensity, steady-state cardiovascular exercise, is what increases energy, elevates focus, and builds health. So, in order to maximize energy, elevate mood, and improve all biomarkers of health, 80% of your focus should be on building a bigger aerobic engine. The remaining 20% can be strength and resistance training, sprint work, and high-intensity interval training (HIIT). This can also be for body composition, building muscle, increasing bone density, and a number of other physiological benefits.

You only have to look at the healthiest and longest-living cultures of the world to recognize that they aren't lifting heavy weights and running wind sprints. Yet members of these cultures tend to exhibit high levels of energy and cognitive function. Even at an advanced age, they are lucid and active. Their activities are aerobic in nature, meaning, literally "with oxygen," and they are performed at a moderate level of intensity sustained over longer periods of time. Think walking, gardening, jogging, yoga, and tai chi.

The widely-known paradox of natural bodybuilding and fitness competitions is that, often, when we look our best aesthetically, we feel our worst. Ask any bodybuilder and they'll tell you, when they're on stage, they're tired, moody, and can't wait to eat some carbs and put weight back on.

To feel superhuman and outperform the competition, aerobic conditioning needs to be a part of your weekly routine. In the next section, I'll teach you how to build a bigger aerobic engine.

Stu Mittleman was an ultra-distance running champion who had set three consecutive American 100-mile road race records in the U.S. National Championships from 1980 to 1982. In 1986, Mittleman won the 1,000-mile World Championship, and even set a new world record by running the distance in 11 days, 2 hours, 6 minutes, and 6 seconds. Just to put things into perspective, that's the equivalent of running 3.5 marathons a day for 11 days straight. In addition to that, one of Mittleman's records was that he ran 577.75 miles in just 4 days. This record still stands today.

In 2008, Mittleman became the sixth American, and only the third American male, to be inducted into the American Ultra-Running Hall of Fame. Mittleman outlines his specific training approach in his book Slow Burn.

In terms of enhancing focus, Mittleman's approach has been shown to have a positive effect on cognitive function including:

- Improved neuronal survivability and function
- Lowered neuroinflammation
- Improved vascularization
- Greater neuroendocrine response to stress
- Decreased brain amyloid burden

His approach has been shown to have positive effects on physiological processes as well, such as glucose-regulation and cardiovascular health, which, when compromised, increases our risk of developing cognitive impairment and Alzheimer's disease. It will also help with fat loss and improve body composition.

Often clients ask about the latest research which shows that steady state cardio doesn't work as well as sprints. It's true, fortunately, the two aren't mutually exclusive.

The truth is that most people aren't physically capable of doing high intensity sprints. Clients come to me and they're doing HIIT (high intensity interval training) 2 to 4 times a week with a trainer. Still, they can't lose weight and feel like something is not optimized.

When I ask them how long they can jog on the treadmill at 6.0 mph, which is only a 10-minute mile, they have no idea. When they say, "I hate cardio!" Well, that's when I know they need it.

That first attempt at a slow, steady state jog is usually a wake up call. The interval training is not translating to improved aerobic conditioning. This will limit your progress and prevent the energetic, cognitive, and physical changes you seek.

By incorporating this type of training into your weekly programming, you can expect these additional, scientifically-validated cognitive benefits:

- Improved attention to detail
- Greater planning and organizational skills
- Elevated ability to multitask
- Improved working memory

This type of training also reduces the energy expenditure that you have when you are working on everyday tasks so you'll have more energy to allocate towards other activities (according to a 1997 study conducted by the American Heart Association).

Best of all, it's simple.

All you have to do is perform 20 to 60 minutes of steady-state aerobic exercise, like jogging or swimming, 3 to 5 times a week. This is best done in the morning, outdoors, with lots of exposure to direct sunlight. If you can't jog, make it a very brisk walk.

There are a few reasons why you would want to do this in the morning. First and foremost, this causes your body to be flooded with oxygen, which is the most vital nutrient that we need for energy, focus, and peak performance. This oxygenation increases a compound called brain-derived neurotrophic factor (BDNF), which is a protein that acts on your peripheral nervous system and central nervous system to encourage the growth of new neurons and new neural connections in addition to helping your existing neurons survive and thrive.

These changes are seen with the dramatic change in blood flow that occurs with aerobic exercise, and they do not occur to the same degree with weight training.

While resistance (weight) training increases the production of growth factors in the muscles, they have a tendency to stay in the muscles, and do not efficiently transport into the brain. So by exercising in the morning and increasing levels of BDNF, you will be able to think faster and have more clarity to handle the intellectual demands of your day.

Morning workouts are also a cornerstone habit, meaning that they have a domino effect on other positive decisions you might make throughout the day. We value those things we invest in and commit to. So by expending energy early in the day, and investing in your health, you are more likely to continue to make additional healthy decisions throughout the day.

Not only is this approach simple, but it is less physically taxing than many other forms of exercise. In fact, you never want to push past a Level 7 on a difficulty scale from 1 to 10. The most accurate way to gauge

Effectiveness of Long and Short Bout Walking on Increasing Physical Activity in Women

Katrina M. Serwe, M.S.,[1] Ann M. Swartz, Ph.D.,[2] Teresa L. Hart, Ph.D.,[2] and Scott J. Strath, Ph.D.[2]

Author information ► Copyright and License information ►

Abstract

Go to: ⊡

Background

The accumulation of physical activity (PA) throughout the day has been suggested as a means to increase PA behavior. It is not known, however, if accumulated PA results in equivalent increases in PA behavior compared with one continuous session. The purpose of this investigation was to compare changes in PA between participants assigned to walk daily in accumulated shorter bouts vs. one continuous session.

Methods

In this 8-week randomized controlled trial, 60 inactive women were randomly assigned to one of the following: (1) control group, (2) 30 minutes a day of walking 5 days a week in one continuous long bout (LB), or (3) three short 10-minute bouts (SB) of walking a day, all at a prescribed heart rate intensity. Walking was assessed by pedometer and self-reported walking log. Before and after measures were taken of average steps/day, resting systolic and diastolic blood pressure (SBP, DBP), resting heart rate (RHR), six-minute walk test (6MWT) distance, height, weight, body mass index (BMI), and hip and waist circumference.

Results

Both walking groups significantly increased PA measured as steps/day compared to controls ($p < 0.001$), and no significant differences were found between LB and SB groups. The LB group demonstrated significant decreases in hip circumference and significant increases in 6MWT distance compared to the control group.

Conclusions

Both walking groups significantly increased PA participation. LB group participants completed more walking at a higher intensity than the SB and control groups, which resulted in significant increases in health benefits.

how hard you should be working is by calculating your aerobic training heart rate. Here's how: First, calculate your maximum heart rate by subtracting your age from 220. So for a 40 year old man, this would be 180 (220 - 40 = 180).

Your aerobic training heart rate is approximately 70% of your maximum heart rate, and it's in between 60% and 85%, depending on your fitness level and any underlying health conditions.

I recommend that most fit men and women stay between 70% and 85% of their maximum heart rate.

To calculate this, you would multiply your maximum heart rate by 0.7 in order to get your lower threshold. In the case of our 40-year-old man, that would be 126.

You multiply your maximum heart rate by 0.85 to get your upper threshold. For our subject in this example, that would come out to be 153 (180 x 0.85 = 153). This means his aerobic training zone is between 126-153 beats per minute.

Five days a week, on weekday mornings, exercise for 20 to 30 in your aerobic training zone.

Remember, it usually takes about five minutes to get your heart rate into your aerobic training zone. So, a 20-minute workout would take around 25 minutes in total. These durations have been shown in scientific studies to be the minimum effective dose for triggering the positive adaptations that increase energy, focus, and all of the other biomarkers of health that have been discussed.

Use a heart rate monitor, with a chest strap, to ensure that you are within your aerobic training zone. I use a Garmin Forerunner 220 heart rate monitor.

And I aim for five 20 to 30 minute workouts per week.

I do not recommend relying on activity tracking wristbands like the FitBit Charge HR as they have a tendency to be less accurate.

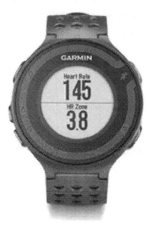 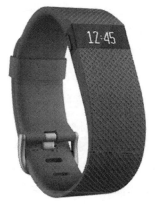

The One Thing:

Beginners: Jog **<u>one minute</u>** *every* morning in your *aerobic training zone [180 - age -10 < Your Heart Rate].*

This does not include the time it takes you to get into your aerobic training zone. For most clients that takes between 1 to 5 minutes.

Once you are within your aerobic zone, you start the clock, and keep your heart rate there or higher for at least one minute. I encourage you to go longer if you're feeling good. The minimum effective dose for beginners to feel a boost in energy is between 1 to 5 minutes.

A Concept II row machine, or squat thrusts (at home), can be substituted instead of jogging.

Early on, consistency should be your focus, not the time. Make it part of your routine, the same way you brush your teeth every morning.

Intermediate and Advanced: Perform **<u>20 to 30 minutes</u>** *of steady-state aerobic exercise 3 to 7 days a week within your aerobic training zone.* This does not include the time it takes you to get into your aerobic training zone.

Again, this should be performed in the morning, ideally outdoors, with your eyes (remove glasses, contacts, sunglasses) and lots of skin exposed to sunlight.

On the other days of the week do at least one minute of jogging, squat thrusts (a.k.a. burpees), or rows on the Concept II row machine in your aerobic training zone.

Here is some of my favorite gear for upgrading your aerobic conditioning workouts:

- The Garmin Forerunner 220 heart rate monitor with chest strap
- The Fitbit Charge HR activity tracker (great for tracking overall daily activity and sleep)

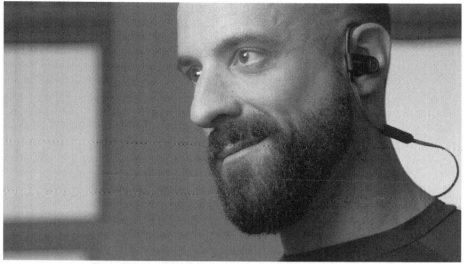

Powerbeats2 Wireless headphones by Dre (now Apple)

- Powerbeats2 Wireless headphones by Dre (now Apple)
- Spotify Running feature of the Spotify smartphone application

Living in Chicago, running outdoors is not always an option. When forced to workout indoors, my first preference is an indoor track. When a track is not available, my favorite treadmill is the Woodway 4Front.

Swimming is also a great way to integrate this type of training. Just make sure that you have a waterproof heart rate monitor. Too much time in chlorinated water may not be the wisest way to spend your time if you're one of the many individuals with a genetic predisposition to suboptimal detoxification.

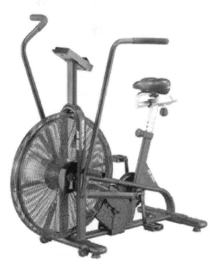

Other valuable aerobic conditioning tools include:

- Assault AirBike
- Concept2 Row Machine
- SR-1 Rogue Bearing Speed Rope
- Stairmaster Stepmill 7,000 PT[7]

THE OTHER 20% OF YOUR TRAINING

So 80% of your training is based on building a bigger aerobic engine (the oxidative energy system), and stretching to improve flexibility and reduce risk of injuries. For the other 20%, I propose that you focus on building strength and muscular endurance. The remaining 20% of your training should include:

- *Strength & Resistance Training (30 seconds to 2 minutes).* Weight training has been shown to decrease levels of C-reactive protein, which is an inflammatory marker, by 32.8% (according to a 2010 study). Hacks include:
  * *Book: "Body by Science"* by Doug McGruff, M.D.
  * *Book: "The Power of 10"* by Adam Zickerman
  * ARX Fit Omni Machine (www.arxfit.com)
  * StrongLifts 5x5
  * BioDensity Strength and Bone Health Machine

- *Mobility, Yoga, Breathing, and Soft Tissue Work.* Hacks include:
  * Trigger Point Roller or Rumble Roller

---

[7] Note: I do not recommend at-home stair climbers or anything that doesn't replicate climbing real stairs.

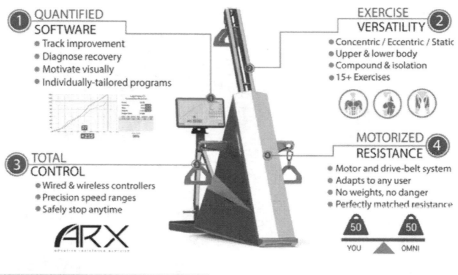

① **QUANTIFIED SOFTWARE**
* Track improvement
* Diagnose recovery
* Motivate visually
* Individually-tailored programs

② **EXERCISE VERSATILITY**
* Concentric / Eccentric / Static
* Upper & lower body
* Compound & isolation
* 15+ Exercises

③ **TOTAL CONTROL**
* Wired & wireless controllers
* Precision speed ranges
* Safely stop anytime

④ **MOTORIZED RESISTANCE**
* Motor and drive-belt system
* Adapts to any user
* No weights, no danger
* Perfectly matched resistance

50 YOU | 50 OMNI

ΛRX

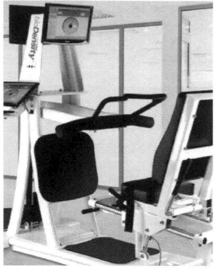

* Lacrosse ball
* Joe DeFranco's "Limber 11" YouTube video. Requires foam roller and lacrosse ball.
* Elevation Training Mask 2.0
* Bas Rutten o2 Trainer
* The Wim Hof Method
* Expand-a-Lung Breathing Fitness Exerciser
* Budokon: Flow & Flexibility DVD
* Stretching in the shower

– *Anaerobic System (3 seconds to 2 minutes).* Hacks include:
  * *"Power Speed Endurance"* by Brian Mackenzie
  * *"Warrior Cardio"* by Martin Rooney
  * The Extreme Kettlebell Cardio Workout DVD
  * The Extreme Kettlebell Cardio Workout 2 DVD

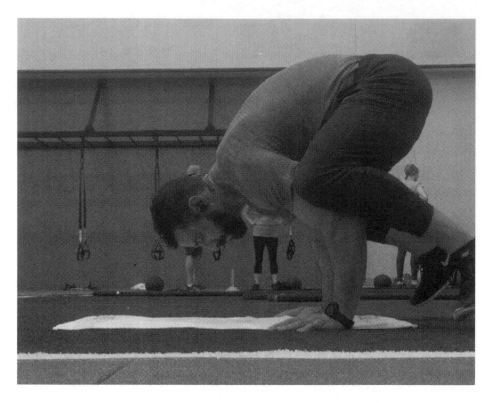

– *Workouts:* CrossFit Grace, CrossFit Fran, CrossFit Filthy 50, CrossFit Murph, CrossFit the Seven, CrossFit ODP (repeatability test), CrossFit 300 FY, CrossFit Angie, CrossFit Annie, CrossFit Fight Gone Bad, CrossFit Helen, CrossFit Cindy. Here are 10 more CrossFit workouts you can do at home or when you're on the road and don't have access to a gym:

* For time: 200 air squats

* 21-15-9 air squats + pushups (do 21 reps of each air squats and pushups, then 15 of each, then 9.)

* 8 rounds for time: 10 situps + 10 burpees

* 10 rounds for time: 10 pushups, 10 squats, 10 tuck jumps (Lift knees as high as possible when you jump, "tucking" into your chest)

* 3 rounds for time: Run 800 meters + 50 air squats (Measure out 800 m ahead of time if you're running down a street, or use a treadmill)
* 10 rounds for time: 10 pushups + 10 sit-ups +10 air squats
* 3 rounds: 50 sit-ups + 400 m run
* For time: 100 jumping jacks + 75 air squats + 50 pushups + 25 burpees
* 5 rounds for time: ten vertical jumps (jump as high as you can) + 10 pushups
* For time: Run 1 mile, stopping to do 10 pushups for every minute that elapses during the run

- *Creatine Phosphagen System (less than 30 seconds).* Hacks include:
   * Maximum-effort sprints. Beginners should start with hill sprints or sprinting on a treadmill at an incline.
   * Powerlifting - explosive, maximal effort lifts (snatch, clean and press, barbell high pull, etc.)

When it comes to steady-state cardio, the pitfalls I see most often are that people are either not doing it at all, or they are doing it too long, or they are doing it at too high levels of intensity.

On the other hand, when it comes to resistance training, high-intensity interval training, and sprint work, I hardly ever see people pushing themselves as hard as they should be. And they're usually resting way too long. All of the scientifically-validated benefits of high-intensity training involve either maximum effort or exercise at 90% to 95% of heart rate maximum.

In working with hundreds of people one-on-one, the consistent pattern that I've seen is that most of us are not at these intensity levels.

We're simply not pushing ourselves hard enough to reap these benefits. As a consequence, our workouts are too long, and this type of "no man's land" training is causing us to stress our biological systems. This has many detrimental effects.

Overtraining increases oxidative damage and inflammation. It weakens the immune system, decreases the metabolism of fat, and disrupts cortisol levels. Cortisol dysregulation promotes an increase in abdominal belly fat and a loss of muscle mass, both of which lead to further weight gain. Worst of all, overtraining has been known to cause neurodegeneration.

It is critical that you keep your glycogenic and phosphagen training extremely high-intensity in nature and tremendously short in duration. That's how you prevent overtraining.

One of the most effective strategies I teach and use myself for incorporating resistance training into my routine is through fractionalized workouts. There are a number of ways that I do this, but two of the simplest are:

1. Commit to one pushup and one prisoner squat each morning as soon as you get out of bed. If you want to do more, you're free to do so, but it's important that you make the commitment to do at least one of each every morning. I encourage most clients to do this the second their feet touch the floor.
2. I also leave a door-mount chin-up bar at the entryway to my bathroom, and do at least one pull-up when I enter and exit. Do more if you are motivated and able.

In a 2015 interview, Jamie Foxx said he starts every morning with pull-ups, pushups, and crunches; crediting pull-ups as the most beneficial muscle-building exercise for staying in shape. He's worked his way up to 100 reps of each.

SITTING IS THE NEW SMOKING

New research has shown that people who sit the most have a 50% higher risk of all cause mortality.

People who sit more than 8 hours a day have a 90% increased risk of type-2 Diabetes.

Sitting for more than eight hours a day is also associated with a:

- 147 percent increased relative risk of cardiovascular events
- 54 percent increased risk of lung cancer
- 30 percent higher risk of colon cancer
- 66 percent higher risk of uterine cancer

Most Americans spend 9 to 10 hours a day sitting down.

People who sit the least have dramatically lower incidents of diabetes, heart disease, obesity, cancer, and all-cause mortality.

Sit less, and move more. To do this will involve integrating some new behavior patterns. A good starting point is to aim for at least 10,000 steps per day.

I recommend using the Fitbit Charge HR activity tracker. The Fitbit may be one of the best biohacking investments you can make. It adds a gamification element of movement that results in greater activity levels. It helps you to become more aware of your patterns, behaviors, and how some of your lifestyle decisions may be impacting you in ways you hadn't suspected.

If you work a job, like most normal people, squeezing in 10,000 steps a day consistently and finding ways not to sit is easier said than done. So, here are some ideas that might help:

- Use your activity band (Fitbit Charge HR, Jawbone Up24, Jawbone Up3) to set inactivity reminders so that you remember to stand up every 30 minutes.

- For every hour you spend sitting, do 50 jumping jacks.
- Get a LifeSpan Treadmill desk and/or a VARIDESK standing desk. I personally work at my kitchen counter with my Macbook Pro elevated using a simple 3M Adjustable Monitor Stand and an AmazonBasics Ventilated Adjustable Laptop Stand. The entire setup was around $36. The Standdesk is another option for a couple hundred dollars that does not require a high counter.
- Find creative ways to go outside. Take calls, schedule meetings, and do anything possible outside, even better, while walking. If the weather doesn't allow for this, do a walking meeting indoors.
- Walk or bike to work. If you live far away, try taking public transportation part of the way and then walking and driving the rest of the distance.

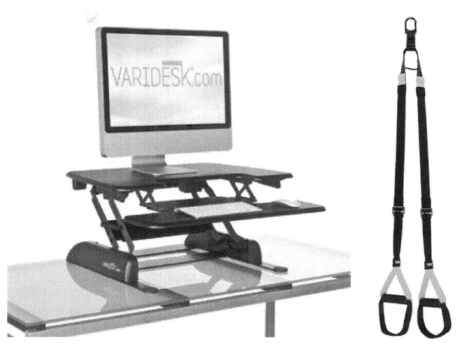

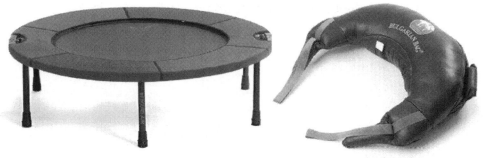

ReboundAir Classic Rebounder   Suples Bulgarian Bag

- Use the stairs whenever possible.
- Do your own chores.
- Get a dog.
- Park further away from places than you usually would.

Some of my other favorite gizmos and gadgets that I use to upgrade my workouts include:

- Jaybird X2 Sport Bluetooth wireless headphones
- Podcasts & audio books (Audible)
- ReboundAir Ultimate Rebounder, Bellicon rebounder, or JumpSport Fitness Trampoline Model 250
- PowerBlock Adjustable Dumbbells
- Vita Vibe MP12 Mini Parallettes Set (for travel)
- Onnit Battle Ropes
- TRX Suspension Trainer
- Suples Bulgarian Bag
- Yoga mat
- Kettlebells of various weights
- Mir Short Weighted Vest (for incline walking)

- Compex Sport Elite Muscle Stimulator (www.shopcompex.com)
- MarcPro Plus (save $47 on the MarcPro Plus at www. BiohackingSecrets.com/marcpro with discount code "biohacks").

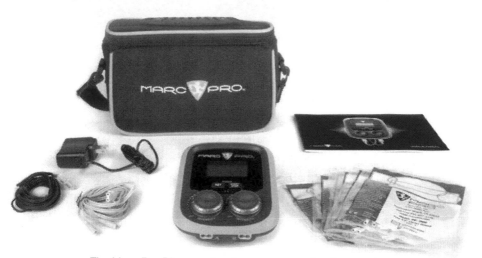

The Marc Pro Plus accelerates recovery and reduces pain.

I'm also a big fan of using music to get myself pumped up and in a state to work out.

FASTER RECOVERY = FASTER GAINS

I utilize and recommend cold thermogenesis (CT) in the form of ice baths, cold plunges (I do mine in Lake Michigan), cryotherapy (Chicago Cryo Spa), and cold showers to accelerate recovery. I end every shower with the water as cold as it can go for 30 seconds to five minutes. This allows you to train more frequently and at higher intensity levels. It also improves your body's ability to adapt and recover.

As mentioned in a previous section, Cryotherapy is now being used by everyone from professional athletes to celebrities. Many high-level business executives use it too. Its benefits include:

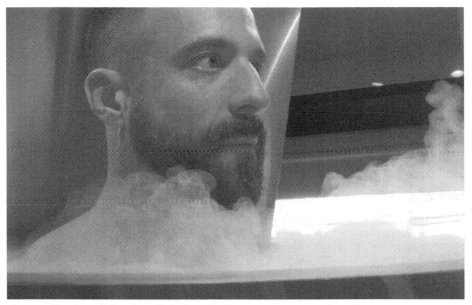

The benefits of Cryotherapy include accelerated muscle and joint repair.

- Anti-aging
- Improved mitochondrial functioning
- Lowering inflammation
- Muscle and joint repair
- Fighting depression

BEFORE YOUR WORKOUT

Here's a fun, inexpensive hack for increasing time to exhaustion, power output, and endurance during your workouts. Take 3 teaspoons of baking soda (I use Arm & Hammer or Bob's Red Mill) with 4 to 8 ounces of water 30 minutes prior to your workout. Why?

Baking soda is a systemic lactic acid buffer in the body. You may be familiar with Beta Alanine which is sold in many supplements. Beta Alanine buffers lactic acid as well, but only in muscle tissue.

Baking soda works throughout the entire body and is pennies on the dollar.

I've used this biohack with my athletes as part of their performance protocol and seen 10% to 25% increases in muscular endurance and delayed onset of fatigue.

It also increases cerebral blood flow in a dose-dependent manner.

But the benefits of baking soda don't stop there. It has also been shown to increase mitochondrial respiration, particularly during longer form exercise (see chart). It is hypothesized this occurs due to increases in the mitochondrial builder protein PGC-1a.

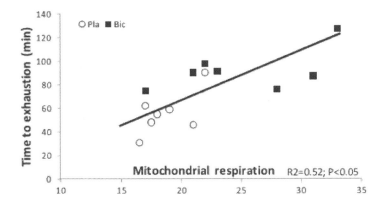

You can simply take 3 teaspoons with 4 to 6 ounces of water (adding organic lemon juice or Bragg Organic Apple Cider Vinegar optional) about 30 minutes prior to exercise. Or you can use it as part of a longer term peak performance protocol like I design for a number of my one-on-one clients.

MOVEMENT BIOHACKS

This is not an all-inclusive summary from this section but will help you get started until you are able to explore in more detail.

The One Thing:

Beginners: Perform one minute of steady-state aerobic exercise every day within your aerobic training zone.

Intermediate and Advanced: Increase the amount of time in your aerobic training zone to 20 to 30 minutes at least three days a week.

Biohack #1: The majority (80%) of your exercises should be aerobic and mobility/flexibility-based. The rest of it (20%) can be strength and resistance training, sprint work, and high-intensity interval training (HIIT). Build a bigger aerobic engine first.

Biohack #2: Optimally, training should address all three major energy systems:

- *The Phosphagen System* (also known as the Creatine Phosphate System, 3 to 30 seconds in duration). This includes power lifting, bursting, and sprinting.
- *The Anaerobic System* (also known as the Glycolytic System, 30 seconds to 2 minutes in duration). Includes resistance and interval training.
- *The Oxidative System* (also known as the Aerobic System, greater than 2 minutes in duration).

Biohack #3: Incorporate more movement into your day. Workout first thing in the morning. This is one of the biggest secrets of high performers. If it doesn't get done in the morning, there's a good chance it won't get done at all. Have a trigger, like having your workout clothes already laid out the night before where you will see them, that reminds you to throw on your gear and get moving.

Schedule your workouts the same way you would schedule anything important. I recommend using Fantastical by FlexiBits (www.flexibits.com/fantastical).

When you're short on time, use a workout DVD (or stream to your ipad) so you don't have to research, plan, or program your workout. No thinking required. Just press play.

Biohack #4: The Marc Pro Plus is intended for muscle conditioning by stimulating muscle in order to improve or facilitate muscle performance. The Marc Pro Plus is also used for temporary relief of pain associated with sore and aching muscles in the shoulder, waist, back, neck, upper extremities (arm), and lower extremities (leg) due to strain from exercise and normal household and work activities (www.BiohackingSecrets.com/marcpro). Mention coupon code "biohacks" at checkout to save $47 on the MarcPro Plus.

STRESS MANAGEMENT

When we wish things were different than they are, we get stressed.

A 2013 "State of the American Workplace Report" found that 70% of those surveyed either hate work or are entirely disengaged. Then, when you take into consideration relationships, financial security, and health, the number of people living with chronic stress is epidemic.

The medical definition of stress is "The perception of a real or imagined threat to your body or your ego."

This could be someone demanding your wallet at gunpoint, or the belief that your spouse is cheating on you (even if he or she is not).

Chronic stress literally wreaks havoc on your body, sending your hormonal systems into disarray, causing digestive issues, insulin resistance, high blood sugar, and obesity. It suppresses the immune system, and inhibits mental processing and focus. Furthermore, it causes depression, anxiety, and mood disorders.

If you actually knew what was happening to you when you were stressed, it would terrify you.

I've worked with dozens of clients who ate clean, exercised every day, slept well, and yet they were still unwell and exhausted. Every last one had some area of their lives that created chronic stress for them.

More than 90% of the time the stress comes from work or their marriage, or some combination of the two. Whatever the source, if you have everything else right but miss this one, you're bound to have huge health, energy, and focus problems.

Some signs and symptoms of chronic stress are:

- Impaired cognitive function
- Changes in memory
- Digestive problems
- Fatigue
- Sleep issues (falling asleep, staying asleep, or getting up in the morning)
- Mood swings
- Anxiety
- Depression
- Cravings for sugar, processed carbohydrates, and caffeine
- A weakened immune system

A great resource is the book *"Why Zebras Don't Get Ulcers"* by Robert M. Sapolsky. Saplosky combines cutting-edge research with practical advice and explains how chronic stress causes or intensifies a range of physical and mental afflictions, including depression, ulcers, colitis, heart disease, and more.

Meditation is one of the most valuable tools to combat chronic stress. The following list of high-achievers all credit meditation with helping them perform at their highest levels: Oprah Winfrey, Kobe Bryant, Jerry Seinfeld, Madonna, Russell Simmons, Hugh Jackman, Clint Eastwood, Nicole Kidman, Russell Brand, Eva Mendes, Gwyneth Paltrow, Paul McCartney, Lady Gaga, Howard Stern, Ellen Degeneres, John Lennon, Martin Scorsese, Steve Jobs, George Lucas, Brian Wilson (of the Beach

Boys), Mick Jagger, Judd Apatow, Eddie Vedder, Dr. Oz, Rick Rubin, Richard Gere, Angelina Jolie, Halle Berry, Rupert Murdoch, and Arianna Huffington.

If you're anything like me, you may have tried meditation in the past and felt like it just wasn't for you or that you weren't any good at it.

I tried meditating for years before I even felt like I had the slightest semblance of what most of us type-A folks would call "success."

You sit down to meditate, and a second later, your mind is racing with thoughts about the cute girl you should have said something to at the grocery store, or the jerk that cut you off on the highway.

That's normal. It's part of the learning curve.

Before diving into some specific strategies and practices to help you manage your stress, let's take a deeper look at both the science behind meditation and some common misconceptions.

THE SCIENCE OF MEDITATION

A 2014 Harvard Study unveiled that meditation literally increases gray matter density in the brain. This 8-week study, conducted by Harvard researchers at Massachusetts General Hospital, found that meditation literally rebuilds the brain's gray matter, particularly in the Hippocampus. This is the part of the brain known to be responsible for learning and memory.

Participants of the study meditated for 30 minutes a day for eight weeks, and the results showed that meditation helped to:

- Increase brain mass
- Increase intelligence
- Reduce anxiety
- Improve quality of life

These results were shown across a number of different assessment scales. *Meditation is good for your brain and makes you smarter.* A 2015 study from UCLA showed that meditation helps to preserve the aging brain. It also confirmed that participants who had been meditating for an average of 20 years had more gray matter volume throughout the entire brain, not just the hippocampus.

Studies have shown that kids who take short meditation breaks in school perform better on standardized tests and have higher perceived intelligence. Neuroscientists have also found that after just 11 hours of meditation, study participants had structural changes in the part of their brain involved in monitoring focus and self-control. And, if that's not enough, another study, conducted at the University of California in 2013, found that just two weeks of meditation improved working memory and focus. It also resulted in a 16% point increase in GRE scores.

Meditation reduces anxiety and reverses depressive symptoms. A meta-analysis involving 163 different studies showed mindfulness meditation to have a dramatic effect on anxiety, stress, and social anxiety. Another study from 2014 at John Hopkins University, found that meditation rivaled anti-depressants in its ability to reduce the symptoms of depression, anxiety, and physical pain.

They've even done meditation studies on people with clinical anxiety, and 90% of them experienced significant reductions in their anxiety levels. Observational studies have also shown meditation to:

- Improve relationships
- Strengthen marital bonds
- Boost confidence
- Strengthen the immune system

The important point that I'm trying to get across is that meditation is not only beneficial because it helps you to feel less stressed. The greatest benefits of meditation occur because of its ability to literally increase the size of your brain and create new neurological connections that bring about permanent changes in your behavior and mental processes.

Many people, and I was one of them, feel like they can't meditate because their brain is too busy. This is especially common with the Type-A folks, but all you need is one minute to feel the benefits.

Meditation make us smarter, happier, and more focused. Perhaps its greatest benefit is a heightened awareness of the patterns of thought, behavior, and emotion we experience.

Meditation clears the mind and brings it back to a state where the brain can work and function at a higher level.

SYNERGISTIC BENEFITS: COMBINING MEDITATION, MOVEMENT, AND NATURE

When it comes to getting rid of stress, scientific research supports three elements more than any other. They are meditation, movement (particularly cardiovascular exercise, as described in the previous section), and spending time outside in nature. For time management purposes, I recommend combining these strategies.

The benefits will be more pronounced, and the results exponentially greater if you practice meditation in the morning. I recommend you start out using the Smartphone application Headspace (www.headspace. com). They offer a 10-day free trial that's perfect for beginners. Other meditation apps I recommend include: Brain.FM (a web-based program), Calm (app), and Omvana (app).

Here's how you can combine meditation, exercise, and time in nature. Three to five day a week, get a 20-30 minute steady-state, cardiovascular workout in your target heart rate zone. It's much more beneficial if you do this exercise outside, with your eyes and skin exposed to direct sunlight. So, just by taking a simple jog a few times a week, you'll have two of the three covered. All you have left to do is integrate meditation.

BrainSync's Kelly Howell has three meditations designed to be listened to during your workouts: The Running Meditation, Breakthrough Training in the Zone: Vol. 1, and Power Training in the Zone: Vol II. I load MP3s onto my phone, and throw in a pair of wireless Bluetooth headphones.

There are two books that I recommend on combining meditation with your jog. The first is *"Running with the Mind of Meditation"* by Sakyong Mipham, and the other is *"Chi Running: A Revolutionary Approach to Effortless, Injury-Free Running"* by Danny Dreyer and Katherine Dreyer. These books teach simple ways to bring mindfulness and body awareness into your workouts.

HOW TO HACK YOUR MEDITATION

The Headspace app is where I recommend most people start because it's simple and easy. Put on headphones, press play, and follow along. Here are some other biohacks you can use to upgrade your meditations and neutralize unwanted stress:

Counting: As you breathe in and out, preferably through your nose, count your inhalations and exhalations. Start by counting one as you inhale, two as you exhale, three as you inhale a second time, and so on until you get to 10. Once you reach 10, start back at one.

You'll want to set the timer on your phone for anywhere from 5 to 30 minutes. Find a comfortable place where you can lay down, a chair with your feet flat on the floor, or a place you can sit cross-legged on a cushion with your back flat up against the wall. I recommend the Bean Yoga cushion or a Biomat (www.BioHackingSecrets.com/Biomat). I enjoy the Biomat because it's like laying on an infrared sauna. It heats up to 160 degrees, and the infrared rays penetrate deep into your body easing muscle tension and helping you relax.

Then, just count and breathe. If you find your mind wandering, that's normal. Acknowledge the thought, and bring your attention back to your breath and the count.

Breathing: A simple breathing meditation exercise is to breathe in and out through your nose (or mouth if your sinuses are congested). As you do, imagine bright white, energizing air filling your throat, and then your chest, and then your belly, and then your lower abdomen, in that order. Then, imagine this bright white light radiating out throughout your entire body, energizing your cells, and grabbing onto toxins, stress, and any negative emotions.

As you exhale, imagine the air leaving, first from your lower abdomen, then your belly, then your chest, and then your throat. This time imagine it as a dull, grey air that contains all of the toxins, stress, and negative emotions you are releasing from your body. If you like, you can even add a simple mantra. What I like to do is think the word "so" as I breathe in, and then I think the word "hum" as I exhale.

Mindfulness Meditation: The goal of this exercise is for you to develop a greater awareness of your body, senses, and environment. As you breathe slowly and deeply in a seated or lying position, start with the top of your head, and then slowly scan down your body one millimeter at a time. At first, you'll want to pay attention to any sensations in the area of the body that you are concentrating on, and then you'll allow that area to fully and completely relax.

Once you've done this for your entire body, which can take anywhere from 2 to 10 minutes, bring your awareness around to the environment that surrounds you. Notice the contact points between your body and the cushion, or your chair, or the floor. Notice areas of more pressure or less pressure. Notice the temperature. Is there a breeze? What emotions are you experiencing in that moment? What sounds can you hear? Are you able to notice any sounds that you didn't recognize earlier? Do you feel sleepy or relaxed? Imagine the game is noticing as many things about your body, environment, thoughts, and emotions as you possibly can.

As you do this, continually let your body become more and more relaxed. Try to feel as good as you can. Breathe in a way that feels good. Sometimes it helps to take a deep breath in and let that breath go with an audible sigh, like you would make at the end of a long day.

BRAIN ENTRAINMENT (FREQUENCY-FOLLOWING RESPONSE)

Scientists have found that the human brain changes its frequency to match the frequency of the dominant external stimulus, like music, sound, light, or pulsed electromagnetic frequencies (PEMF). This is what it is referred to as "frequency following response."

You can hack your meditation by using sound frequencies to induce a deeper meditative state, delivering more benefits in less time.

Here's a quick breakdown of the different brain wave frequencies and what goes on in each state:

- *Delta Brain Waves (0.1-3.9 Hz):* A delta state is associated with dreamless sleep. It's also where we release the greatest amounts of human growth hormone. The delta state is also often

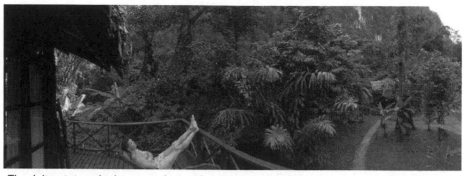

The delta state, which occurs during deep sleep, helps the body recover and re-energize.

associated with slow wave sleep (SWS). It is during this stage that the blood rushes from the brain to the muscles, initiating physical recovery, recuperation, and a re-energizing of the body. This state also supports healthy immune function and normal glucose metabolism during the day.

- *Theta Brain Waves (4-7.9 Hz):* A theta state is associated with dreaming and REM (rapid eye movement) sleep. In the theta state, we experienced an increased production of catecholamines, which play an important role in memory and learning. It is also in this state that we achieve increased levels of creativity. Deep meditation, guided visualization, and trances (which can be induced via hypnosis) also activate the theta state and allow us to access the unconscious mind.

- *Alpha Brain Waves (8-13.9 Hz):* Alpha brain waves are associated with a relaxed focus, improved learning abilities, and increased serotonin production. We achieve an alpha state via meditation and also right when we go to sleep. This is also the state that we are in when we first wake up in the morning. In the alpha state, we also begin to access the unconscious mind.

- *Beta Brain Waves (14-30 Hz):* A beta state is associated with increased alertness, concentration, and cognitive function.

Higher levels of a beta state can have negative consequences, including anxiety and over-activation of the sympathetic nervous system, like the fight or flight response.

Most of us spend our lives primarily in a beta state. This means that, generally, we are alert, aroused, concentrating, but also stressed.

When we lower the brain wave frequency to alpha, which is what happens during meditation, we increase our capacity to perform high-level tasks, learn new information, analyze complex situations, and experience the state that athletes commonly refer to as "the zone."

Lower brainwave frequencies are also correlated with increases in "feel-good" neurotransmitters like:

- Dopamine
- Norepinephrine
- Serotonin
- GABA
- Endorphins (the same chemicals responsible for what people call "runner's high")

The most commonly used frequencies for FFS, or brain entrainment, are binaural beats. Not everyone responds favorable to binaural beats. As a general rule of thumb, if using a guided audio or binaural beat makes you feel good, then continue to utilize it as a tool in your meditative practice. However, if it doesn't, trust your body's response and try something else.

There are literally hundreds of binaural beat audios out there. What we've found is that the human brain quickly adapts to an external stimulus, resulting in diminishing returns. To prevent adaptation,

I recommend a variety of audios and technologies to enhance your meditative practice.

Some of the audios listed below utilize binaural beats and some do not. Here are a few of my favorites:

- Brain.fm (I use the guided meditations)
- The HeadSpace (app)
- Holosync by Centerpoint "The Dive"
- Dr. Jeffery Thompson's neuroacoustic CDs (These are available on Spotify)
- "The 6 Phase Meditation" (Omvana app)
- Overnight Riches: A Flow Dream Meditation (Omvana app)
- Amplifying Your Money Magnetism by Matthew Ferry
- "Retrieve Your Destiny" by Kelly Howell (BrainSync)
- "Running Meditation" by Kelly Howell (BrainSync)
- "The 7-Minute Vacation" by Kelly Howell (BrainSync) - I start many clients here
- "Breakthrough Training in the Zone: Vol. 1" by Kelly Howell (BrainSync)
- "Power Training in the Zone: Vol II" by Kelly Howell (BrainSync)
- "Meditate with the Himalayan Masters" by Swami Veda Bharati and Paul Scheele
- Sam Harris also has two free meditation audios on his website. One is a 9-minute mindfulness meditation, and the other is a 26-minute meditation called "Looking for the Self." Both of them can be downloaded from his website, www.SamHarris.org.
- Calm the Mind: How to Balance the Autonomic Nervous System

The autonomic nervous system involuntarily and reflexively controls our breathing, heart rate, digestion, and internal organs.

It includes both the sympathetic and parasympathetic nervous systems.

The biohacks and technologies in this section act like a reset button by balancing the autonomic nervous system, calming and focusing the mind, and allowing your body to recover from stress.

PULSED ELECTROMAGNETIC FIELDS (PEMFS)

The beneficial therapeutic effects of selected low-energy, time-varying magnetic fields, called PEMFs, have been documented with increasing frequency since 1973. PEMFs work to:

- Reduce pain, inflammation, the effects of stress on the body, and platelet adhesion.
- Improve energy, circulation, blood and tissue oxygenation, sleep quality, blood pressure and cholesterol levels, the uptake of nutrients, cellular detoxification and the ability to regenerate cells.

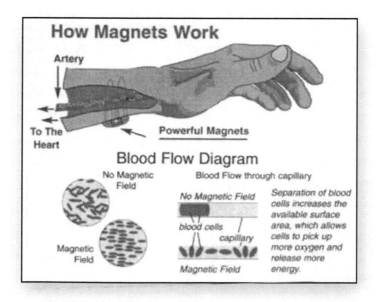

- Balance the immune system and stimulate RNA and DNA.
- Accelerate repair of bone and soft tissue. Benefits reported specifically in individuals with osteoarthritis.
- Relax muscles and decrease stiffness.
- Reduce brain fog and elevate mental clarity

Emerging research suggests PEMFs may improve brain function by reducing neuroinflammation.

Similar to the process that occurs while we sleep, PEMFs may stimulate glial cells within the brain's glymphatic system allowing accumulated toxins to be flushed out and eliminated. It's suspected that individuals with cognitive decline, dementia, Alzheimer's, and Parkinson's may have poor glymphatic function. A lack of sleep, leaky blood brain barrier (BBB), or a sluggish glymphatic system all impair brain neuron's ability to function.

Clients have reported PEMF therapy to help with urinary incontinence, carpel tunnels, peripheral neuropathy, and a wide range of other challenges.

I asked one of the world's foremost experts on Pulsed Electromagnetic Fields to explain how they work and the science behind this emerging therapy, William Pawluk, MD (www.drpawluk.com):

J Neurosci Res. 2014 Jun;92(6):761-71. doi: 10.1002/jnr.23361. Epub 2014 Feb 12.

Pulsed electromagnetic fields potentiate neurite outgrowth in the dopaminergic MN9D cell line.

Lekhraj R[1], Cynamon DE, DeLuca SE, Taub ES, Pilla AA, Casper D.

⊛ Author information

Abstract

Pulsed electromagnetic fields (PEMF) exert biological effects and are in clinical use to facilitate bone repair and wound healing. Research has demonstrated that PEMF can induce signaling molecules and growth factors, molecules that play important roles in neuronal differentiation. Here, we tested the effects of a low-amplitude, nonthermal, pulsed radiofrequency signal on morphological neuronal differentiation in MN9D, a dopaminergic cell line. Cells were plated in medium with 10% fetal calf serum. After 1 day, medium was replaced with serum-containing medium, serum-free medium, or medium supplemented with dibutyryl cyclic adenosine monophosphate (Bt2 cAMP), a cAMP analog known to induce neurite outgrowth. Cultures were divided into groups and treated with PEMF signals for either 30 min per day or continuously for 15 min every hour for 3 days. Both serum withdrawal and Bt2 cAMP significantly increased neurite length. PEMF treatment similarly increased neurite length under both serum-free and serum-supplemented conditions, although to a lesser degree in the presence of serum, when continuous treatments had greater effects. PEMF signals also increased cell body width, indicating neuronal maturation, and decreased protein content, suggesting that this treatment was antimitotic, an effect reversed by the inhibitor of cAMP formation dideoxyadenosine. Bt2 cAMP and PEMF effects were not additive, suggesting that neurite elongation was achieved through a common pathway. PEMF signals increased cAMP levels from 3 to 5 hr after treatment, supporting this mechanism of action. Although neuritogenesis is considered a developmental process, it may also represent the plasticity required to form and maintain synaptic connections throughout life.

Q: What are PEMFs and how do they work?

A: Science teaches us that everything is energy. Energy is always dynamic and, therefore, has a frequency; it changes by the second or minute, for example, at the very least.

All energy is electromagnetic in nature. All atoms, chemicals and cells produce electromagnetic fields (EMFs). Every organ in the body produces it own signature bioelectromagnetic field.

Science has proven that our bodies actually project their own magnetic fields and that all 70 trillion cells in the body communicate via electromagnetic frequencies. Nothing happens in the body without an electromagnetic exchange. When the electromagnetic activity of the body ceases, life ceases.

Physics, that is, electromagnetic energy, controls chemistry. This in turn controls tissue function. Disruption of electromagnetic energy in cells causes impaired cell metabolism, whatever the initial cause. This happens anywhere in the disease process.

PEMFs address impaired chemistry and thus the function of cells - which in turn, improves health. PEMFs deliver beneficial, health-enhancing EMFs and frequencies to the cells. Low frequency PEMFs of even the weakest strengths pass right through the body, penetrating every cell, tissue, organ and even bone without being absorbed or altered! As they pass through, they stimulate most of the electrical and chemical processes in the tissues. Therapeutic PEMFs are specifically designed to positively support cellular energy, resulting in better cellular health and function.

Devices that produce PEMFs vary by a number of important features: frequency, waveform, strength, and

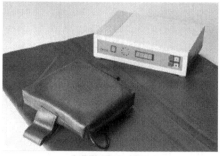

A PEMF device.

types of stimulators. Frequencies can be simple or complex; and high, medium or low. Intensity can also be high, medium or low.

No "one-size" treatment fits all situations. Most PEMF devices help to varying degrees depending on the problem or condition, but selecting the wrong device may produce unsatisfactory results. Since the body is complex, PEMFs are ideal devices to be able get good results without needing a myriad of different treatments.

Q: Aren't some EMFs bad for you?

A: They can be. Evidence is mounting that a new form of pollution called "electrosmog" is a very real threat because it is disruptive to cell metabolism. Manmade, unnatural EMFs come from electrical wiring and equipment, for example, power lines, communications towers, computers, TVs, cell phones - everything from the wiring in our homes to fluorescent lighting to microwave ovens, hair dryers, clock radios, electric blankets and more.

Electrosmog EMFs are not designed with the body in mind. They can be a strong inducer of stress in the body and, therefore, drain our energy. Electrosmog includes "dirty" electricity, ground currents, microwaves

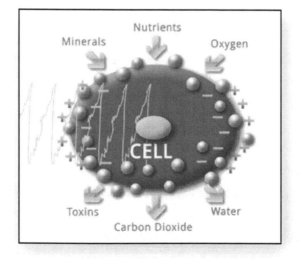

and radio waves. Microwaves are not only from leaky microwave ovens, but also from cell towers, cell phones and wireless equipment.

Electrosmog is all around us and can only be partially blocked. One of the best solutions is to take measures to decrease your exposure. With therapeutic PEMFs, one can purposely add beneficial balancing frequencies to the body to decrease the burden of the negative effects of electrosmog.

Q: PEMFs and Magnets: What's the difference?

A: PEMFs are frequency-based, applied to either the whole body or parts of the body. PEMFs may only be needed for short periods of time, while the effects last for many hours, setting in motion cellular and whole-body changes to restore and maintain balance in metabolism and health. The body does not acclimate, or "get used to" the healthy energy signals of therapeutic PEMFs, even if used for a long time, compared to magnets.

Stationary (or "static"), non-varying, magnetic fields from magnets have fixed strengths. They are used in mattresses, bracelets, knee wraps and the like. Most have very shallow penetration into the body, resulting in a very limited ability to affect deeper tissues, and they rarely treat all the cells of the body simultaneously. Only skilled practitioners may guide you to get the best results from these approaches.

Q: What types of PEMFs systems are most effective?

A: There are quite a number of PEMF systems available now in the US, for daily in-home use, that can help meet your unique needs. Some are FDA-approved and many more are available over-the counter or from various experienced practitioners. Some whole-body systems have been available in the US for over a decade and have been used in Europe by tens of thousands of people for a wide variety of problems without significant negative effects for over 20 years. One PEMF system has been studied through NIH-supported research at the University of Virginia for Rheumatoid Arthritis. These whole body systems have been used worldwide, not only by health-conscious individuals for health improvement and maintenance, but also by world-class and Olympic athletes for increased endurance, enhanced performance, and faster recovery.

Dr. William Pawluk is a Board Certified Family Physician, Holistic Health Practitioner, and Former Assistant Professor at Johns Hopkins University School of Medicine and University of Maryland. Dr. Pawluk is the creator of www.drpawluk.com, an authoritative informational source on PEMFs. Dr. Pawluck offers a number of PEMF machines to rent and purchase.

Here are some of the PEMF machines I've used, owned, or had recommended by clients:

- *Ondamed:* For therapeutic purposes, I currently use the Ondamed more than any other PEMF machine. It has proven beneficial in a wide range of physical, emotional, autoimmune, and infection-related conditions. Within a week of doing a specific daily protocol

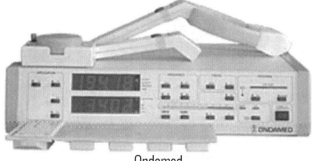

Ondamed

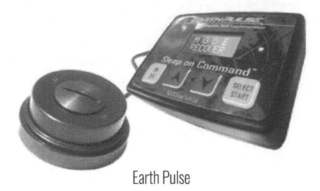

Earth Pulse

of one hour treatment sessions, I saw a marked improvement in mobility and flexibility accompanied by less stiffness. In fact, I almost did the splits for the first time in my life! It is the most expensive device and requires some orientation and training.

- *MicroPulse:* The most economical PEMF option; created by scientists responsible for NASA research on PEMFs.
- *EarthPulse:* My favorite for tissue regeneration, increased ATP, and accelerated recovery. Put it under your mattress and pillow

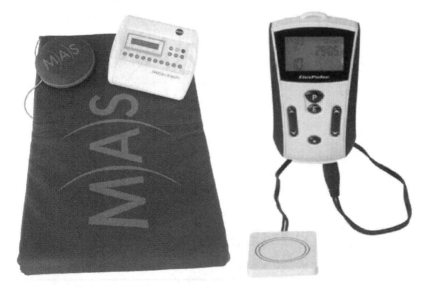

while you sleep. After sleeping on this for one week I was able to increase my static breath hold time by 37 seconds. Here's a special page they set up for biohackers: www.BioHackingSecrets. com/earthpulse

- *Parmeds Super*
- *Parmeds Ultra 3D:* Dr.Pawluk's top recommendation if you have the coin.
- *PEMF-120:* Specifically for back pain; using a combination of my protocols for pain and PEMF I've had clients experience as high as 50% to 80% reductions in back pain within the first month working together.
- *MAS PEMF mat*
- *OrthoCor Medical PEMF brace for knee pain*
- *FlexPulse:* Focus, concentration; portable; similar to MicroPulse but with more settings and power capabilities.

Here's how to select the right frequency for your PEMF therapy:

- *10 Hz for cellular stimulation:* NASA research found this frequency resulted in a nearly 400% increase in neural stem cells and turns on 160 genes responsible for growth and regeneration.
- *10 Hz / 100 Hz oscillations for cellular repair:* Muscles in the body oscillate at different frequencies, the most common being 10 Hz and 100 Hz. The former is found in larger muscle groups, the intestines and blood vessels. The latter is observed more commonly in the upper body, particularly the shoulders and upper chest.
- *3 Hz for deep relaxation and sleep:* This delta frequency is beneficial for deep relaxation and assistance with sleep onset

and maintenance. I have used both the EarthPulse and the FlexPulse to help decrease time to sleep onset and ensure deep, rejuvinatize sleep. When I use the FlexPulse I place both coils under my pillow and run the device at this 3 Hz frequency.

– *7.8 Hz for balance and restoration:* Considered the average Schumann resonance and the basic fundamental resonance of the atmosphere of planet Earth. This is the theta brainwave frequency. The brain, in theta, is considered to be like a sponge, allowing larger amounts of information to be learned and retained. Theta frequencies can facilitate creative breakthroughs and help overcome writer's block. Long time meditators and monks spend extended periods of time in the theta state. As I write this, at 3:08am on a Saturday night, I have a FlexPulse coil affixed to each side of my head just above the ears.

– *23 Hz for alertness:* Considered the alertness, or beta, frequency. We are in beta most of the day when we are mentally active and attentive. Beta stimulation improves mental function and physical efficiency. People who have mid-day energy slumps have often shifted their brainwaves out of beta and into theta or alpha. That, or they consumed any variety of immunogenic and allergenic foods with lunch. That too will hit you like a glass of warm milk and a Tylenol PM.

– *1000 Hz for mood balancing:* Recent research has found that square wave 1,000 Hz stimulation to the brain was effective in treating acute depression, even in those on medical therapies. This frequency has benefits for those with high levels of stress, low mood, and seasonal affective disorder (winter blues).

To find out what PEMF devices I'm currently using myself and with clients go to www.BioHackingSecrets.com/PEMF.

As a part of our body's autonomic nervous system, the heart at rest was once thought to function much like a metronome, producing a steady, consistent rhythm. By studying heart rate variability (HRV), scientists now know this is far from true.

Rather than being monotonously regular, the rhythm of a healthy heart, even under resting conditions, is surprisingly irregular, with the time interval between consecutive heart beats constantly changing. It is this beat to beat variation in heart rate that we refer to as heart rate variability (HRV). Tools for tracking HRV are:

- emWave2 by HeartMath (www.heartmath.com)
- Jaybird Reign wristband (www.jaybirdsport.com)
- BioForce HRV (www.bioforcehrv.com)
- SweetBeat HRV smartphone application (www.sweetwaterhrv.com)

When we examine the scientific literature of allostasis (the process of achieving stability, or homeostasis through physiological or behavioral

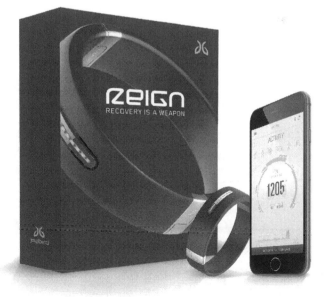

change), HRV may be the most accurate data point we have to give physical and psychological stress a tangible value.

Essentially, HRV is an assessment of the balance between your sympathetic nervous system (which stimulates the body's "flight or fight" response) and your para-sympathetic nervous system (which stimulates the body's "rest and digest" or "feed and breath" response). It's a snapshot of our body's ability to cope with sympathetic-dominant stress.

Simply put, less variation in your heart rhythms is indicative of compromised nervous system performance and suboptimal cognitive function. It may also be a sign you're overtraining, or under-recovering (from your workouts).

Professional athletes in mixed martial arts, boxing, major league baseball, NBA, and the NFL are now using HRV monitoring to assess whether their nervous system has recovered from an intense competition or training session.

Less variation may be indicative of over-training and the necessity for more rest and recovery. There are many factors that impact the activity of the autonomic nervous system and, therefore, influence heart rate variability. These include our breathing patterns, exercise, and thoughts.

Research at the Institute of HeartMath has shown that one of the most powerful factors that affect our heart's changing rhythm is our feelings and emotions. In general, emotional stress, including emotions such as anger, frustration, and anxiety, gives rise to heart rhythm patterns that are irregular and erratic. Scientists call this an "incoherent heart rhythm pattern." In contrast, positive emotions send a very different signal throughout our body.

When we experience uplifting emotions such as gratitude, appreciation, joy, care, and love, our heart rhythm becomes more ordered and takes on a smoother, more harmonious wave. This is referred to as a "coherent heart rhythm pattern."

It is also known that when we consciously generate positive emotions and thoughts, a more coherent heart rhythm is generated, creating balance between the two branches of the autonomic nervous system and greater homeostasis throughout the body.

This state of increased harmony and order in both our psychological (mental and emotional) and physiological (bodily) processes is known as psychophysiological coherence. Since the dawn of time, humans have understood the impact that positive emotions and thinking have on how we feel and perform. The difference is that we now have access to technology that gives us the ability to monitor the impact of our emotional and psychological state through HRV.

Research shows when we intentionally activate psychophysiological coherence, we experience greater emotional stability, increased mental clarity, and improved cognitive function. Simply put, our body and brain work better, we feel better, and we perform better. The HeartMath tools teach us how to self-activate, and eventually sustain positive, productive emotions, in order to rapidly access a state of coherence and spend more time there throughout our day.

A recent study, assessing improvements in mental and emotional well-being, looked at over 5,500 people using HeartMath training and technology for periods varying from six to nine weeks. Using this HRV training, participants reported:

- 50 % decrease in fatigue
- 46 % drop in anxiety
- 60% lower levels of depression
- 24% increase in focus
- 25% improvement in listening ability
- 30% improvement in sleep quality and duration

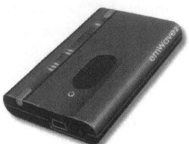

John Gray, author of *"Men Are From Mars, Women Are From Venus,"* states "On mornings, when I have a little bit more time, I will grab a blank journal to have nearby, power up my emWave, and use it to get myself into coherence before I meditate."

Many people use their emWave for 20 to 30 minutes, however, benefits can be derived in as little as just five minutes. For more information on HRV training, or to see what HRV monitor I'm currently using, go to www.BioHackingSecrets.com/hrv.

THE MIND ALIVE, DAVID SMART

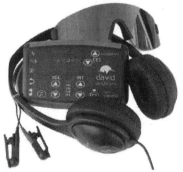

The DAVID Smart utilizes a futuristic-looking pair of glasses and headphones in order to deliver a unique fusion of audio and visual entrainment (AKA frequency following response).

Sessions on the DAVID Smart are designed to improve academic performance, reduce stress, boost mood, and improve concentration and memory in college students. They also include a proprietary randomization process, which helps encourage dissociation and brain frequency tracking to the stimulus. There are five categories of sessions featured: Energize, Meditate, Brain Brightener, Sleep, and Mood Booster. Each category has two selections of varying lengths.

A few months back, I was wiped from a packed day and looking down the barrel of at least 3 to 4 hours of writing ahead of me. I decided to fire up the DAVID Smart that had arrived earlier that afternoon. I threw on the headphones and glasses, which looked a lot like the Oakley's outfielders used to wear in the 80's, and selected the 20-minute meditation session. Laying down on my Biomat, I let the sound waves and multi-colored flashing lights go to work. The session flew by. When I took off the headset, I felt much more relaxed, and focused.

To save 10% on the DAVID (Digital Audio Visual Integration Device) Delight Pro and DAVID Smart call 1-800-661-MIND and use discount code "biohacks."

NUCALM

Originally developed by a neuroscientist named Dr. G. Blake Holloway, the NuCalm device was intended to treat patients with post-traumatic stress disorder (PTSD) who suffered intense anxiety, stress, and cognitive impairment. The system includes four main components.They are:

- A proprietary chewable supplement containing relaxing neural transmitters to counteract adrenaline
- A Cranial Electrotherapy Stimulation (CES) device
- Proprietary neural-acoustic software
- Blackout glasses

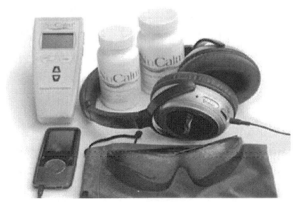

NuCalm works by organically entraining brainwaves to a frequency that promotes relaxation and calm. However, unlike other systems that use binaural beats, the NuCalm system uses an exclusive algorithm wherein the frequency periodically changes in order to prevent brain adaptation. The NuCalm system quickly takes the user from the beta state that people are typically in when they are awake to the first phase of sleep, the alpha state.

The unique combination of these four components gives this system the ability to interrupt and override our body's stress response. Once this is done, the system quickly guides the user into a more productive state.

NuCalm entrains the brain to move to the alpha and theta ranges without effort, creating homeostasis and deepening meditative practices. This also triggers neural muscular release and overall relaxation.

The NuCalm system has been used by the Chicago Blackhawks for the last three years. In those three years, they have won the Stanley Cup twice. The only year that they didn't win, they lost to the Los Angeles Kings in Game 7, which had gone into overtime.

THE BIOMAT 7000MX PRO

The Biomat 7000MX serves a few different therapeutic purposes.

It provides many of the benefits of an infrared sauna (www. BioHackingSecrets.com/sauna) without the inconveniences. The most common frustration clients report with at-home infrared saunas is that they take a long time to heat. So you have to plan ahead.

The Biomat's medical and therapeutic properties are based on Nobel Prize winning research on ionic channels (transfer of free electrons). It uses the same infrared technology that NASA identified as the safest

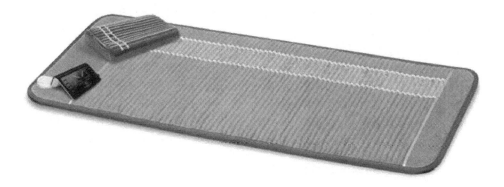

and the most beneficial type of light wave. Right at this moment, as I am working on this book, I have an infrared light over my feet and another on a chair next to my bed, which is shining on my face and chest.

The combination of deep penetrating infrared waves and negative ions (like we get when barefoot in contact with the earth or swimming in the ocean) help to heal the body on a cellular level. I have many of my clients do their treatments on the Biomat because of its ability to induce relaxation, relieve stress, and stimulate the body's detoxification pathways.

Here are some of the specific benefits of the Biomat 7000MX:

- Increases circulation
- Reduces stress and fatigue
- Smooths and relaxes muscles
- Eases joint pain, aches, and stiffness
- Strengthens the immune system
- Improves sleep
- Reduces inflammation
- Increases oxygenation of the tissues
- Temporary relief of back pain, strains, aches, tightness, stiffness, aches, and muscle spasms

HYPERTHERMIC CONDITIONING: SAUNAS AND ULTRA BATHS

Two other tools that are very effective at reducing stress, in addition to improving detoxification and inducing a deeper night's sleep, are ultra baths and dry saunas.

An ultra bath involves filling the bathtub with water that is as hot as you can physically tolerate. Then, add 2 cups of Epsom salt and 1 cup of baking soda. Some optional additions are 1 cup 35% food grade hydrogen peroxide, and 12 to 15 drops of therapeutic grade lavender essential oil.

You can use regular Epsom salt for this, which is available at any drug store. Dr. Teal's also has an Epsom salt soaking solution that contains lavender. I use regular Arm & Hammer baking soda when I occasionally include hydrogen peroxide. I use the One Minute Miracle brand hydrogen peroxide. For the lavender oil, I use Majestic Pure Cosmeceuticals, therapeutic grade.

Raising your body temperature induces relaxation and triggers your body's natural detoxification pathways. It reduces tension both physically and psychologically.

When you add 2 cups of Epsom salt, you are essentially bathing your body in magnesium. This is a vital nutrient that about 60% of the population are deficient in. The baking soda is sodium bicarbonate, and this will help you to absorb even more of the magnesium and provide alkaline-balancing effects. Both of these reduce stress and allow you to achieve a deeper night's sleep.

The Japanese are one of the longest-living cultures on earth. There's a Japanese tradition known as "ofuro" which involves hot baths taken at night time before going to bed. In addition to the stress relief, relaxation, and detoxification benefits, these hot baths have also been known to increase melatonin production. Mice given daily melatonin live longer.

I also recommend ultra baths to those clients who come to me with chronic pain or inflammatory conditions. I have them take an ultra bath early in the day, and they often experience a profound reduction in their symptoms, increased comfort, and greater quality of life throughout the day.

Here are some of the benefits that you can expect from taking consistent 20 to 30 minute ultra baths:

- Relaxation of your nervous system and lower cortisol levels, both of which increase weight loss and dampen inflammation
- Enhanced detoxification through the sulfur and magnesium contained in the Epsom salt
- Enhanced sleep because of the relaxation effects of heat, magnesium, and elevated endogenous melatonin production
- Alkalization of the body by way of the sodium bicarbonate (baking soda)
- Increased circulation and elevated heart rate, which mimics the effects of exercise. (This is especially beneficial for individuals who are physically incapable of exercising due to injury or other underlining health issues.)
- Decreased blood pressure
- Increased insulin sensitivity
- Increased heart rate variability
- Increased elimination of toxins through the skin, the body's largest organ

The dry sauna carries many similar benefits. Some of the benefits of dry saunas and infrared saunas over ultra baths, and even steam rooms, are that the saunas do not expose the body to fluoride, chlorine, pharmaceutical drugs, and many of the other chemicals commonly found in tap water.

So, if you're one of the many people who do not have a reverse osmosis water filtration system for your home, the disadvantage of an ultra bath is that you are taking in some of these toxins while you bathe.

In a steam room, you're not only taking in these toxins through your skin, but you're also breathing them into your lungs.

It's also important to be aware that individuals with a high toxic burden often feel lousy when they first start using these saunas as the body liberates these toxins. Listen to your body and start small, even if you just use the sauna for a few minutes at a time at first. Each time,

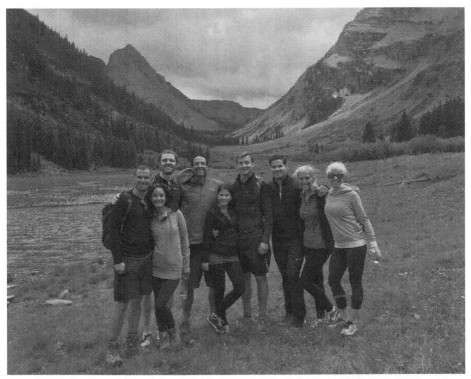

Spending time in nature is another powerful tool to help reduce or eliminate stress.

bring yourself to the point where you start to experience discomfort, and then exit the sauna, and take a 2-minute cold shower. Stay consistent and gradually work your way up to 20 to 30 minute sessions.

In one study, folks who hit the sauna for 30 minutes post-workout just twice a week for three weeks, increased their cardiovascular conditioning (as measured by time to exhaustion) by over 30%.

Other physiological changes elicited by hyperthermic conditioning (i.e. dry sauna) include improved:

- Cardiovascular conditioning
- Body temperature regulation
- Detoxification
- Red blood cell count
- Glycogen utilization
- Oxygen transport and utilization

Research has shown saunas increase levels of norepinephrine, which is a hormone involved in our body's stress response. This helps to support concentration and focus.

They also have been known to increase prolactin, which may promote myelin growth. This helps repair damage to nerves and it helps your brain to process at faster speeds.

Lastly, dry saunas have been shown to boost feelings of wellbeing. In fact, animal studies have shown exposure to heat stress significantly increases endorphin release.

Other useful tools for reducing stress include:

- Acupuncture
- Yoga Nidra
- Hypnosis

- Sensory deprivation tanks
- Spending time in nature (camping, hiking, water sports, boating)
- Massage (deep tissue and trigger point work; Turkish and Russian massage)
- The Art of Living Foundation (www.artofliving.org)
- NanoVi (www.eng3corp.com): Produces the same biological signal your body makes to repair cell damage brought on by free radicals (also known as reactive oxygen species or ROS)

HOW TO CONQUER FEARS, PHOBIAS, AND STRESSFUL EMOTIONS

Neuro-linguistic programming is based on the fundamental dynamic between the mind (neuro) and language (linguistic), and how their interplay affects our body and behavior (programming).

According to the science in this field, you can use Disassociation to reduce stress-inducing emotions, fears, and phobias. Here's how:

Step 1: Identify the emotion that you want to change. This could be just about anything. An example might be a fear of snakes, or maybe you have some apprehension about encountering a certain person. For example, you may have a dislike of visiting your mother-in-law's house.

Step 2: Imagine yourself sitting in a movie theater. On the movie screen you see yourself going through the situation you are trying to avoid or are in fear of. Since you are sitting in this theater, you are viewing this scenario as an observer.

Step 3: Still watching the screen, imagine playing the movie backwards. Then, fast forward it, and then play it backwards again. If

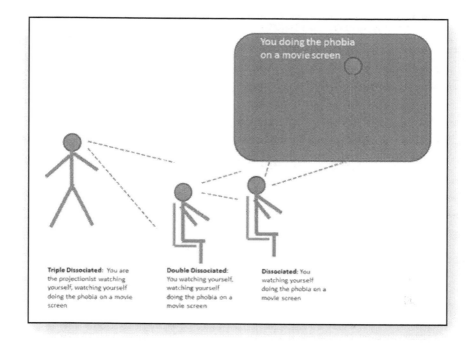

it's a situation that does not involve another person or communication with others, play it backwards again, but this time add funny music. If it's a situation that does involve interaction or communication with another person, change their voice to that of a funny cartoon character or a small child. The point is that you will want to change the picture up on the screen to something that makes you laugh and feels non-threatening.

Step 4: Repeat the process of playing this movie backwards and fast forwarding it three to four times with the added sounds and/or vocal elements.

Step 5: Now step into the version of yourself on the screen so that you see the situation through his or her eyes and no longer as an observer. You may notice that your stress levels and emotions towards the stimulus have changed and perhaps even disappeared entirely. If your stress and negative emotions persist, keep repeating this process until these negative feelings have subsided.

SUPPLEMENTS FOR STRESS MANAGEMENT

There are a number of supplements that I recommend to clients for mitigating stress. I have used many of them myself, and all of the ones listed are supported in scientific literature. They include but are not limited to:

- *Cytozyme-AD by Biotics Research Corporation:* This supplement contains bovine Neonatal Adrenal Complex, superoxide dismutase, and catalase.
- *InterPlexus Seriphos:* This is as a phosphorylated serine adaptogen and adrenal support complex.
- *L-Theanine (Suntheanine form):* This is an amino acid that has been shown to induce a calming effect on the body. It also induces alpha brain waves, which are associated with a relaxed state of heightened focus and concentration. These are the same brain waves that we experience during meditation. This supplement also provides neuro-protection and restoration of the neurotransmitter GABA (gamma-aminobutyric acid), which increases its clinical efficacy and relaxation effect. A number of studies have shown that l-theanine is also able to stimulate similar effects, feelings, and benefits as meditation, massage, and aromatherapy, independent of these practices.
- *GABA:* This is a major inhibitory neurotransmitter that reduces the excitability of neurons and interrupts the body's stress response. Over-stimulated and overactive neurons can cause

chronic fatigue, low mood, and in some cases, insomnia. GABA is naturally produced from the amino acid glutamine. It's concentrated in the hypothalamus and plays an important role in healthy pituitary function.

- *Lithium Orotate:* I have used lithium with clients struggling with low mood, stress, anxiety, depressive, and bipolar disorders. I have also used it as part of a protocol for clients suffering from migraines and cluster headaches. There are over 100 medical conditions that benefit from lithium supplementation. It is an essential trace mineral like sodium, potassium, calcium, and magnesium. It is not technically a drug but rather, a mineral, similar to salt. Studies have shown lithium orotate benefits mood and brain health. One study found that, in just 3 weeks, adults given lithium increased brain cell volume by 3%.
- 5-HTP
- Magnesium Glycinate
- Phosphatidylserine
- Adaptogens
- Ashwagandha
- Rhodiola
- Panax Ginseng

Individuals who are often stressed or fatigued (or rely on stimulants to avoid fatigue) frequently have dysregulation of the hypothalamic pituitary adrenal axis (HPA). By restoring balance in the HPA axis, we are able to balance hormones and improve their endogenous synthesis in the body, improve sleep cycles, and more effectively regulate homeostatic body temperature.

GABA is the only amino acid capable of crossing the blood-brain barrier (when taken orally). GABA receptor sites are located in the same areas of the brain as the receptor sites for barbiturates, alcohol, and benzodiazepines.

I have used the adrenal health formula from Gaia Herbs with many clients (www.BioHackingSecrets.com/coaching) to help them recover from adrenal fatigue and increase natural energy levels.

This complex contains Siberian Rhodiola, holy basil, Ashwagandha, Schisandra berry, and a number of other therapeutic adaptogenic herbs.

STRESS MANAGEMENT BIOHACKS

The One Thing: Commit to meditating for at least five minutes every day for the next 28 days.

Biohack #1: Meditating 5 to 30 minutes daily has been shown to:

- Increase brain mass
- Increase intelligence
- Reduce anxiety
- Improve quality of life

Meditate for at least 5 minutes every morning for 30 days. I recommend beginners start with the Headspace smartphone application.

Biohack #2: Stress management tools recommended include:

- HeartMath, using emWave2 or Inner Balance IOS app
- The Mind Alive, DAVID Smart & DAVID Delight Pro
- NuCalm System
- The Biomat 7000MX infrared mat
- NanoVi by Eng3 Corp

- Ultra Baths
- Dry Saunas (hyperthermic conditioning)
- Listening to classical music with headphones.

Biohack #3: The types of meditation and yoga I advise you to try are:

- Pranayama Yoga & Pranayama Yoga Meditation
- Vipassana Meditation
- Transcendental Meditation: The clinical trials on Transcendental Meditation are literally better than nutrition studies as it pertains to improving overall health.
- Kundalini Yoga
- Primordial Sound Meditation
- Mindfulness Meditation

Biohack #4: Supplements and other forms of treatment for stress management include:

- Acupuncture
- Yoga Nidra
- Hypnosis
- Sensory deprivation tanks
- Spending time in nature (camping, hiking, water sports, boating)
- Massage
- Russian and Turkish-style bath houses (contrast hydrotherapy, dry saunas, massage)
- The Art of Living Foundation
- Cytozyme-AD by Biotics Research Corporation
- InterPlexus Seriphos
- L-theanine (Suntheanine form)

- GABA
- 5-HTP Magnesium Glycinate
- Phosphatidylserine
- Ashwagandha
- Rhodiola
- Panax Ginseng
- Ancient Minerals Ultra Magnesium Oil with OptiMSM (after showers or baths)

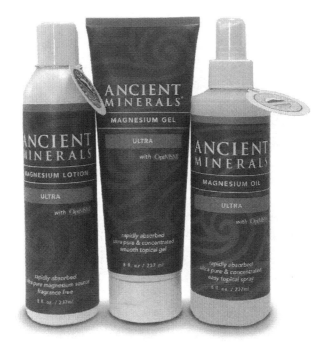

Biohack #5: Other tools that I recommend include:
- *"Why Zebras Don't Get Ulcers"* by Robert M. Sapolsky.
- Brain.fm (I use the guided meditations)
- The HeadSpace (app)
- Holosync by Centerpoint "The Dive"
- Dr. Jeffery Thompson's neuroacoustic CDs on Spotify

- *"The 6 Phase Meditation"* (Omvana app)
- Overnight Riches: A Flow Dream Meditation (Omvana app)
- *"Amplifying Your Money Magnetism"* by Matthew Ferry
- BrainSync's Kelly Howell meditations
- *"Meditate with the Himalayan Masters"* by Swami Veda Bharati and Paul R. Scheele
- Sam Harris' 9-minute mindfulness meditation, *"Looking for the Self"* and *"Waking Up."*
- Dr. Joe Dispenza's "Tuning Into New Potentials" and "Reconditioning the Body to a New Mind" mediations

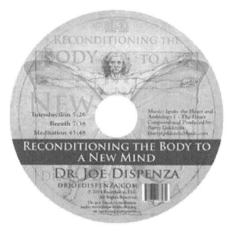
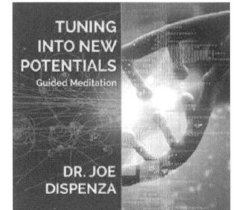

SLEEP

At 65 years old, Jay Leno still manages to tour on the comedy circuit, averaging over 150 gigs a year in addition to his hosting The Tonight Show. He sleeps only about five hours a night.

Herb Kelleher, co-founder of Southwest Airlines, slept only four hours a night during the time he was running this continuously profitable airline.

At 74 years old, Martha Stewart's company produces four magazines, a TV show, radio show, and product lines in Staples and Michael's. She sleeps less than four hours a night.

President Barack Obama and former president Bill Clinton are both renowned for sleeping only 5 to 6 hours a night.

Yet, according to the documentary Sleepless in America, 40 percent of Americans are sleep deprived, with many getting less than 5 hours of sleep per night. Insomnia has reached epidemic proportions. 1 in 3 Americans have trouble sleeping every night. The number of adults using prescription sleeping pills doubled from 2000 to 2004 and has reached an all time high.

This is no surprise in a society that values activity and productivity above all else.

SLEEPING HABITS OF THE
RICH & FAMOUS

We're always told the importance of getting a regular, solid eight hours' sleep when it comes to being productive and successful, but not everyone follows this seemingly sound advice. Some of the most famous, successful and driven people throughout history have had some very strange sleeping habits - from micro-kips to sleeping in phases, we've got the oddest rich and famous sleeping habits in this new infographic, brought to you by Big Brand Beds.

KEY:

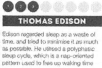

The blue bar shows the hours slept by the individual (on average)

The overall number of hours slept by the individual in a 24 period (on average)

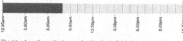

WINSTON CHURCHILL

Naps were so important to Churchill that he kept a bed in the House of Parliament and believed napping was the key to his success leading the country through the Battle of Britain

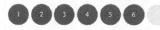

NIKOLA TESLA

Tesla's odd sleeping pattern caused him to have a mental breakdown at the age of 25. He managed to pull himself together and continued well into his old age, working another 38 years

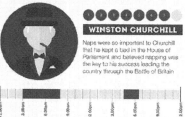

THOMAS EDISON

Edison regarded sleep as a waste of time, and tried to minimise it as much as possible. He utilised a polyphasic sleep cycle, which is a nap-oriented pattern used to free up waking time

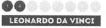

LEONARDO DA VINCI

Da Vinci followed an even more extreme polyphasic sleep cycle than Edison, called the Uberman sleep cycle, which consists of taking a 20 minute nap every four hours

WOLFGANG MOZART

Mozart would often continue composing until 1.00am, then would sleep for only five hours before getting up again at 6.00am and continuing composing throughout the morning

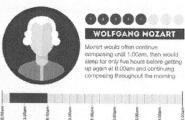

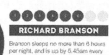

RICHARD BRANSON

Branson sleeps no more than 6 hours per night, and is up by 5.45am every morning to ensure he gets a head start on his day. He tries to exercise each morning and spend time with his family

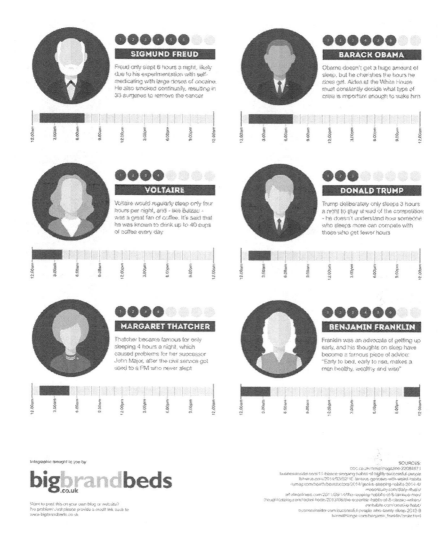

We look at examples of successful people who don't need a lot of sleep and assume, because we are both human, we have similar biological needs. If the leader of the free world can operate on 5 to 6 hours of sleep a night, so can we - right?

But the more we uncover about sleep, the more we realize that we don't know much at all.

To help decode the mystery of sleep, enter David Dinges, head of the Sleep and Chronobiology Laboratory at the hospital at the University of Pennsylvania. Dinges has the distinct honor of depriving more people of sleep than perhaps anyone in the world.

In what was the longest sleep-restriction study of all time, Dinges and his lead author, Hans Van Dongen, made an interesting discovery. They studied the effects of sleep deprivation over a two-week period by limiting the subjects to time ranges between 4 to 9 hours of sleep. What did they find?

Sleep durations under seven hours correlated with decreases in physical and cognitive performance along with a lack of energy production. Now, that's probably no surprise to you. The subjects who were sleeping less than 7 hours reported that they were slightly sleepy. That's not surprising either. Despite their slightly sleepy state, after a couple of weeks these participants believed they had adjusted and their lack of sleep didn't decrease their performance. However, the psychomotor vigilance task (PVT), which was considered the gold-standard of sleepiness measures, painted a very different picture. In fact, the PVT showed that their performances tanked.

Therein lies the problem. This is one of the reasons why so many of us fail to change our sleep patterns. We are unable to objectively recognize the negative implications lack of sleep is having on our performance. In reality, we are far less sharp than we think we are. This leaves us in a dilemma. We lack the ability to objectively recognize and quantify the downside of our lack of sleep.

There are a small percentage of people who can maintain performance levels with 5 hours of sleep per night or less, but they only make up about 5% of the population. This is because of a genetic predisposition; it's not something that you can be trained to be able to do.

There are also a small percentage of people who require 9 to 10 hours of sleep. The rest of us need the standard 7 to 9 hours.

Now, what do we know about people who don't get enough sleep?

We know that insufficient sleep levels are associated with chronic inflammation. As I have previously stated, chronic inflammation is the primary driver behind all modern degenerative diseases. Therefore, lack of sleep can be linked as a major factor in, if not the root cause of, many different conditions, including:

- Insulin resistance
- Diabetes
- Obesity
- Heart disease
- Cognitive impairment
- Increased cortisol
- Chronic stress
- Weakened immune function
- Psychiatric disorders (a long list of them, including anxiety and depression)

INADEQUATE SLEEP IS ASSOCIATED WITH LOW ENERGY

To begin, it is a well-known fact that inadequate amounts of sleep causes lower amounts of energy. Sleep deprivation elevates thyroid-stimulating hormone (TSH), and this is inversely related to serum thyroid hormone levels. Our body increases levels of TSH when our serum hormone levels are low. Thyroid hormones are key drivers for energy production and metabolic health, including the regulation of body weight. Take note that elevated TSH levels are often observed in overweight and obese patients.

COGNITIVE IMPAIRMENT VIA LACK OF SLEEP

Lack of sleep interferes with the generation of nerve cells and impairs both short and long-term memory. All of this compromises our ability to focus, solve problems, think clearly, and react quickly. Inadequate sleep decreases activity and worsens a number of psychiatric conditions, ranging from depression, to anxiety, and even PTSD.

Many of these changes affecting our body's hormonal balance, cognition, and energy, can be seen in just a matter of days. One study found that inadequate sleep increased the body's stress hormone, cortisol after only 6 days of restricting test subjects to 4 hours of sleep per night. This increase in cortisol further exacerbates sleep problems.

Cortisol and the hormone melatonin, which is responsible for helping us achieve the onset of and sustaining sleep, oppose one another. In other words, as cortisol goes down, melatonin levels increase, and we are able to fall asleep at night. Through insufficient sleep and our modern diet and lifestyle, these elevated cortisol levels further suppress melatonin production.

LACK OF SLEEP CAN KILL YOU

Normal rats live between two and three years. However, a recent study, that prevented rats from falling asleep, found that the rats denied REM sleep were dead within five weeks. Rats that were denied sleep altogether were dead within three weeks.

The scientific literature is clear. *There are no benefits to sleep deprivation.*

Some people function better on lower levels of sleep than others, but interestingly, the research suggests that these people die younger.

We cannot train ourselves to function better on a lack of sleep. There are no up-regulated enzymes or adaptive changes you can make. You become less intelligent and mental processing slows.

The biggest impediment to making behavioral changes necessary for us to get adequate sleep is our own inability to recognize the negative impact of its absence.

Funny enough, the Guinness Book of World Records has stopped letting people deprive themselves of sleep because it is too dangerous, while setting records for things like swallowing glass and swords are still fair game.

THE #1 BIOHACK FOR UPGRADING YOUR ENERGY AND FOCUS

Lions sleep 18 to 20 hours a day, yet are one of the most clinical and precise hunters on the planet.

Allocating at least 7 ½ hours in bed each night is the single greatest biohack you can implement for upgrading energy and focus. Still not convinced? Recent studies have shown:

- One night of good sleep can improve your motor skills by 20%.
- Eight hours of quality sleep increases your ability to gain new insight into complex problems by 50%.
- Sleep increases testosterone levels: A 2008 study showed that men who slept four hours a night had 60% lower testosterone levels than men who slept eight hours a night. This correlated to a 50% increase in testosterone for every additional hour slept.

The question is, how do we get leverage on ourselves in order to change our sleep patterns and set aside more time for this performance-enhancing habit?

Former Navy Seal, Dr. Kirk Parsley, has a solution. He calls it the "7-Day Sleep Challenge" in which he asks people to give themselves 9 hours of time in bed (sleep period) for just one week. This will result in 8 to 8 ½ hours of actual sleep (sleep duration). By day 6 and 7, people are happier, healthier, faster, stronger, and smarter. For many people

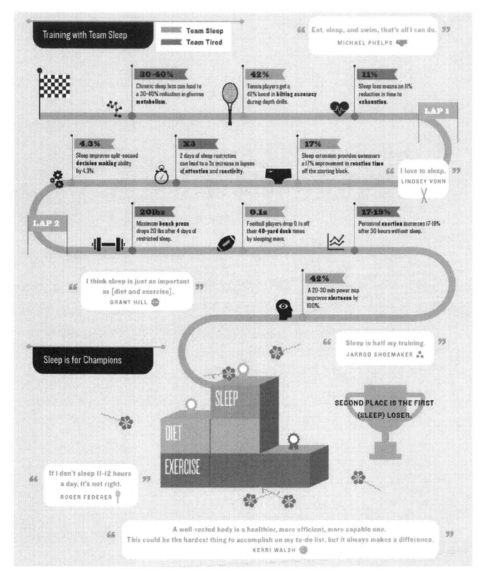

this begins far before day 6. This is one of the best ways that you can support your trademark work effort and maximize productivity.

Parsley says, "...because I promise you that if you're cutting sleep in the name of being more productive, it's not working." On days 6 and 7, he asks that you find ways to quantify your performance, mood, mental clarity, and strength. This can be as simple as rating your energy, mood, focus, creativity, intelligence, and any other important traits on a scale of 1 to 10. If there are any important tasks that you do on a daily or weekly basis for your career, find a simple way to measure and assess your performance there as well.

This approach is powerful because it motivates using both the carrot and the stick. We get the carrot when we physically and emotionally experience the benefits of sufficient sleep. Then, by quantifying our performance on days 6 and 7, we become more objective in recognizing the detrimental effects that sleep deprivation can have on our energy, focus, and quality of life. After we have optimized our sleep and taken everything to the next level, we won't want to downgrade ever again.

For some of us, 9 hours sounds like an impossible amount of time when we consider our busy schedule. Parsley shares a story which might give you a new perspective. He says, "My Navy Seals instructors and leaders used to ask, 'If I gave you a million dollars to do X by a certain time, could you do it?' Most of the time the answer was 'yes,' and once they sucked you in, they would reply, '...then you can do it without a million dollars.'"

I challenge you to set aside at least 7 ½ hours per night for time in bed (sleep period). This will allow you to get the minimum 7 hours of sleep we require to keep energy and cognitive performance intact. I recommend setting two recurring alarms on your smartphone as well. One should go off an hour before you get in bed, reminding you to shut down all of your electronics, including your TV, cell phone, and computers. The second one should go off when it's time for you to get in bed.

Work backwards by figuring out what time you need to get up in order to do your morning workout and whatever other important activities set you up to win the day. This will help you determine when to set your first alarm. For example, if you know that you need to wake up at 6:30 am, your alarm telling you to shut off all your electronics would go off at 10:00 pm. Then, your alarm telling you to get into bed would go off at 11:00 pm. These alarms serve to interrupt our old behavior patterns until new habits are fully ingrained.

For already healthy individuals, there are no biohacks which compensate for insufficient sleep. However, there are many biohacks and lifestyle changes that can increase sleep quality, yielding better results in shorter amounts of time.

The One Thing: Set aside at least 7 ½ hours per night for time in bed (sleep period). This will allow you to get the minimum 7 hours of sleep (sleep duration) we require to keep energy and cognitive performance intact.

HOW TO HACK YOUR MATTRESS FOR A BETTER NIGHT'S REST

One of the best things that you can do to improve the quality of your sleep is to invest in a great mattress.

If you spend 8 hours a night in bed, that equates to nearly one third of your life. Therefore, finding the greatest possible bed for your sleep is one of the supreme decisions you can make. It needs to be perfect for you so that you can't wait to crawl into bed.

SLEEP

Mark Ford and his research team at the Palm Beach Letter conducted research which analyzed all of the important qualities of a great mattress. These included comfort, overall quality, and durability. In the fourth chapter of his book, *"Living Rich: How to Live as Well as a Millionaire on a Middle-Class Budget,"* Ford provides the top mattress picks in a number of different categories.

The selections that were made came about from over 100 hours of dedicated research conducted by a whole team of individuals. Mark and his team of researchers scoured through reports from sleep experts, mattress countries, specific mattress warranties, consumer reports, and hundreds of customer satisfaction reviews to compile the data.

Below, I have included their top mattress recommendation in each category.

Top Innerspring Mattress Picks:
- Serta, Trump Home series
- Stearns & Foster, Silver Dream collection
- Sealy Posturepedic, Supreme Tociano
- Simmons Beautyrest, World Class Braithwaite
- Simmons Beautyrest Elite, Legend

Top Memory Foam Mattress Picks:
- Tempur-Pedic Tepur-HD collection, Rhapsody
- Simmons ComforPedic Phenom
- Serta iComfort Gel Memory Foam

Top Picks for Latex
- Habitat Furnishings Latex
- OrganicPedic Terra Latex

Top Inflatable Airbed Picks

- Habitat Furnishing's Arise airbed system
- Comfortaire
- Select Comfort's Sleep Number m7 bed

...*And The Winner Is:* Tempur-Pedic Tempur-HD collection's Tempur-Rhapsody. This mattress received the top PBL score in its category. Taking into account the price, the exceptional warranty period, and consistent positive reviews, the value cannot be beat. At a price of $2,900 with a warranty of 20 years, you'll be paying a mere $145 per year to sleep like a billionaire.

The Habitat Furnishings natural latex mattress was a close second.

For individuals with signs of toxic overload (see Troubleshooting), I recommend Mountain Air Organic Beds (www. MountainAirOrganicBeds.com). They are free from the Formaldehyde, flame retardants, and petroleum that has been found in many commercial mattresses. This is sage advice for anyone really. None of us want to find out our body has been absorbing these poisonous chemicals while we sleep.

3 COMPONENTS TO A GOOD NIGHT'S REST

There are 3 major components of sleep that a good night's rest is dependent upon. We will also further incorporate biohacks and strategies that address factors that could interfere with rest and recovery. First, let's address these 3 critical factors:

Sleep Quantity: This is what is being referred to when we describe how many hours of sleep we need per night. What people get confused about is the difference between sleep period and sleep duration. Sleep period is the amount of time that's spent in bed, and sleep duration is the amount of time that one actually spends sleeping. The minimum amount of sleep quantity required to keep cognitive and energetic functions intact is 7 hours of sleep time, which would require no less than 7 ½ hours in bed (sleep period).

Sleep Quality: We pass through five different stages of sleep, Stage 1, 2, 3, 4 & REM (rapid eye movement) sleep. These stages progress in a cycle from Stage 1 to 4 followed by REM sleep. These cycles can last anywhere from 90 to 110 minutes.

We spend almost 50% of our total sleep time in Stage 2 sleep and 20% in REM sleep. The remaining 30% is spread throughout stages 1, 3, and 4. All of these stages of sleep are important. Although we spend a great deal of time in Stage 2 and REM sleep, we derive a great deal of our neuro-regenerative benefits, recovery, and restoration from Stages 3 and 4 of our sleep cycles. Individuals with sleep disorders such as insomnia, sleep apnea, restless leg syndrome, narcolepsy, and older adults tend to spend less time in these more vital stages of sleep and more time in Stage 1, which is the lightest stage of sleep.

Sleep Timing: This refers to the time that sleep onset and sleep offset occurs - in other words, what time you go to bed and what time you wake up.

Not all sleep is created equal and a number of studies indicate that following a consistent sleep schedule that more closely coincides with the rising and setting of the sun is far more beneficial than if sleep were obtained at other times throughout the day.

Many sleep experts have observed that an hour of sleep before midnight is worth approximately two hours of sleep after midnight.

ROADBLOCKS TO A GOOD NIGHT'S SLEEP

You now know the 3 most important factors to getting proper sleep, let's discuss the 3 biggest challenges that can get in our way. They are:

Discipline: We all live busy, hectic lives with demands to meet concerning our career, family, social activities, and our own health. Allowing for adequate sleep durations and sleep periods can be difficult, but you have to treat it like anything else that's important.

Practicing key habits when we don't want to, but knowing that we should, is perhaps the greatest habit of all.

Endocrine Disruptions: Our modern lifestyle creates a great deal of problems, many of which are hard to escape. We often must deal with:

- A lack of resources for proper nutrition (if we are even looking for them)
- A lack of time and opportunities for physical activity (if we are even looking for them)
- Chronic stress
- Inadequate amounts of sleep
- Unnatural light
- Odd working hours (including night shifts)

Because many of us deal with so much, are always stressed, feel at loss for time, and believe that we need to keep going whether we get adequate amounts of sleep or not, we may be tempted to turn to stimulants. Whether these stimulants are natural or artificial, they disrupt the delicate balance of our body's hormonal systems.

Dysregulation of the HPA axis is one of the most common challenges we face today. Through a number of pathways, we artificially induce our body's fight or flight response. This has a tendency to trigger chronically-elevated levels of cortisol, depressed melatonin production, and a wide array of other hormone-related complications.

Overstimulation of Our Brain & Nervous System: While this is a separate issue, it shares many common etiologies responsible for hormonal dysregulation. These include:

- Exposure to computers, TVs, cell phones, and artificial lights
- The use of stimulants and prescription drugs
- Unnatural work shifts
- Exercising too close to the time of sleep onset

Now, let's go over some of the most effective tools, techniques, and biohacks that will help you to optimize your sleep for upgraded energy and focus.

ANCESTRAL SLEEP HACKS FROM MODERN DAY HUNTER GATHERERS

In the pursuit of peak performance, it only makes sense to study those who are already performing at world class levels. The secret is to uncover the things that they do consistently and then apply those same habits ourselves.

Roger Federer and LeBron James both sleep an average of 12 hours a night.

Federer owns an all-time record of 17 Grand Slam titles. He says, "If I don't sleep 11 to 12 hours a night, it's not right."

LeBron James is one of the best professional basketball player in the game today, and an argument could even be made for all-time. He's won or been awarded:

- Two NBA championships (2012, 2013)
- Four NBA Most Valuable Player awards (2009, 2010, 2012, 2013)
- Two NBA Finals NVP awards (2012, 2013)
- Two Olympic Gold Metals (2008, 2012)
- One NBA scoring title (2008)
- One NBA Rookie of the Year Award (2004)

He's also been selected for 11 NBA All-Star teams, 11 All-NBA teams, 6 All-Defensive teams, and is the Cleveland Cavilers' all-time leading scorer. He achieved all of this by the time he was 30 years old.

Steve Nash is a two-time NBA League Most Valuable Player. He sleeps 10 hours a night. He also naps every game day. Nash comments on his career saying, "You have a busy, stressful schedule, but it's something you have to make a priority."

Usain Bolt (the first man to win six Olympic Gold Medals in sprinting), Venus Williams, and Maria Sharapova all get 10 hours of sleep per night.

Rafael Nadal owns 14 Grand Slam titles. By winning the 2014 French Open, Nadal became the only male player to win a single Grand Slam tournament nine times and the first to win a Grand Slam tournament for 10 consecutive years. The Spaniard reportedly sleeps 8 to 9 hours per night.

Our modern lifestyle is overrun with unnatural variables that interfere with our quality of sleep. Many theories as to what "natural" sleep looks like have existed for decades, but a groundbreaking study published by Professor Jerry Siegel of UCLA in the journal of Current Biology lends new insights.

In the study, Professor Siegel analyzed the sleep habits of three modern hunter/gatherer societies. Not only did they analyze external factors like ambient temperature, season, and natural light, but they also utilized tracking bracelets to gather diurnal activity levels and behavior patterns. The three groups examined in the study were the Hadza of Northern Tanzania, the San people of the Kalahari, and the Tsimane of Bolivia.

Again, these are all hunter/gatherer societies, and they were all close to the equator, which is the latitude from which scientists believe that early humans evolved.

The study found that the sleep period, the amount of time they spent in bed, was between 6 hours and 54 minutes and 8 hours and 30 minutes.

When it came to the sleep duration, which was the actual time spent in a state of sleep, they spent between 5 hours and 42 minutes and 7 hours and 6 minutes in slumber. It's important to remember that when we review studies recommending 7 to 9 hours of sleep, they are almost always referring to sleep period and not sleep duration.

Both the San people and the Tsimane slept about an hour longer in winter compared to summer. These hunter/gatherer people are free from many of the modern lifestyle factors that can interfere with adequate sleep, including:

- Artificial light
- Processed foods
- Sedentary lifestyle
- Stimulants and prescription drugs
- Unnatural work shifts
- Chronic stress

Contrary to what evolutionary biologists had expected, these indigenous tribes did not go to sleep and wake with the rising and setting of the sun. On average, they went to bed (sleep onset) between 2 ½ and 4 ½ hours after sunset.

They would use this time to sit around the fire and tell stories (social bonding) or to dance (movement).

The Hadza and Tsimane groups woke up (sleep offset) about one hour before sunrise. The San people woke up before sunrise in the winter and about one hour after sunrise in the summer. The study found that neither their sleep nor waking onset correlated with the levels of light emitted by the sun. They were more closely tied to changes in ambient temperature.

At night, the drop in temperature would trigger the onset of sleep. In the mornings, as the temperatures began to rise, so did the study participants.

The researchers also observed a vasoconstriction of the extremities, which forces more blood into one's core and brain. It is hypothesized that this vasoconstriction also increases temperature around the brain and vital organs, preparing the body to awaken.

The National Sleep Foundation recommends that people get between 7 and 9 hours of sleep. Again, they are referring to "sleep period" and not "sleep duration" because that is what the majority of people understand.

Siegel's study found that modern hunter/gatherers had sleep periods ranging from 7 hours to 8 ½ hours, which is in line with the range recommended by the National Sleep Foundation.

These indigenous people go to sleep roughly three hours after sunset and wake somewhere just before or just after sunrise, depending on the time of year and the specific tribe that they were in.

These sleep patterns are consistent, and these indigenous people experience a greater quality of sleep because they are not exposed to the myriad of factors that can disrupt endocrine function and over-stimulate the brain and central nervous system.

SLEEP HACKING: THE ART & SCIENCE OF SLEEPING

Now let's put all of this research into some actionable lifestyle shifts to optimize your sleep quantity, quality, and timing.

1. Go to Bed Earlier: When you fall asleep, your body goes through a 90-minute sleep cycle, followed by REM sleep. Earlier in the night, the majority of those sleep cycles are spent in non-REM sleep (Stages 3, 4 and very little REM sleep). Later in the night, things shift and more time is spent in Stage 2 and REM sleep (the stage associated with dreaming).

What's important to take away is that much of our body and brain's restoration process take place during deep Stage 3 and Stage 4 sleep.

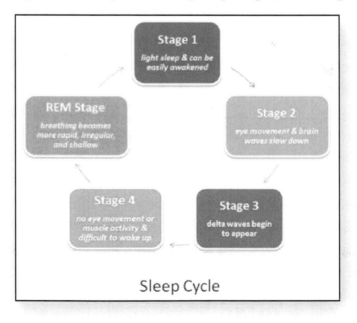

Therefore, when we stay up too late, we deprive our body and mind of these beneficial levels of sleep.

Most clients find it easiest to start with the time they have to get up the next morning and subtract 8 ½ hours. This is when they set a recurring alarm to shut down electronics.

Then, 7 ½ hours before their morning alarm clock, they set a recurring alarm to remind them to get in bed. This allows for the minimum 7 hours of sleep required to avoid depredated physical and cognitive function. To optimize performance, I recommend 8 ½ to 9 ½ hours in bed which will yield about 30 to 60 minutes less in sleep duration.

2. Have a Consistent Schedule for Sleep Onset, Wake Onset, and Meal Timing: The human body craves routine and relies heavily on consistency to optimize healthy hormone levels (melatonin, lepton, ghrelin, and testosterone). Have a routine that prepares your body and mind for rest. Over time these behavioral triggers will notify your body and brain that it is time for bed.

We've already touched on a few of these possible routines, including shutting off all electronics one hour before bed, taking a hot ultra bath or an ice bath, reading a book, or making love with your significant other.

3. Get a Sleep Study: Sleep apnea is a problem that prevents many people from getting adequate rest. It can cause damage to the immune system, increase risk of cardiovascular problems, zap energy, and negatively impact cognitive processes. It's important to note that getting closer to your ideal body weight is one of the simplest fixes for correcting sleep apnea. If you find out that you have apnea, and it needs to be treated, most people get better results with an APAP machine as opposed to a CPAP machine.

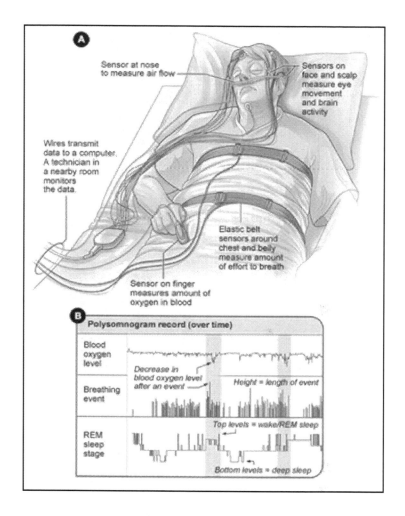

Use 20-30 minute afternoon naps or meditation to rejuvenate the mind. When using naps, it's imperative that you not sleep longer than 30 minutes because you can end up waking up during a deeper sleep cycle. This will cause you to feel worse than you would if you had never taken a nap in the first place. With that said, even if you do this, you'll still experience the performance-enhancing benefits of getting more sleep. So, even sleeping longer than 30 minutes and interrupting your sleep cycle is better than depriving yourself of sleep.

It is recommended that you work with your body's cycles (90 to 110 minutes). In other words, if you are going to nap longer than 30 minutes, then you should make sure that it's at least 90 minutes that you sleep. Further, if you are going to nap longer than 110 minutes, you should make sure that you sleep for at least three hours.

4. *Bank Sleep in Advance:* A 2009 study provides some good news. Leading up to a tiring event, you can "bank sleep" by sleeping more in advance. The study took two groups of people. One group was allowed to increase their sleep leading up to the study. The other group had to maintain their current sleep patterns.

Both groups were then restricted to just three hours of sleep per night, and a variety of performance and cognitive tests were measured. The group that was able to bank sleep showed less performance deterioration, and they were "more resilient during the sleep restriction." They had better reaction times and alertness, and they even recovered faster the week following the sleep deprivation compared to the group that was not allowed to bank sleep.

5. *Sleep in a Cold Room:* Set the temperature of the room that you sleep in to between 67 and 69 degrees Fahrenheit. A great biohack, especially for hot summer months, is a ChiliPad (www.Chilitechnology.com). This is a mattress pad with a cooling and heating temperature control system.

This can be a powerful tool in lowering the ambient temperature of your bed and inducing sleep onset. Other clients have used the Elasto-Gel Hypothermia Cap. In a study from the University of Pittsburgh School of Medicine, wearing a cooling cap helped insomniacs sleep almost as well as healthy folks with no sleep issues.

I've also recommended them to help lessen the severity of migraines with a couple female clients.

6. *Avoid Potential Interruptions:* Make sure that your room is pitch-black. This involves the use of blackout shades, taping over all electronics, and a sleep mask. I advise that you use the Dream Essentials Contoured Sleep Mask or the Sleep Master Sleep Mask.

To eliminate noise interruptions, I also recommend using ear plugs (3M E-A-Rsoft FX ear plugs; 3M OCS1135 Ear Soft Yellow Neons). If you're concerned about missing your alarm clock, you can use the vibrating alarm feature on the Fitbit Charge HR or the Jawbone UP3 activity tracker wristbands.

You shouldn't consume any stimulants within 8 hours of bedtime.

Work out in the morning instead of night to prevent overstimulation. If you do workout at night, make sure that you are done at least 2 hours prior to getting into bed. Working out during the day has been shown to improve quality of sleep, particularly if you practice the steady state cardiovascular workouts done outdoors in the sun (as suggested in the "Movement" section).

Be sure to turn off all electronics at least one hour before going to bed. This includes your TV, cell phone, and computer. It is also advised that you put your phone on "Airplane Mode" to help you resist the temptation to check it before bed and until after you've meditated and written in your journal in the morning.

The artificial blue light that's emitted from all electronics and many light bulbs have been shown in scientific studies to suppress the body's endogenous production of melatonin. Some additional steps that you can take to reduce your exposure to blue light include:

- *Using Blue Light Blocking Glasses:* You can use the Gunnar Intercept or Haus (www.BioHackingSecrets.com/gunnar), or you can use amber-tinted glasses with similar functionality for around $7 on Amazon. I have the Uvex S1993X model.

– *Blue-Light Blocking:* F.lux is free software that you can install on your computer. The way this works is you enter in your geographic location, and it adjusts the amount of blue light emitted from your screen based on the rising and setting of the sun. Additionally, some people use screens to block blue light from their computers. I personally haven't used these, but some of my clients have found it helpful.

7. Consider Inversion Therapy: It is well-documented that hanging upside down can help you to fall asleep faster and sleep more soundly. This technique has been shown to help the muscles relax, improve circulation, increase oxygenation, and stimulate the lymphatic system (this helps to strengthen immune response and remove toxins). All of this makes it easier to fall asleep and improves quality of sleep.

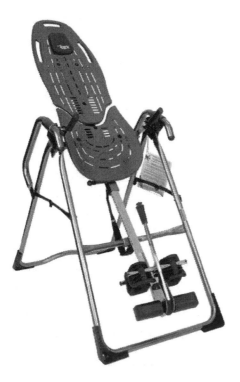

Many people utilize inversion therapy, using either inversion boots or an inversion table, to help reduce back pain as well.

For inversion tables, I recommend the IronMan Gravity 4,000 or the Teeter EP-960 with back pain relief kit. You can also get a pair of Teeter Hang Ups Gravity Boots for around $100, and they work with any chin up bar.

Inversion therapy is also shown to improve blood circulation. According Dr. Robert Martin, author of The Gravity Guiding System: Turning the Aging Process

Upside Down, the brain functions with a 14% increase in accuracy when the body is inverted. Other benefits of inversion therapy include:

- Boosts mood
- Enhances immunity
- Decreases muscle tension by 35%
- Improves posture
- Reduces stress

8. *Bridge the Gap:* The science is clear. Almost all humans experience compromised cognitive performance and physical health with less than 7 hours of sleep.

However, how we feel and our attitude the next morning is determined to a much larger degree by the thoughts and beliefs we hold about sleep and how we expect to feel when our alarm goes off.

Do you believe you need 7 hours of sleep to feel good? Or do you expect to feel incredible when your alarm goes off and are you excited for the possibilities of the day ahead?

I've experimented with everything from 4 to 10+ hours of sleep. And, most of the time, I found myself waking up kinda meh.

It wasn't until I started taking a few seconds at night, before shutting down, to tell myself that I was about to get the perfect amount of sleep and that I was going to feel amazing in the morning, that I noticed a dramatic improvement in my energy levels upon waking up. You see, how you believe you will feel when your alarm goes off has an even bigger impact on your energy levels than the amount of sleep you get.

Before you retire for the evening, take a few seconds to think about something you're excited to jump out of bed for in the morning; something you can't wait to do because it's going to move you one step closer to the life you deserve to live.

Put your alarm clock across the room so you aren't tempted to hit the snooze button. None of us are thinking clearly those first few seconds of the morning. So it's imperative to set yourself up for success. And that means forcing yourself to get up, out of bed, to turn the alarm off. Because once you're up, it's ten times easier to stay up and get in the shower or start your morning routine.

Swiss psychiatrist and psychotherapist, Carl Jung, said, "What you resist, persists." Meaning, when we wish an aspect of our life were different than it is, we give that situation more energy.

This does not mean we shouldn't desire and take actions that will produce a life of greater abundance, health, and happiness. Rather it means we want to move forward towards an even better life, in a state of acceptance and gratitude. When we are thankful for everything we already have, it amplifies our ability to attract the things we want.

Your time is now. It will always be now. The belief that you should not experience happiness and appreciation for your life until everything is where you want it to be is like running a race with tunnel vision on a moving finish line. You'll never get there. And you'll end up missing all the awesome stuff along the way.

Think of it this way, when you hit the snooze button you're resisting your life. You're choosing to stay unconscious rather than being thankful for another day you have the opportunity to live, love, laugh, and create. Maybe there's more to the old saying, "You snooze, you lose" than we thought. Make it fun and inspiring to wake up from the second your alarm goes off.

In fact, start with your alarm. Most of us use alarm tones we can't stand. The very sound of which immediately puts us in a bad mood before we've even gotten out of bed.

Why not do the opposite? Choose a song that inspires you or gets you fired up as your morning alarm clock.

I recommend changing songs every few weeks, or couple of months, because we start to develop diminishing returns to the effect a song has on us when we hear it repeatedly. Once your song is no longer getting you fired up, change it for a new one that does. This is easy to do on the iPhone and most smartphones.

Additional bio hacks to improve sleep quality may include:

- Put your alarm clock across the room so you have to get up to turn it off. Once you're on your feet, refuse to let yourself get back in bed.
- Place the FlexPulse PEMF coils under your pillow at 3 Hz and let them run on "continuous" throughout the night. Or use the EarthPulse in "recovery" mode or manual set at 9.6 Hz. Just be sure to set your sleep time for at least 15 minutes less than you plan on sleeping so that you're not groggy when your alarm goes off. Both will assist the glymphatic system in the removal of brain toxins. Other PEMF devices I use, or have used, include the MicroPulse, Ondamed, Parmeds Super, OrthoCor (for knee pain), and PEMF-120.
- If you're particularly sluggish in the morning, immediately jump in a hot shower. Elevated temperatures wake us up. Then end with a 2 to 10 minute cold shower to increase energy production, reduce inflammation, improve circulation, and trigger downstream biochemical reactions that will help you to Carpe Diem (seize the day).
- The Rest Assured program (SounderSleep.com/marketplace) helps to reduce stress using simple, easy to follow breathing and movement exercises that improve daytime relaxation and ensure a good night's sleep. I've used this with a number of different clients who report that it has helped them immensely.

- *Pro Biomat 7000MX:* Without going into too much detail on the relaxation and energetic benefits of infrared light and grounding (the beneficial flow of electrons between your body and the earth) the biomat provides both of these elements and when used throughout the day can improve sleep. Swimming in lakes, rivers and the ocean is, and will always be, the best forms of grounding.
- Spoonk Acupressure & Sleep Induction Mat
- *Fitbit Charge HR or the Jawbone UP3:* These will help you to track sleep and wake cycles, including restfulness and restlessness.
- *Fisher Wallace Stimulator (www.fisherwallace. com):* This is a wearable neuro-stimulation device that has been shown to support healthy mood and sleep. It is available for purchase without a prescription in Canada and

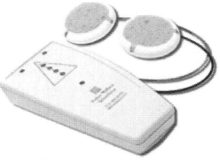

Fisher Wallace Stimulator

Europe and with a prescription in the US. When it is prescribed for depression, anxiety, insomnia, and pain, patients are able to get the cost of the prescription reimbursed by their insurance companies more easily.
- EarthPulse PEMF device (I keep mine under my mattress and run it while I sleep). Some nights I'll put the two FlexPulse pads under my pillow and run them at 3Hz instead. Learn more at www.BioHackingSecrets.com/earthpulse.
- *The Ketogenic Diet:* This has been shown to increase levels of inhibitory neurotransmitters like GABA.
- *DAVID Delight Pro:* This unique system combines auditory, visual, and cranial electronic stimulation (CES) to help guide the body into

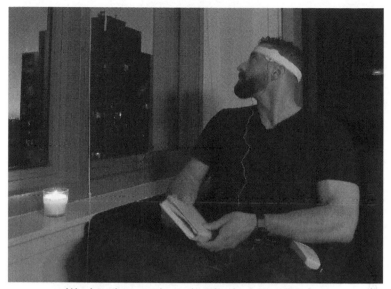

Winding down at the end of the day with the Fisher
Wallace Stimulator and the 5 Minute Journal.

a deep state of rest. I've used the DAVID Smart device a number of times, I enjoyed it so much that I'm investing in a DAVID Delight Pro for my own personal use. It contains the additional benefit of CES, which is not available in the Smart model.

– The NuCalm System (See "Stress Management" section)

– *Nuk Medic Pro (L) Adult Pacifier:* Almost everyone can remember when their parents made them stop using a pacifier. For many it was a traumatic experience. I still remember screaming and crying all night in defiance. As weird as it may sound, many clients sleep much better using one of these Nuk Medic Pro adult pacifiers to help them at night. Reported benefits using this unconventional biohack include reduced time to sleep onset, in addition to decreased snoring and less nighttime restlessness.

– *Earthing Starter Kit:* Helps keep our body's electrical frequency close to that of the earth where we experience optimal health and biological function. When you can't go barefoot or swim in oceans, lakes, and rivers, grounding/earthing is the next best option. This is especially important after long flights (www. BioHackingSecrets.com/Earthing).

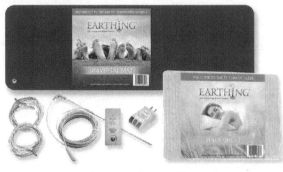

Earthing Starter Kit

- *EarthRunners Circadian X Conductive Leather Sandals:* Earth Runner's barefoot technology allows for energy flow between the foot and Earth. Both their copper inserts and conductive laces ground you electrically by allowing electron transfer from the planet to your body (www.earthrunners.com).
- *SomniResonance Delta Sleeper:* Decades of clinical and academic research have helped to identify the frequencies naturally

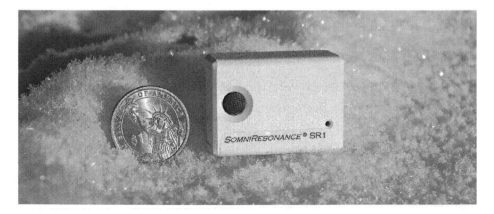

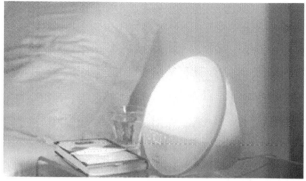

Sunrise Alarm Clock

produced by the brain during the process of falling asleep. The SomniResonance device works by gently mimicking the natural brain frequency patterns produced in the normal stages of falling asleep. The SR-1 is pressed onto your chest over the Brachial Plexus, below the middle of the collar bone where these frequencies are emitted and gently guide the brain into more restful brainwave patterns. It functions similar to frequency following response (FFR), despite the dominant external stimulus being pulsed electromagnetic fields (PEMF) rather than sound frequencies. Many individuals find this helps them fall asleep more easily. To save 5% enter discount code "biohacks" at deltasleeper.com.

– Philips Sunrise Alarm Clock

There are also a number of smartphone sleep applications I've used and recommend:

– Sleep Cycle
– Pzizz
– Dormio
– SleepStream
– Omharmonics
– Brain.fm

For auditory brain entrainment, I recommend:

- Binaural Beats (there are many; some good, some not-so-good)
- Music by Steven Halpern (Sleepscape Delta)
- Hypnosis audios by Benjamin Bonetti
- Sphinx of Imagination hypnosis audio by Hypnotica
- Yoga Nidra with Dr. Deirdre
- Kelly Howell audios (try starting with The Secret Universal Mind Meditation)
- Dr. Jeffrey Thompson audios (the Delta Sleep System is a good primer)

The last 2 listed are a couple of my favorites. It can be quite uncomfortable sleeping with headphones, and that's why I recommend using Tooks Headphone Headband with integrated removable headphones.

Here is a list of supplements that can be helpful for improving sleep:

- GABA
- Phenibit (phGABA)
- 5-HTP: This is a precursor to the hormone melatonin that you can use without creating a negative feedback loop.
- Tryptophan
- Low-dose Naltrexone
- Magnesium Glycinate
- Magnesium L-Threonate
- Low-dose Sublingual Melatonin
- Organic chamomile tea
- L-Theanine (SunTheanine form)
- Potassium Ornithine

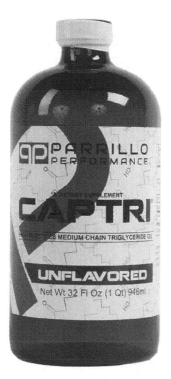

You may consider Human Growth Hormone (HGH). While not technically a supplement, HGH has been shown to improve sleep quality along with the enhancement of the rejuvenating processes that take place during sleep. When it makes sense for clients, we may start with 0.2 mg Genotropin HGH, which should be taken only every other day at first, right before bed. This depends on the person's age, hormonal levels, and health status, however.

If you find yourself hungry before going to bed, I recommend 1 to 2 tablespoons of raw organic virgin coconut oil, or pure Caprylic acid MCT oil as found in Parrillo CapTri or Bulletproof Brain Octane.

Most nights I take 100 mg of 5-HTP and 4 mg of Low-dose Naltrexone before bed. Occasionally, I'll also take 500 mg of GABA and/or 0.5 mg of Sublingual Melatonin.

One of the questions that I get often is whether or not a person should get up early in the morning to exercise if that means compromising time in bed. It depends on a number of different factors such as an individual's goals (physique enhancement vs. health and mental clarity), hormonal balance, genes, and underlining health conditions.

In most cases, the best solution for this problem is to just plan better and find a way to get to bed earlier so that you still get the required amount of sleep. If that's not an option, I recommend still making sleep your focus, when you absolutely have to choose, and then finding ways to be more active throughout the day. For instance, you may begin using

25 minutes during your lunch break to go for a quick jog. You could also walk or bike to work, get a standing desk or treadmill desk, and/or do jumping jacks throughout the day.

Ideally, you'll want exercise in the morning and go to bed earlier to get at least 7 ½ hours of time spent in bed. It would be even better if you can find ways to stay physically active throughout your day as well. Of course, everyone has limitations, but try your best to find ways to fit at least the minimum amount of sleep and exercise into your schedule each day in order to keep your body healthy as well as stay energetic and focused.

SLEEP BIOHACKS

This is not an all-inclusive summary from this section but will help you get started until you are able to explore in more detail.

The One Thing: Set aside at least 7 ½ hours per night for time in bed (sleep period). This will allow you to get the minimum 7 hours of sleep (sleep duration) most of us require to keep energy and cognitive performance intact.

Biohack #1: Tempur-Pedic Tempur-HD collection's Tempur-Rhapsody was found to be the number one mattress when assessed by Mark Ford and his research team. For a more in-depth explanation of how this mattress was picked, read *"Living Rich: How to Live as Well as a Millionaire on a Middle-Class Budget."*

Biohack #2: Factors that can interfere with adequate sleep include: Artificial light, Processed foods, Sedentary lifestyle, Stimulants and prescription drugs, Unnatural work shifts, and Chronic stress.

Biohack #3: Tools and programs which can help you achieve adequate amounts of sleep include:

- Rest Assured
- Pro Biomat 7000MX
- Spoonk Acupressure & Sleep Induction Mat
- Fitbit Charge HR or the Jawbone UP3
- Fisher Wallace Stimulator
- Philips Sunrise Alarm Clock
- The Ketogenic Diet
- DAVID Delight Pro
- The NuCalm System
- Ondamed, Flexpulse, and EarthPulse PEMF devices
- Sleep mask
- Tooks Headband Headphones
- Earplugs
- ChiliPad (www.chilitechnology.com)

Biohack #4: Recommended smartphone sleep applications:

- Sleep Cycle
- Pzizz
- Dormio
- SleepStream
- Omharmonics
- Brain.fm
- For auditory enhancements, I recommend:
- Binaural Beats
- Music by Steven Halpern (Sleepscape Delta)
- Hypnosis by Benjamin Bonetti

– Sphinx of Imagination by Hypnotica
– Yoga Nidra with Dr. Deirdre
– Kelly Howell audios (try The Secret Universal Mind Meditation)
– Dr. Jeffrey Thompson audios (start with his Delta Sleep System)

Biohack #5: Consider the following hormones and supplements: GABA, Phenibit (phGABA), 5-HTP, Tryptophan, Genotropin HGH (0.2 mg), Low-dose Naltrexone, Magnesium Glycinate, Magnesium L-Threonate, Low-dose Sublingual Melatonin, L-Theanine (SunTheanine form), Potassium Ornithine.

SUPPLEMENTS

Two time Nobel Prize winner Dr. Linus Pauling said, "Nearly all disease can be traced to a nutritional deficiency."

Humans living in a pristine, natural environment and living an ancestral lifestyle, would likely do just fine without supplements. The reality is that, today, the intersection of these two scenarios exist only in the rarest of cases.

Even still, there exists the possibility that, by providing these ancestral people with the right supplements, they too may experience enhanced energy, focus, mood, performance, and quality of life.

The reality is that our modern world is profoundly different from the environment of our ancestors. Our external environment has undergone radical changes in the past 250 years. The Industrial Revolution (1760-1840) gave birth to environmental pollution as we know it today.

Our internal environment, the human genome, has changed very little in that same time period. Subsequently, our genes are ill-equipped to handle many of the environmental stressors we face today. It is this mismatch that is largely responsible for the cellular energy crisis, rampant nutrient deficiencies, and chronic degenerative conditions we face today.

ARE SUPPLEMENTS NECESSARY?

The right supplements may help us to level the playing field when lifestyle and behavioral modifications are not possible. By intelligently supplementing a whole food diet with the right nutrients, we are often able to counteract the multitude of genetic-environmental mismatches facing modern man. Our Neolithic ancestors had a number of things working in their favor us modern humans do not. For example:

– Produce and meat are most nutritious when they are the freshest. In almost all cases, the food in our grocery stores is weeks old by the time it makes it to our shelves. It has come from Mexico and other foreign countries with lower production costs, and been subjected to radiation, coatings, and genetic modification to extend shelf life and increase profit margins. Invisible pesticides, herbicides (glyphosate - Roundup), chemicals, and hormones present in non-organic foods further increase the risks associated with their consumption.

– A decrease in the diversity of vegetables and fruit species consumed and the addition of toxins like pesticides, herbicides, hormones, vaccines, and antibiotics in our food.

– A "dilution effect" showing an inverse relationship between crop yields and nutrient content.

– Environmental toxins in the air we breathe and the water we drink and bathe in.

– Heavy use of antibiotics, birth control, and other prescription medications can overtax the liver, stress the kidneys, and damage the gut (microbiome). Our greatest exposure to antibiotics is the consumption of animal protein from non-organic sources, not prescriptions from your doctor. 80 percent of antibiotics used in the United States are fed to livestock.

Declining Fruit and Vegetable Nutrient Composition: What Is the Evidence?

Donald R. Davis[1,2,3]

Biochemical Institute, The University of Texas, Austin, TX 78712; and Bio-Communications Research Institute, 3100 North Hillside Avenue, Wichita, KS 67219

Additional index words. nutritive value, history, dilution effect, genetic dilution effect, agriculture, grains

Abstract. Three kinds of evidence point toward declines of some nutrients in fruits and vegetables available in the United States and the United Kingdom: 1) early studies of fertilization found inverse relationships between crop yield and mineral concentrations—the widely cited "dilution effect"; 2) three recent studies of historical food composition data found apparent median declines of 5% to 40% or more in some minerals in groups of vegetables and perhaps fruits; one study also evaluated vitamins and protein with similar results; and 3) recent side-by-side plantings of low- and high-yield cultivars of broccoli and grains found consistently negative correlations between yield and concentrations of minerals and protein, a newly recognized genetic dilution effect. Studies of historical food composition data are inherently limited, but the other methods can focus on single crops of any kind, can include any nutrient of interest, and can be carefully controlled. They can also test proposed methods to minimize or overcome the diluting effects of yield whether by environmental means or by plant breeding.

- An increase in chronic stress and a decrease in sleep quality and duration add to these tolls. The average person sleeps 60 to 90 minutes less than we did just 50 years ago.

- Use of cosmetics and chemicals used for cleaning expose us to parabens, BHA, BHT, phthalates, formaldehyde, lead, perchloroethylene (dry cleaning), and other carcinogens. If you eat organic, but you expose your largest organ - your skin - to these chemicals you're overburdening your body's detoxification pathways and increasing your risk of genetic mutations.

- We are less connected with our natural environment than we ever have been throughout history. By and large, people spend less and less time outdoors as time progresses. As you probably know, we require sunlight to synthesize Vitamin D. Natural sunlight lowers inflammation, reverses autoimmunity, fights disease, and charges our human battery. Conversely, our increased exposure to artificial light can inhibit melatonin production and interfere with sleep.

- The average American worker might spend 13 to 15 hours sitting a day, and many studies have shown that sitting actively promotes dozens of chronic diseases, including obesity and Type 2 Diabetes.

– Our culture has moved away from having the same types of tight-knit social groups that used to be commonplace. This lack of love and social connectedness has had a devastating impact on our health and nervous system. None of these problems are likely to go away soon, and, in fact, are most likely to continue getting worse. So it's up to you to make the best efforts towards health.

These are just some of the more obvious variances between those of us living in modern industrialized societies and the indigenous hunter/ gatherer tribes of the past. These contrasts may explain why many clients find a personalized supplement program to be the "missing link" in reaching their physical and genetic potential.

THE HIDDEN DANGERS OF VITAMINS AND SUPPLEMENTS

The diet and exercise industry is littered with products where marketing quality far surpasses product quality. 9 out of 10 supplements contain some form of a known toxin, genetically-modified ingredient, dangerous filler, or allergenic compound that can offset and negate any potential benefit.

Let's say, for example, that you are currently taking a whey protein supplement or pre-workout supplement. If this is true, you should grab the container and look at it.

The whey protein should be specified as "non denatured, bioactive whey protein from grass-fed cows." Otherwise, you're essentially consuming the runoff from the cheese manufacturing process, using

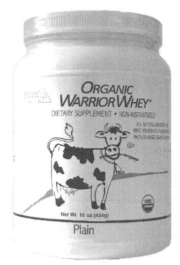

The only whey protein I use and recommend to clients. Non-denatured, bioactive whey protein from grass-fed cows has been shown to increase endogenous glutathione, the body's master antioxidant.

dairy from cows fed genetically-modified ingredients, chicken feces (as mentioned in the "Nutrition" section), and given chemicals, hormones, vaccines, and antibiotics. All of these are concentrated in the whey that's in that container.

You should also take note that whey protein has been identified as one of the top gluten cross-reactants by Cyrex Labs. That means if you are one of the many people who are sensitive to gluten, then you are also likely sensitive to whey since it mimics the effects of gluten on our digestive and immune system. Furthermore, many people are unknowingly sensitive to all forms of dairy, including whey, and whey protein often triggers immunogenic and allergenic responses in the body that make us less healthy and zap our energy.

We haven't even touched on the fact that the majority of whey protein products also contain artificial sweeteners like Sucralose, Aspartame, and Acesulfame. These artificial sweeteners kill the good bacteria in your gut, worsen insulin sensitivity, and cause Diabetes and weight gain to a greater degree than regular sugar. Artificial sweeteners are also a common cause of headaches and migraines for many individuals. Moreover, a 2012 meta-analysis of the Health Professional's Follow-Up Study (HPFS) and the Nurse's Health Study (NHS) looked at epidemiological data gathered on a 22-year period. These studies found artificial sweeteners like aspartame to significantly increase the risk of many cancers like Non-Hodgkin lymphoma, leukemia, and myeloma.

There are also problems that come with using soy proteins, added sugar, trans fats, and refined oils (like canola, vegetable oil, soybean oil, etc.), MSG, wheat, gluten, and artificial colors.

That's just what you can be exposed to when consuming whey protein. Similar threats can be found in supplements of all forms. Here's a short list of the many potentially harmful ingredients that can be found in a large majority of supplements:

- Invisible GMO ingredients (i.e. Aspartame, ascorbic acid, sodium acerbate, vitamin C, citric acid, sodium citrate, ethanol, "natural" and "artificial" flavors, lactic acid, maltodextrins, molasses, monosodium glutamate, sucrose, high fructose corn syrup, hydrolyzed vegetable protein, textured vegetable protein, xanthan gum, vitamins, yeast, soy and soy derivatives, canola oil, and amino acids)
- Hydrogenated oils and vegetable oils
- Artificial colors
- Magnesium stearate
- Titanium oxide
- Carrageenan
- Heavy metals (e.g. Fluoride, arsenic, and lead)
- Acrylamides

- Sodium benzoate and BHT
- Cupric sulfate and boric acid

Additionally, there are a number of synthetic ingredients that should also be avoided. Whereas the natural bioactive forms of these vitamins come with health benefits, the synthetic forms can come with health risks and unwanted side effects. These include:

- *Vitamin A:* colic acetate, palmitate
- *Vitamin B1:* thiamine mononitrate, thiamine hydrochloride
- *Vitamin B2:* riboflavin, pantothenic acid, calcium D-pantothenate
- *Vitamin B6:* pyridoxine hydrochloride
- *Vitamin B12:* cyanocobalamin
- *PABA (para-aminobenzoic acid):* aminobenzoic acid
- *Folic acid*
- *Choline:* choline chloride, choline bitartrate
- *Biotin:* D-Biotin
- *Vitamin C:* ascorbic acid and "vitamin C" (almost all forms of vitamin C on the market are manufactured from genetically-modified corn).
- *Vitamin D:* Calciferol, irradiated ergosterol
- *Vitamin E:* dl-alpha tocopheryl, dl-alpha tocopheryl acetate or succinate (the "dl" form of any vitamin is synthetic)

SUPPLEMENTS YOU SHOULD BE TAKING

I get asked all the time "If you could only use one supplement what would it be?"

Which is hard to answer because the one supplement I'd recommend for a person with brain fog is not necessarily the supplement I'd recommend for someone who needs more energy. I would have to know certain things about them, such as their:

– Health status
– Goals
– Genetic mutations and predispositions
– Gender
– Age
– Body composition
– Lifestyle
– Predispositions

Having made that clear, below are the foundational supplements most people should be taking for focus, energy, and overall performance:

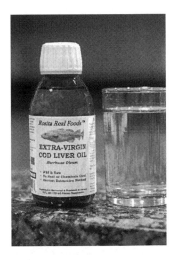

– *Wild, raw, extra-virgin cod liver oil* (high in vitamin A, vitamin D, EPA, and DHA)
– *Vitamin D3 liquid*
– *Magnesium Glycinate:* Magnesium is one of the most important nutrients required by our bodies. It is necessary for more than 300 biochemical reactions, and it is essential to human life. Glycinate is the most bioavailable form, followed by magnesium malate.
A few of the benefits of magnesium include: Maintaining healthy nerve and muscle function, Maintaining cardiovascular function, Maintaining a healthy immune system, Strengthening bones, Regulating blood sugar, Supporting energy production and

protein synthesis, and Maintaining normal blood pressure levels.

- *Probiotic* (Prescript Assist, VSL3, AOR Probiotic-3, etc.), *vitamin D3, and a low-carb vegan protein powder* (www.BioHackingSecrets. com/protein) that is free from dairy, gluten, grains, legumes, vegetable oils, artificial sweeteners, artificial colors, and genetically-modified organisms (GMOs).

Here are some of the supplements I would recommend for enhancing energy production:

- *A bioactive B vitamin complex which includes:* Methylfolate (around 3 mg, ideally as L-5-methyltetrahydrofolate), Vitamin B6 (as pyridoxal 5-phosphate, around 50 mg), Riboflavin (as riboflavin 5-phosphate, around 100 mg), Vitamin B12 (as methylcobalamin, around 3 mg), and Betaine anhydrous (as trimethylglycine, around 2 grams).
- *CoQ10 (coenzyme Q10, ubiquinol form, 100-300 mg):* Our bodies require CoQ10 to convert energy from fats and sugars into usable cellular energy. It is an indispensable component of healthy mitochondrial function and a potent antioxidant that helps protect our cells and vital organs from free radicals and oxidative stress. CoQ10 levels decline with age by as much as 72%, and these reductions are even higher among individuals taking statin drugs, which are used to lower LDL and cholesterol. The ubiquinol form of CoQ10 absorbs eight times greater than ubiquinone. Also, the ubiquinol form has been shown to be 94% more effective and bioactive.
- *D-Ribose (5-15 mg per day blended into smoothie):* Adenosine triphospate (ATP) is a coenzyme and energy carrier in the body. It is composed of three chemical groups, one of which is D-Ribose.

It is directly involved with energy synthesis and can be used to increase and restore cellular energy levels. While D-Ribose is technically a sugar, it is not burned by the body in the same way.

- *Nicotinamide riboside (NAD+)* is an enzyme that promotes cellular energy production and has been shown to slow the aging process in humans. It also enhances mitochondrial efficiency, supporting optimal energy levels and peak performance, cognitive function and neuronal health, and activation of sirtuins, especially SIRT1[8] and SIRT3 genes, which have been associated with an increased lifespan. Effective doses of nicotinamide riboside range from 300-500 mg a day. Many people do not experience the benefits of this novel compound because they do not take enough. At this time it is quite expensive, and this can be cost-prohibitive for some individuals. I take 300 mg per day.

- *Taurine* has been shown in scientific studies to boost cognitive and neuronal function in addition to promoting the generation of new brain cells, particularly in the areas of the brain associated with memory and learning. I recommend 800-1,000 mg of L-taurine daily.

---

[8] "Sirtuin 1 (SIRT1) is an evolutionarily conserved NAD+-dependent deacetylase that is at the pinnacle of metabolic control, all the way from yeast to humans. SIRT1 senses changes in intracellular NAD+ levels, which reflect energy level, and uses this information to adapt the cellular energy output such that it matches cellular energy requirements. The changes induced by SIRT1 activation are generally (but not exclusively) transcriptional in nature and are related to an increase in mitochondrial metabolism and antioxidant protection. These attractive features have validated SIRT1 as a therapeutic target in the management of metabolic disease and prompted an intensive search to identify pharmacological SIRT1 activators. In this review, we first give an overview of the SIRT1 biology with a particular focus on its role in metabolic control. We then analyze the pros and cons of the current strategies used to activate SIRT1 and explore the emerging evidence indicating that modulation of NAD+ levels could provide an effective way to achieve such goals."(Pharmacological Reviews January 2012 vol. 64 no. 1 166-187)

– *Pyrroloquinoline quinone* (PQQ, 10-20 mg per day): Research has shown PQQ to stimulate the growth of new mitochondria and activate genes associated with mitochondrial protection.

Other supplements I have found to be helpful for focus, cognitive function and energy production, which I might recommend to some clients, depending on their circumstances, include:

– Liposomal glutathione
– NADH (sublingual)
– Creatine monohydrate (CreaPure) and creatine hydrochloride (creatine HCL forms)
– Acetyl l-carnitine arginate
– Sublingual or intramuscular Vitamin B12 (Methylcobalamin or hydroxocobalamin forms; test to see which elicits a better response)
– Rhodiola Rosea
– Vinpocetine
– Phosphatidylserine
– Bacopa
– Apoaequorin (Prevagen)
– Docosahexaenoic acid (DHA)
– L-theanine (SunTheanine form)
– Uridine
– Phosphatidylcholine (from sunflower lecithin)
– Alpha-GPC
– Piracetam
– Aniracetam

Inventor, famed futurist, and author (Transcend and The Singularity is Near), Ray Kurzweil, is one of the original biohackers. For years, he took over 250 pills a day. Recently, he whittled that number down to around 150.

Kurzweil uses supplements to keep his mind sharp, stay focused, and to, hopefully, live long enough to usher an era he has coined Singularity. The Singularity Movement refers to the moment in time when humans and machines merge. Kurzweil predicts accelerated growth rate of computer technology will soon enable nanorobots to program our cells and extend human lifespan indefinitely.

Suzanne Somers has managed to defy aging, exhibiting the physical characteristics of someone 20 years younger. She takes daily human growth hormone injections and 80 to 90 supplements a day. This regimen has not only helped her to maintain her physical youth on a cellular level, but, by keeping her mind sharp, she has been able to consistently publish a bestselling book every two years. Her most recent publication was *"TOX-SICK: From Toxic to Not Sick,"* which was released in 2015.

Somers refers to her extensive supplement regimen as her "age management" protocol. I've not counted the number of bottles or pills that I go through on a daily basis because those numbers fluctuate according to my goals and the specific experiments I am running. However, I can tell you that my numbers are probably not that dissimilar from those of Kurzweil and Somers.

In 2007, I was on vacation in Cabo San Lucas with a group of my close friends. We were spending a lot of our time on the beach during the day in the hot sun and then going out at night to enjoy the Cabo nightlife. As usual, I had brought a veritable medicine cabinet of supplements with me in order to offset the detrimental effects of high alcohol consumption, lack of restful sleep, and time spent on the beach without sufficient hydration. I wanted to make sure that I maintained high levels of energy.

SUPPLEMENTS

On day 3, one of my friends, Matt, came to my room as I was taking my post-meal supplements and said, "Alright man, I'm dying here, You've got to give me something or I'm not going to make it out."

In a process that has now become customary on our trips, I put together a small cocktail of nutraceuticals and gave them to Matt. He thankfully took them and washed them down with some water. While he was doing so, I inserted a small scoop into one of my bottles of ginseng. I proceeded to toss these into the back of my mouth and then rinse them down with some water.

For those of you who have not tasted pure ginseng powder, it is particularly bitter and packs a potent punch. I have done this hundreds of times and must have made it look easy because Matt looked at me and said, "What was that? Let me get some of that, too." I tried to warn him, but he insisted. I readied a scoop for Matt and handed him the water and the ginseng, Without hesitation, he catapulted the ginseng into his mouth, and what transpired was hilarious.

The ginseng must have shot all the way to the back of his throat because he immediately choked and sprayed a giant cloud of ginseng all over my room. He desperately grasped for the water and tried to chug it down. His eyes watering, and his hands on his knees, Matt choked out the words, "Dude, how the fuck do you take that every day? That has to be the worst thing that I've ever tasted in my entire life."

Matt survived. Today we even laugh about the incident.

The important thing for you to remember is, most supplements are not made to be tasty. They're made to be effective. If you find one a bit too intense, simply start slow and build up. It's worth it, I promise.

Heck, Matt can, and does, even eat ginseng power today.

CASE STUDY: DETOX PROTOCOL FOR NICK

Nick lives in Cairo, Egypt. He was struggling with many signs of gut dysbiosis, toxic overload, and chronic fatigue. Unfortunately, Egypt has limited access to many lab tests as well as many of the supplements and tools available in the states. Fortunately, he came to visit his family over the holidays, which gave him the opportunity to stock up before returning back home.

Nick was experiencing extreme food sensitivities, which made it hard for him to eat anything. Most of the supplements that he was taking were triggering adverse reactions as well. This was limiting his ability to apply more advanced strategies.

After thinking a lot about the things he told me were going wrong with him, I gave Nick a call. There were a number of different solutions I felt would not only help him, but be gentle on his system. I first advised that we order anything that he didn't have access to in Egypt so that we could get it in the mail before he flew out again. I was careful to make sure I chose supplements that were affordable and entirely natural.

Another recommendation I made was that he come and stay with me for a couple of days so I could thoroughly explain and walk him through the process I follow when I am detoxing my system. In other words, I wanted to go over the products and how to implement each of them. Here are some of the products that I recommended to him:

Liquid chlorophyll: World Organic, 16-Oz bottle

I recommended that Nick drink this daily. It's great for binding to toxins and protecting your cells and DNA from the damage that some intestinal pathogens can create. It's the organic compounds known as porphyrins in chlorophyll that bind to heavy metals and chelate them from the body. Chlorophyll also activates the PPAR-receptor of cells which is responsible for the transcription of DNA, opening of the cell wall (allowing cellular detoxification to take place), and enhance insulin sensitivity. Prescription drugs that activate the PPAR-receptor (like Pioglitazone; brand name Actos) have been shown to be effective in the treatment of prostate and breast cancers.

Raw, Organic Extra Virgin Coconut Oil

I usually use the version of this made by Carrington Farms. However, as long as the coconut is raw, organic, virgin oil, meaning that it's completely unadulterated, just about any brand will work. I taught Nick how to do a three-day coconut oil cleanse. He wasn't eating much anyway, so I figured it was a great opportunity to detox his body with this treatment.

If you want to use coconut oil for detox, integrate it into your nutrition program. Start small to get your body used to it a little at a time. Again, it is very important that the oil is raw, unprocessed, organic coconut oil.

This detox lasts for a period of 1-3 days. Three days will work best, if you can do it. If you have reached a point, like Nick has, where you're not eating a lot anyway, then you might as well go the whole three days. What you would do is start the day off with two tablespoons of coconut. You can just drink this with some lemon water or some filtered water. Throughout the day, you might take another tablespoon or two. You can take up to twelve tablespoons per day.

As you go about this, be sure to drink as much water as possible. There's an easy way to know how much water you should be consuming. All you do is take your current body weight and multiply it by 0.7. During this time, try to stay away from caffeine and other things that may dehydrate you. Now, if you are one of those people who can't function without caffeine, don't sweat it. Just try to go with good sources. For example, you might try to drink teas like green tea and Guayusa. If you do drink coffee, try to go organic.

Keep in mind, a lot of people are sensitive to coffee, especially those with gut issues. It mimics the effects of gluten on the body, so many times people who have sensitivities to grains and gluten don't feel that good after they drink coffee. One of the indicators that you may be one of these people is having an increase in energy and then having a fairly rapid crash where the energy has not been sustained. Some people will experience the jitters. This can be tied to a magnesium deficiency, or it's just the way that their body processes caffeine.

Some people notice stiffness, back pain, and joint pain as well. All of these are signs that coffee may not be the best thing for you. There are other options for you if you are used to using caffeine to function, such as Prolab Advanced Caffeine. This is a 200 mg capsule, and you would want to take this in accordance to what your normal caffeine intake is. For instance, you might want to bite one of these capsules in half rather than taking the whole thing.

You can just take this supplement along with a bunch of water. This is actually a lot better for you in many ways because the proteins found in coffee can be problematic. People often assume it's the caffeine that's causing issues, but it's actually the proteins in the coffee that mimic gluten and cause some of these symptoms.

Organic Coffee Enemas

There are organic therapy coffee roasts you can get, which really can help your system out a lot. The best value that I came across was from a company called Cafe Mam. They have a 5-pound therapy roast that you can order for a fairly reasonable price. Another product you could possibly use is PureLife's Coffee Enema Kit. You can get one pound of this for around $30, whereas the Cafe Mam gives you five pounds for around $50. So, it's a lot more bang for your buck.

You're probably cringing at the very thought of enemas. It may help you to know that enemas have been used for centuries, and they actually originated in Egypt. It's also a foundational element of the Gerson protocol, which is a natural cancer treatment therapy. I know a girl who had terminal cancer, diagnosed at Stage 4, and she wasn't expected to live. She took the traditional routes of treatment, and the cancer continued to come back.

It wasn't until she switched to the Gerson protocol and started doing daily coffee enemas as well as juicing with green vegetables and switching to a plant-based diet, with fats only coming from plant-based sources, that she started getting better. In fact, the cancer went away, and it never came back. Even better, she wasn't supposed to have kids and she now has a two year old daughter. She's now as healthy as she's ever been.

It's more of a psychological hurdle to use this treatment than anything else. The benefits of the regimen are primarily related to the detoxification of the liver. You have some people with a genetic predisposition for which this type of treatment is less effective. If you combine that with something like gut dysbiosis, which may be caused by parasites, bacteria, or fungi, it can further increase the body's toxic burden. When this happens, your liver starts getting clogged up. Some of the signs of a clogged liver are decreased energy production, increased body fat, and cognitive brain fog. Things will just keep getting worse and worse. You end up being exposed to other environmental toxins, and your body can't get rid of them. All of this just causes a downward spiral.

What a coffee enema does is stimulate the liver's ability to detoxify. So, it's basically like giving your liver a massage. This has also been known to increase the endogenous production of glutathione, your body's most important anti-oxidant. It is involved in a number of enzymatic reactions and the quenching and elimination of free radicals. In addition, this reduces oxidative stress. As a matter of fact, glutathione is found to be low in people who have Parkinson's, Alzheimer's, and dementia.

This is a "chicken before the egg" type of scenario, meaning that it's not really certain if glutathione is low because the liver function is compromised, or if, because liver function is compromised, the glutathione is low. We don't really know for sure because it's a case by case situation. However, you can use these coffee enemas to address the problem. This helps to stimulate the body's ability to get this stuff out. It just frees your body of some of the toxins it has been exposed to and starts moving things along in the other direction.

After talking with a number of people who had essentially cured themselves from terminal cancer. I decided to try it myself. At first it's kind of hard, and your body rejects it. So, you have to give it a few tries, especially if you have small intestinal bacterial overgrowth and things like that. It might be difficult to hold enemas at first, but it comes with practice. I remember that I struggled with it for the first 5-10 times I tried. But then, it gets everything moving, and you get an immediate increase in energy. I dropped like 5 or 10 pounds, just from having my liver functioning better and being able to clean everything out.

The best approach is to do these coffee enemas back to back. You'll need an enema bucket and Cafe Mam coffee. You'll also need a water filter so you don't absorb all of the fluoride, chlorine, and so forth in tap water. I recommend structured, ozonated water for colon cleansing and enemas. Adding structure to the water decreases particle size and makes the water easier for cells to absorb. This improves detoxification and hydration.

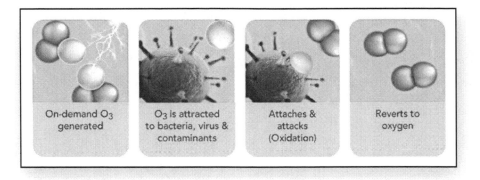

Ozone (O3) rapidly oxidizes organisms like bacteria and viruses it comes into contact with, then converts safely back into Oxygen (O2). By oxygenating the water used for enemas and colon cleansing with ozone, it helps to rid the body of yeast infections, bacteria, and parasites. These pathogens thrive in low oxygen environments.

Ozonated water also lowers inflammation in the walls of the colon and intestines; this inflammation is common in individuals with digestive disorders like Crohn's, colitis, celiac disease, and IBS.

Some symptoms I've seen improved or reversed by enemas and colon cleansing with ozonated water are:

- Coated tongue
- Constipation
- Backache
- Bad breath
- Body odor
- Bloating
- Fatigue
- Bad gas
- Headaches
- Indigestion
- Loss of concentration

- Lung congestion
- Sinus congestion
- Skin problems
- Nail fungus
- Yeast infections (and associated symptoms)

I have a number of different enema "recipes" I recommend to clients depending on their goals and health status. Folks who are dealing with high levels of accumulated toxins usually feel worse before they feel better. Guys who are athletic and generally healthy find frequent enemas give them an edge that otherwise alluded them. And they usually lose 5-10 additional pounds without changing any aspects of their diet or exercise routine.

Personally, I find I feel best when I do an enema at least three times a week. I'll usually combine it with PEMF therapy, meditation, photobiomodulation, or just use that time to respond to emails and texts that have come through while my phone was in airplane mode.

Here are a couple of the enemas I use on the regular (WARNING - I've worked up to these levels since 2013 so give your body time to acclimate):

- *Coffee Enema:* 8-16 ounces of coffee and 24 ounces of filtered water. Hold for 15-20 minutes (or whenever my meditation ends or I feel like the time is right.
- *Gerson Special:* 8-16 ounces of coffee, 24 ounces of water, 2-3 tablespoons of organic castor oil, 1/2 teaspoon of ox bile. Mix ox bile, castor oil, and coffee first. Then add to water. Oil and water may separate. This is normal and can be remedied by swishing a bar of natural coconut-based soap or black african soap in the solution. Do not use commercial soaps which contain chemicals, fragrances, and other compounds best avoided.

- *Probiotic Enema:* 24-32 ounces of filtered water and a blend of probiotics I rotate for ecological diversity.
- *Ozonated water colon hydrotherapy*

This can be a really huge thing for your health. I do them about 3-5 times a week now, just because I feel better when I do. My energy is higher and my skin looks better. I just have a more youthful appearance overall, I have better cognitive function, and I'm leaner as a result. When I don't do them, I start to notice less definition in my midsection. It's fat that's almost resistant to diet and exercise. Once I take care of my liver, it comes right off.

Another enema treatment is the Bentonite detox. You take half a cup of Bentonite clay (Sonnie's #7 Detoxificant), which you can get on Amazon. This is also something that you can use daily to help bind the toxins in your intestines and clear them out. The coffee enemas should be done daily, and some people even do them multiple times a day. For my friend Nick, I recommended that he do two coffee enemas, once a day, back to back. So, he would do his enema and release it into the toilet and then do another coffee enema, lying on his left side with both of these. This allows it to get into your colon, small intestine, and large intestine.

You use the Bentonite clay orally on a daily basis, and then once a week as an enema. Whereas the coffee enema binds to toxins in the liver and helps stimulate the elimination of these toxins through the liver, the Bentonite enemas are effective at binding to toxins in the intestines and clearing those out.

If you are doing them both, you can do them on the same day, but you will want to do the Bentonite last. If you do the coffee afterwards instead, it will just rinse away the Bentonite clay. You want this to remain and be given the opportunity to work the way it's supposed to.

Organic Lemon Water

I use the Hydro Flask, a 64 ounce water bottle, and told Nick to use the same thing. Fill this up with filtered water, and then juice either half or a full organic lemon. Squeeze the lemon and add the juice to the water. Throw in anywhere from a pinch to a tablespoon of Himalayan sea salt. Shake it up and drink. Try to do this 2-3 times a day for a gentle detox which is really going to help get things moving. By the way, if you're into juicing, I recommend the Vitamix high performance blender (www.BioHackingSecrets.com/blender).

There are a few people who had symptoms as severe as Nick's who made huge strides but hit a wall and just couldn't get past it. They increased their energy, focus, and mental clarity, but just couldn't get over the hump they needed to because of parasites. Parasites are pretty tricky to get rid of, and sometimes pharmaceuticals are needed. When they got on a specific prescribed protocol that addressed some of these parasitic gut pathogens, everything cleared up for them.

Before taking this route, however, explore the more common causes of gut dysbiosis, like small intestinal bacterial overgrowth (SIBO),

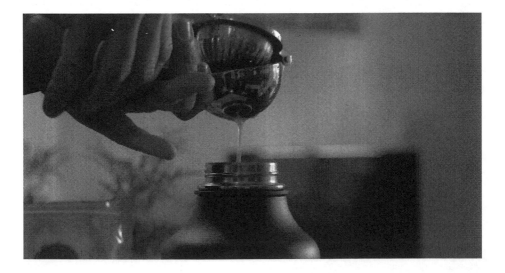

Candida, and yeast. Also try an herbal approach to getting rid of parasites. For an herbal approach, what I would recommend is getting Nature's Way Cayenne Extra Hot. This just costs around $6 a bottle, so it is really, really inexpensive. You can usually find this product on Amazon.com. There's also a product called Scram, which is made by a company called HealthForce. It is an herbal parasite cleanse that is quite effective for a lot of people.

Combine the Nature's Way Cayenne Extra Hot with the HealthForce Scram. You would take one of the cayenne supplements a day, and then you would work up to the point where you take them three times daily. Be sure to take them with your meals. At the same time, follow the protocol on the Scram bottles, which basically works up to 10 capsules a day. You would need at least two bottles of the Scram.

That, along with all of these other strategies, may be all you need to get things working the way they need to again. Hopefully, it's not a pathogen that is causing your ailment, but if it is, then you'll need to get rid of it as soon as possible.

There were other things that I advised Nick to try, such as integrating the use of saunas. I told him that if he has access to a sauna anywhere close to where he lives, he should use it daily. Twenty minutes in a sauna, followed by a two-minute cold shower, is a great treatment which facilitates your body's ability to move stuff out through the skin. If you can do this daily, that will help a lot, and if you can repeat this process twice in a row, that's even better. You'll get faster results this way.

Two other things that a person in this type of situation might integrate into their treatment are raw apple cider vinegar and the Dr. Hidemitsu Hayashi's Hydrogen Rich Water Stick. Many people with toxic overload and slow intestinal motility do well with this combo.

I recommended Bragg Organic Apple Cider Vinegar to Nick. Also, take note that organic aloe Vera is great for healing the intestinal track.

Lilly of the Desert has an aloe Vera juice that is wonderful. These are all products that you could pick up if you have the budget for them. Everything I've recommended in this section is pretty inexpensive though. Here's a quick overview of some of the things that you will need:

- An enema bucket ($5-$7)
- World Organic Liquid Chlorophyll (2-3 16-Oz bottles)
- Bragg Organic Apple Cider Vinegar (2, 32-Oz bottles)
- Sonne's No. 7 Detoxificant for the bentonite enemas
- Carrington Farms pure, unrefined, cold-pressed Organic coconut oil (1-2 54-Oz bottles)
- Hydro Flask (64-Oz)
- Pink Himalayan Sea Salt (There are all kinds, but I use the one that Onnit makes)
- Organic Lemons
- Scram by HealthForce (2 bottles, if parasites are suspected)
- Reese's Pinworm medicine, Pin-X, or other Pyrantel Pamoate anthelmintic
- HealthForce Intestinal Movement Formula
- Nature's Way Cayenne Extra Hot
- Pectasol-C
- Dr. Hidemitsu Hayashi's Hydrogen Rich Water Stick

As far as enema buckets go, the plastic ones are fine to use as most are BPA-free, but metal is always better. Nowadays, most people know that these can be harmful, but all plastic bottles and containers leach chemicals beyond what should be ignored and the extent of which we are just now beginning to discover. We are starting to understand how these unnatural substances affect our bodies, especially when they are combined with heat.

SUPPLEMENT BIOHACKS

This is not an all-inclusive summary from this section but will help you get started until you are able to explore in more detail.

The One Thing: Consider the following stack for improved energy production and mental clarity:

- 1,000 mg magnesium glycinate (with food)
- 5,000-10,000 mcg methylcobalamin B12 sublingual lozenge (daily with or without food)
- 900 mg Docosahexaenoic acid (DHA) (daily with food)
- 100-300 mg of CoQ10 as Ubiquinol (with food)
- 10 mg of D-Ribose (daily in shake)
- A bioactive B vitamin complex which includes:
  * Methylfolate (around 3 mg, ideally as L-5-methyltetrahydrofolate)
  * Vitamin B6 (as pyridoxal 5-phosphate, around 50 mg)
  * Riboflavin (as riboflavin 5-phosphate, around 100 mg)
  * Vitamin B12 (as methylcobalamin, around 3 mg)
  * Betaine anhydrous (as trimethylglycine, around 2 grams)

Biohack #1: Get nutrients from food as much as possible.

Biohack #2: Take nutrients in the natural form and try to avoid synthetic versions.

Biohack #3: Avoid supplements that contain added sugar (in any form), grains (wheat, corn, or other grain by-products), dairy (whey, casein, or other dairy by-products), soy (in any form), artificial colors or chemicals.

HYDRATION, OXYGENATION, & LIGHT

Proper hydration, oxygenation, and exposure to full-spectrum sunlight charge the human battery and drive nearly all biochemical processes in the body.

You can drink plenty of water, and still be dehydrated on a cellular level. You can workout regularly, and still have poor blood oxygen (O_2) saturation and inefficient generation of ATP. Sunlight is used to synthesize vitamin D, facilitate electron transfer, and upregulate mitochondrial production of adenosine triphosphate (ATP).

And then, there's the interplay between all three. For example, when a cell is dehydrated the way it is influenced by light is also altered.

In this section, you'll learn how to best utilize each to optimize your mental clarity, energy, and wellbeing.

HYDRATION

Water is an essential ingredient for life.

It is everywhere: plants, animals, rivers, oceans, air, and sky.

99% of Your Molecules are Water

The estimated gross molecular contents of a typical 20-micrometre human cell

Molecule	Percent of Mass	Mol.Weight (daltons)	Molecules	Percent of Molecules
Water	65*	18*	1.74e14*	98.73*
Other Inorganics	1.5	N/A	1.31e12	0.74
Lipids	12	N/A	8.4e11	0.475
Other Organics	0.4	N/A	7.7e10	0.044
Protein	20	N/A	1.9e10	0.011
RNA	1.0	N/A	5e7	3e-5
DNA	0.1	1e11	46*	3e-11

*Water: Obviously the amount of water is highly dependent on body composition and amount of fat. In adults in developed countries it actually averages ~53% water. This varies substantially by age, sex, and adiposity. In a large sample of adults of all ages and both sexes, the figure for water fraction by weight was found to be 48 ±6% for females and 58 ±8% water for males

http://en.wikipedia.org/wiki/Composition_of_the_human_body

99% of the molecules in your body are water (not to be confused with the statistic that, by weight, the average adult male is about 60% water). We accept our need for water because it is involved in countless biological and chemical reactions. The omnipresent nature of our most precious resource has caused us to take it for granted. Consequently, water has become, perhaps, the most misunderstood element on Earth.

Our need for water runs much deeper than cellular biology and chemistry. It can be traced down to the quantum electrodynamic level (atoms, protons, electrons).

An oxidation-reduction (redox) reaction is a type of chemical reaction that involves a transfer of electrons between two species. An oxidation-reduction reaction is any chemical reaction in which the oxidation number of a molecule, atom, or ion changes by gaining or losing an electron. Redox reactions are common and vital to some of the basic functions of life, including photosynthesis, respiration, combustion, and corrosion or rusting.

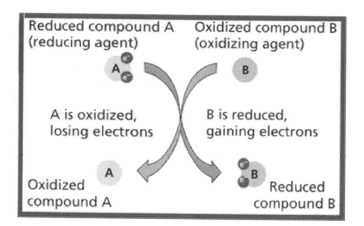

The movement of electrons between chemical species is reduction (for the electron acceptor) and oxidation (for the electron donor). Reduction and oxidation always exist together, one cannot occur without the other, which is why these are referred to as "redox" reactions.

Redox reactions underly all energy transduction in living creatures. Electrons move in accordance to the reduction/redox potential of a substance. The greater a substance's redox potential, the stronger its affinity for electrons. Substances with high (positive) redox potentials accept electrons from hydrogen, becoming reduced. Higher redox potential is associated with greater health and improved energy production. Substances with low (negative) redox potentials donate electrons to hydrogen, becoming oxidized. Lower redox potential is associated with poor energy production, illness, and even cancer.

There are many things you can do to increase your redox potential, and therefore energy. One of them is to drink structured, or hexagonal, water (also known as "living" water).

Live blood analysis with dark field microscopy offers the unique ability to view the blood in real time. Trained professionals are able to note the presence of conditions in the blood that contribute to sickness and disease. In the photo above, you can see an actual live

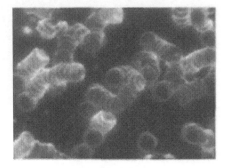 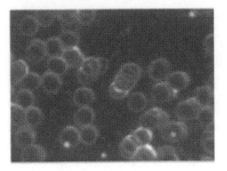

Before   After

Actual live blood sample before and after consuming hexagonal water.

blood sample before consuming hexagonal water. Note the clumping of red blood cells which is associated with inflammatory conditions, cancer, and disease.

The after photo was taken of the same individual, 10 minutes after drinking 16oz. of hexagonal structured water. Note the separation of the red blood cells-for improved oxygen and nutrient uptake.

Living, structured water, which is different than water from your tap, carries a negative charge. This negative charge allows it to store energy, much like a battery. When structured water donates these negatively charged electrons throughout the body, it produces energy.

The important thing to understand at this point is that not all water is created equal. And this is part of the reason many of the studies on water have produced inconsistent findings.

For example, research from the Journal of the American Society of Nephrology investigated four of the most commonly purported health benefits of water. After an exhaustive review of all of the evidence examining the benefits of water consumption, the two physicians spearheading the study concluded, "There is no clear evidence of benefit from drinking increased amounts of water." With all that we know and understand about water, how could this be?

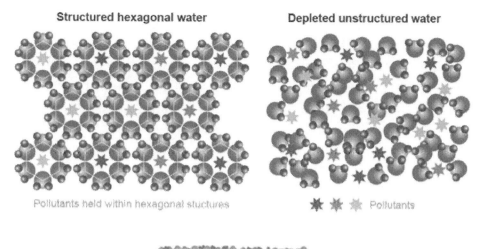

Structured hexagonal water

Depleted unstructured water

Pollutants held within hexagonal stuctures

✳ ✳ ✳ Pollutants

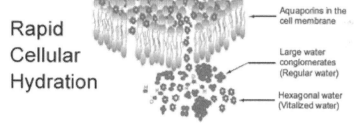

Rapid
Cellular
Hydration

Aquaporins in the
cell membrane

Large water
conglomerates
(Regular water)

Hexagonal water
(Vitalized water)

I'll admit, for years I recommended clients get at least 55% to 70% of their body weight in ounces of water daily, especially when focusing on weight loss. I did so without taking into consideration the source of that water. But as with our food, water quality matters more than quantity. A study conducted using fluoridated tap water from your municipality may produce different findings than a study conducted using clean, natural spring water from an aquifer deep within the Earth.

So what variables should be considered when choosing the best water for energy, mental clarity, and health? The two most important variables to consider when choosing your water sources are:

- *Toxicity:* Does it contain environmental toxins and chemicals?
- *Hexagonal Structure:* Water is a network of hydrogen-bonded

molecules. The most recent scientific findings indicate that biological organisms prefer the six-sided (hexagonal) ring-structure, found naturally in snow water. Hexagonal "living" water carries a negative charge that will allow it to donate electrons and improve energy transduction within the body.

Other, slightly less significant, variables that can influence the properties of water include:

- Oxygenation (ozonation)
- Electrolysis (i.e. ionizaiton)
- Electrolyzed reduced water (alkalized water)
- Electrolyzed oxidized water (acidic water)
- Hydrogen-enrichment

IS YOUR WATER MAKING YOU SICK?

Most of our cities' water supplies are polluted with toxins. City water contains large amounts of chlorine, fluoride, bromide, prescription medications (not removed through the water reclamation process), disinfection bi-products, chemicals, radiation, and heavy metals.

Remember the 2011 Fukushima nuclear accident where a tsunami caused three nuclear reactors to spill radioactive chemicals into the Pacific ocean? It was the worst nuclear accident since the Chernobyl disaster of 1986. These chemicals have now been detected in more than a dozen U.S. municipal water supplies.

Then there's fluoride.

City tap water contains fluorosilicic acid (FSA), which is not real sodium fluoride used in original tooth decay studies. FDA is a toxic waste by-product of making phosphate fertilizer. FSA has been shown to compete with iodine absorption in the thyroid, breast tissue and bone. Affective disorders like depression, cognitive deficits and behavior disorders have all been linked to what we refer to as "fluoride" (FSA) in tap water.

I didn't realize how many of us are still under the impression that fluoride is good for our teeth and has a place in our drinking water.

Just last week, I was with one of my executive coaching clients Joe and his pregnant wife, Ashley. We were going over ways to get them clean, safe drinking water in light of the coming addition to their family.

Environ Health Perspect. 2012 Oct; 120(10): 1362–1368.
Published online 2012 Jul 20. doi: 10.1289/ehp.1104912
Review

PMCID: PMC3491930

Developmental Fluoride Neurotoxicity: A Systematic Review and Meta-Analysis

Anna L. Choi,[✉1] Guifan Sun,[2] Ying Zhang,[3] and Philippe Grandjean[1,4]

Author information ► Article notes ► Copyright and License information ►

Abstract

Go to: ⌄

Background: Although fluoride may cause neurotoxicity in animal models and acute fluoride poisoning causes neurotoxicity in adults, very little is known of its effects on children's neurodevelopment.

Objective: We performed a systematic review and meta-analysis of published studies to investigate the effects of increased fluoride exposure and delayed neurobehavioral development.

Methods: We searched the MEDLINE, EMBASE, Water Resources Abstracts, and TOXNET databases through 2011 for eligible studies. We also searched the China National Knowledge Infrastructure (CNKI) database, because many studies on fluoride neurotoxicity have been published in Chinese journals only. In total, we identified 27 eligible epidemiological studies with high and reference exposures, end points of IQ scores, or related cognitive function measures with means and variances for the two exposure groups. Using random-effects models, we estimated the standardized mean difference between exposed and reference groups across all studies. We conducted sensitivity analyses restricted to studies using the same outcome assessment and having drinking-water fluoride as the only exposure. We performed the Cochran test for heterogeneity between studies, Begg's funnel plot, and Egger test to assess publication bias, and conducted meta-regressions to explore sources of variation in mean differences among the studies.

Results: The standardized weighted mean difference in IQ score between exposed and reference populations was –0.45 (95% confidence interval: –0.56, –0.35) using a random-effects model. Thus, children in high-fluoride areas had significantly lower IQ scores than those who lived in low-fluoride areas. Subgroup and sensitivity analyses also indicated inverse associations, although the substantial heterogeneity did not appear to decrease.

Conclusions: The results support the possibility of an adverse effect of high fluoride exposure on children's neurodevelopment. Future research should include detailed individual-level information on prenatal exposure, neurobehavioral performance, and covariates for adjustment.

I was specifically discussing fluoride because infants are most at risk to the dangerous threats of this toxin.

Ashley asked, "If fluoride is bad why would they put it in our water?"

Good question. Let's take a step back for a quick second.

Dentists and chemical experts have admitted that any benefits derived from the administering of fluoride are topical, meaning from the outside in. Fluoride is absorbed on the surface by the tooth. There is no benefit whatsoever to ingesting fluoride, only risks.

Even the World Health Organization has conceded that there is no difference in tooth decay between countries drinking fluoridated water versus those who do not.

There have been over 30 human studies and over 100 animal studies linking fluoride to brain damage, impaired cognitive function, hypothyroidism, and cancer.

Additionally, these studies have shown that fluoride toxicity can cause a host of other health problems, including:

- Increased absorption of toxic heavy metals
- Compromised collagen synthesis
- Chronic fatigue
- Dementia
- Arthritis
- Inactivation of vital biological enzymes
- Compromised immune function (prevents the formation of antibodies)
- Infertility and damaged sperm
- Cellular damage and death

Commercial water filters do not remove fluoride.

This includes many of the most popular charcoal-based brands, like

Brita, PUR, and Culligan. While these filters do remove chlorine and a number of other toxins, fluoride content remains intact. The same is true for filtered bottled water, and we now know that filtered bottled water also exposes us to a number of chemical toxins beyond the widely recognized Bisphenol A (BPA).

From this standpoint, excess water consumption beyond the biological needs of the body does come with consequences.

So whether drinking larger quantities of water will benefit an individual or expose them to greater environmental toxins depends entirely on the source of that water.

In order to determine if your water is filled with toxins you don't want to ingest, test it using AquaChek strips. These handy strips test for Free Chlorine, pH, Total Alkalinity, and Stabilizer. And the AquaChek 7-Way Strips Measure: Free Chlorine, Total Chlorine, Bromine, Total Hardness, Total Alkalinity, pH and Cyanuric Acid

HOW TO REMOVE TOXINS IN YOUR WATER

Here's what we do know...

Our bodies are around 70% water, roughly the same amount that covers the earth's surface.

Water is central to every function of our cells. In fact, it's so important that humans die after just 3 days of its absence.

People dealing with certain health issues, athletes, people prone to excessive sweating, people who are very physically active, people at high altitudes, and people who live in dry or hot climates require larger quantities of water.

The most practical way to remove fluoride is by installing a reverse osmosis water filter. You can also purchase reverse osmosis bottled water. Essential 9.5pH drinking water is one brand I've recommended.

It still comes in plastic but we're going for progress here, not perfection.

Along with impurities, reverse osmosis removes important minerals we need. So be sure to add those back in using a product like Trace Minerals ConcenTrace and/or BioPure Matrix Electrolyte powder (or Trace Minerals ENDURE).

Electrolytes (sodium, potassium, magnesium, calcium) help transport wastes across the extracellular space to the lymphatic system where they can be removed from the body.

Keep in mind, our skin is the body's largest organ, and we absorb large amounts of chemicals on a day to day basis through our skin, not just the water we drink. So, if your budget allows for it, I recommend installing a whole-house water filtration system, which will remove 98% to 99% of all contaminants. Of course, this can entail a significant investment on your part, so you are encouraged to do your own research before taking such a step.

Much like our food, water may be a substance wherein the quality helps to determine the quantity. If your water has been filtered through a reverse osmosis water filtration system, you'll want to drink around 70% of your current body weight in ounces of water per day. However, if you do not have access to this technology and the water that you drink comes from bottled sources, the tap, or limiting charcoal filters, you may want to keep it closer to 50% of your bodyweight in ounces of water per day, increasing that number based on your levels of thirst.

HOW TO BIOHACK YOUR WATER

Pioneering research by Dr. Gerald Pollack has shown that the water inside our cells has a different chemical structure than regular water.

In school, we learn about the three phases of water: solid (ice), liquid (water), and gas (water vapor, steam).

Dr. Pollack has identified a fourth phase of water - rather than H_2O it's H_3O_2. He refers to it as living water or EZ water. It's more alkaline and conductive than regular water. And this fourth phase of water, which I will also refer to as "structured water" throughout this guide, can store and deliver energy similar to a battery.

Where can we get structured water?

- *Spring Water:* Water under pressure (deep in the ground) becomes structured. Find-A-Spring is a great online resource that will help you find springs in your local area.
- *Glacial Melt:* Ice turns into Structured Water (EZ water) when melting. The phase between liquid and solid is structured water.
- *Organic Vegetables and Fruits:* When these still contain their natural water content, the water inside the cells of these plants is naturally structured.
- *Vortexing:* A vortex occurs naturally, as in streams, rivers, and waterfalls. The vortex is a kind of mechanical perturbation or agitation. Vortexing is a very powerful way of increasing

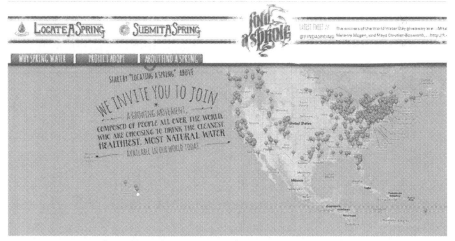

Go to FindASpring.com to locate springs near you.

structure. There are devices on the market which vortex water. One such device is the Natural Action Structured Water Unit (www.naturalactiontechnologies.com).

- *Juicing:* Another way to access the naturally structured water in organic plants. I use and recommend Brevelle juicers. Focus on juicing water-rich, organic, green vegetables as opposed to fruit. Adding organic cilantro, lemon, and liquid chlorophyll to your juice will help your body chelate heavy metals and toxins.

- *Antioxidents:* Most of the tissues in our body are negative. Our cells are a negative charge; oxidants are a positive charge. Antioxidents maintain the negative charge in our body.

- *Sunlight:* Critical to our health, light builds Structured Water (EZ water).

- *Circulation:* Red blood cells work their way through capillaries; light is the driver of flow. Add light and flow increases.

- *Infared Light:* Energy is generated everywhere. It drives the processes in your body. Conversely, UV light can inactivate structured water over time. So it's important to make sure you do not store water where it is exposed to sunlight.

There's a growing body of anecdotal evidence supporting the use of Kangen Water SD501 electrolysis/ionization machines (www.biohackingsecrets.com/kangen). This machine is part of the Robert Wright Cancer Protocol, and there are studies from 2008, 2009, and 2010 showing the effectiveness of electrolyzed water as well as hydrogen-rich water in fighting cancer and improving anti-oxidant status. The Kangen SD501 machine is also used by many celebrities, business moguls, and professional athletes.

Recently I invested in a Kangen SD501 Platinum water machine and noticed immediate improvements in a number of areas.

The first thing I observed was the taste. Kangen water tastes clean. It's hard to describe unless you've experienced it yourself. When a colleague tried explaining it to me the first time I remember thinking he was talking babble.

Where the health benefits really came into play was when I combined the ionized, alkalized Kangen water with a few other strategies I use to upgrade my

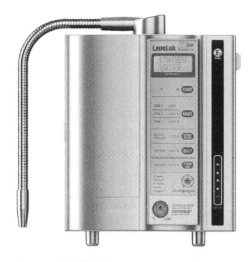

Kangen SD501 Platinum water system

hydration (see below). There was an immediate boost in mental clarity. I remember being severely sleep-deprived and yet I felt great. Well, far better than I should have given my state.

Over the next few weeks my energy, which was good to begin with, continued to rise. I felt less stiffness and recovered faster from my workouts. And there were some unexpected improvements in other areas us men can appreciate.

J Clin Biochem Nutr. 2010 Mar;46(2):140-9. doi: 10.3164/jcbn.09-100. Epub 2010 Feb 24.

Effectiveness of hydrogen rich water on antioxidant status of subjects with potential metabolic syndrome-an open label pilot study.

Nakao A[1], Toyoda Y, Sharma P, Evans M, Guthrie N

⊕ Author information

Abstract

Metabolic syndrome is characterized by cardiometabolic risk factors that include obesity, insulin resistance, hypertension and dyslipidemia. Oxidative stress is known to play a major role in the pathogenesis of metabolic syndrome. The objective of this study was to examine the effectiveness of hydrogen rich water (1.5-2 L/day) in an open label, 8-week study on 20 subjects with potential metabolic syndrome. Hydrogen rich water was produced, by placing a metallic magnesium stick into drinking water (hydrogen concentration; 0.55-0.65 mM), by the following chemical reaction; $Mg + 2H_2O \rightarrow Mg(OH)_2 + H_2$. The consumption of hydrogen rich water for 8 weeks resulted in a 39% increase (p<0.05) in antioxidant enzyme superoxide dismutase (SOD) and a 43% decrease (p<0.05) in thiobarbituric acid reactive substances (TBARS) in urine. Further, subjects demonstrated an 8% increase in high density lipoprotein (HDL)-cholesterol and a 13% decrease in total cholesterol/HDL-cholesterol from baseline to week 4. There was no change in fasting glucose levels during the 8 week study. In conclusion, drinking hydrogen rich water represents a potentially novel therapeutic and preventive strategy for metabolic syndrome. The portable magnesium stick was a safe, easy and effective method of delivering hydrogen rich water for daily consumption by participants in the study.

KEYWORDS: drinking water; hydrogen; magnesium; metabolic syndrome; oxidative stress

I now make this water for many of my executive coaching clients when they're in Chicago and teach them how to do it themselves so that they can experience these benefits. It may be one of the most powerful biohacks I utilize to help clients experience less pain, greater mental clarity, enhanced focus, more energy, and even overcome health issues that have plagued them for decades.

If you invest in a Kangen SD-501, enter my name and distributor ID number 7305654 at checkout, and I'll include 3 special bonus gifts along with a one-on-one Strategy Session (limited time offer) with me.

You can order by going to enagic.com and then clicking "Shop" in the navigation bar or simply go to www.BiohackingSecrets.com/Kangen. After your order is complete, email your receipt to anthony@thehealthblurprint.com to claim your bonuses.

I also use, or have used a Rainshower filer and Natural Action Technologies Dynamically Enhanced Shower Head for my showers. The former removes chlorine and a number of other toxins in tap water. The later removes toxins and adds structure to the water via vortexing.

For a water bottle, I recommend using the 64-Oz Hydro Flask. Using a water bottle is a visual reminder that we need to drink more water. It is also one of the easiest ways to increase your daily water consumption.

HOW I FILTER, IONIZE, AND STRUCTURE MY DRINKING WATER

I have a process that starts with either:

A. Clean spring water from a deep aquifer that's rich in calcium carbonate, iron, and magnesium. This water naturally has a high pH. I have it delivered to my home every month.
B. High pH ionized Kangen water from my SD501 machine.

I then enhance the water by running it through two devices that add oxygen and structure via:

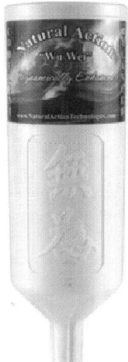

    a. Vortexing, and then...

    b. A device that mimics the natural action of water flowing over rocks, down waterfalls, and moving through twists and turns as it actively descends a mountain. This is one of the ways water is structured in nature. Through this process, the molecular structure of water is changed to reflect less surface tension, neutralize toxins, and add balance on a particle level.

    C. Lastly, I further oxygenate the water using a Sota Water Ozonator depending on the purpose and desired objective. In some cases I will add hydrogen using a hydrogen rich water stick or two capsules of Dr. Patrick Flanagan's Mega Hydrate.

I advise that you front load your water as soon as you wake up, because your body is dehydrated from the night before, and drinking 16 to 32 ounces of filtered water (ideally from a natural spring source, reverse osmosis filter, or structuring device) with your empty stomach vitamins. Then, continue to sip from and refill your water bottle throughout the day. Keep it somewhere in sight as a behavioral trigger, reminding you to stay hydrated.

Prescription medications and supplements are best taken away from Kangen water as the high pH can affect absorption.

OXYGENATION

"250 million years ago oxygen levels on earth = 35%. In 1850, oxygen levels = 22%. Today's levels now hover around 19% or less in most westernized cities. This assumes, of course, these cities are at sea level. O2 levels required for healthy humans = 19.5%. This proof is found on an oxygen dissociation curves of hemoglobin. That's not a good development for our mitochondria."

- Dr. Jack Kruse, neurosurgeon, author
"Epi-Paleo Rx: The Prescription for Disease Reversal and Optimal Health"

Mitochondria are little, bacteria-like organelles inside your cells which produce energy. These tiny energy factories exist in the greatest amounts within your muscles, heart, and brain. They are the metabolically active parts of your body, responsible for your metabolism.

Most of the mass of the human body is oxygen. As you probably know, our bodies require oxygen to produce energy. Oxygen is so vital, in fact, that being denied it for just three minutes results in death.

The way that your metabolism works is your body takes the oxygen that you breathe and the food that you eat and breaks them down to form ATP. The byproducts are carbon dioxide (CO_2) and water (H_2O). This process is known as cellular respiration. When our cells do not get an adequate supply of oxygen, we feel tired, lethargic, foggy-headed, and achy. It also affects our ability to burn body fat. Our bodies require a continuous supply of oxygen to:

- Build and maintain cellular structure
- Transport nutrients
- Manufacture vital enzymes and biological components
- Move, grow, and reproduce

The efficiency and effectiveness of our body's ability to produce energy from oxygen depend on a number of factors. They include, but are not limited to:

- Oxygen intake (volume, breathing patterns)
- Intake rate and consistency (mouth intake = inconsistent, nose intake = consistent)
- Oxygen consumption (the amount of oxygen utilized by the body per minute)
- Oxygen deliverability (the body's ability to deliver oxygen to its cells)

Oxygen deliverability and oxygen consumption will both improve as you implement the nutrition, physical activity, stress management, sleep and supplemental recommendations of this guide.

By developing the ability to breath in (or in and out) through your nose, you will improve your rate of oxygen intake, thereby improving homeostasis in your body. Breathing properly by using your diaphragm, belly, and all of your lungs will cause your body to instinctively move towards the oxygen volume that supports optimal energy and focus.

Let's do an exercise to demonstrate what a complete breath feels like. Sit tall, or stand up, and put your hands on your belly. As you inhale through your nostrils, see that air first filling up your chest, then your upper abdomen, and then your belly.

You should feel your belly expanding as your lungs fill with air, and this should make your hands move out away from your spine. Then, as you exhale, you should feel that air start to leave through your lower belly, and you should feel your hands moving back towards your spine, your upper abdomen, and your chest until the air has fully left your body.

This is the type of deep, diaphragmatic breathing that supports optimal energy production and the oxygenation of your cells. *If you do nothing else to improve the supply of oxygen, and thereby your body's ability to produce ATP, practice deep, diaphragmatic breathing until it becomes your default.*

Also, be sure to breathe through your nose. Now, why is that important? Breathing through your nose helps to normalize breathing volume. Our body requires stability and uses a complex array of systems to maintain homeostasis. Breathing through your nose is part of making these systems work optimally.

During cellular respiration and energy production, we breathe in oxygen, which our cells use along with the food that we eat to produce energy and also the byproduct water and CO_2. This CO_2 is an acidic waste product that we expel through the lungs as we exhale. Many of you are probably aware of the acid/alkaline hypothesis, which to crudely summarize, implies that when we eat acid-forming foods we get sick and when we eat alkaline-forming foods, we'll be healthy and protected from disease.

However, few people are aware that the carbon dioxide exhaled by the lungs is the single biggest source of acid elimination in the human body. This is one of the main reasons why complete diaphragmatic breathing, with full inhalation and complete exhalation, is so important.

Excess amounts of CO_2 in the body have an acidifying effect on our pH, and it has been implicated in adverse cardiovascular effects and nerve damage.

Breathing through the nose ensures a more steady, consistent flow of oxygen and elimination of CO_2, which in turn prevents unwanted disturbances in blood gases. When we breathe through our mouths, especially during exercise, oxygen intake and the release of carbon dioxide are much less consistent. That means the body has to work harder to try to maintain balance.

There are other benefits to nose breathing as well. For one, our noses contain nitric oxide. So, when we nose breathe, we breathe in this beneficial gas in small amounts, too. Nitric oxide causes bronchial dilation (an opening of the airways), vasodilation (an opening of the blood vessels), and has antibacterial properties that help to fight infections and kill pathogenic bacteria.

Additionally, the nose is a smaller opening than the mouth. So our lungs have to work harder to take in the required amount of oxygen. This is especially true when $O2$ demands increase, as they do during exercise. By breathing through the nose, you strengthen your inspiratory and expiratory muscles. Resisted breathing enhances your endurance by increasing your ventilatory capacity (lung size).

THE WIM HOF METHOD

One of the most effective practices I've found to improve the supply of oxygen and support energy production and focus for me and my clients is the Wim Hof Method.

Wim Hof, aka "The Iceman," holds 20 world records. Most of these achievements relate to his ability to withstand extreme temperatures. He has climbed Mt. Everest, a feat more than 250 people have died trying to accomplish. Wim Hof did it, wearing nothing but shorts and climbing boots.

He also reached the summit of Mt. Kilimanjaro in just two days wearing only shorts.

He's run a full marathon in the Namib Desert without water.

Additionally, one of his world records is the Guinness World Record for the longest ice bath ever taken. He was able to withstand the freezing cold water for an amazing 1 hour, 52 minutes, and 42 seconds.

I tried the Wim Hof Method (www.WimHofMethod.com) for the first time in 2015. Jason Ferruggia had invited me to Santa Monica to join one of his 3-day Breakthrough programs and discuss some mutual business ventures.

Jason took me to meet Dr. Trisha Smith, affectionately known in the industry as Doc Trish, a sports therapist and rehabilitation specialist in Los Angeles. Doc Trish shared a story about the Dutchman, and his attempt to break the world record for the longest swim submerged beneath the icy surface of a frozen lake. Only seconds into the swim, the extreme temperatures froze both of Wim's retinas and he was effectively blind.

Fortunately, because of his training, he had a sense for how many strokes and how long it would take him to get to the exit hole. When he got to where he felt the hole should be, there was no hole to be found.

Running out of air, he frantically swam left, then right, looking for his escape. As he lost consciousness, Wim was able to make out a circle that was slightly brighter than the surrounding dark, blue mass. He swam towards the light and was pulled onto the ice just as he lost consciousness.

Wim narrowly escaped the incident with his life, and a number of additional world records he had not set out to capture.

When asked about the experience, and the condition of his eyes after the swim, he casually responded that he was fine and that his eyes thawed after a few minutes.

Doc Trish asked us if we wanted to try it, and we were all in. First, she had us lay on our backs and instructed us to take a deep breath, pulling as much air into our lungs and belly as our bodies would allow. Then, we were to just let it go. There was no need to fully exhale, just let the air and pressure release, making room for the next inhalation.

It's important that each breath is as deep as possible and that your belly is expanding in all four directions: forward, back toward the spine, and out on each side as you breathe in. This process is then repeated for three cycles of 30 to 35 breathes. Within the first cycle, I was already experiencing some of the common physiological symptoms of hyper-oxygenation. There was numbness in my fingers and toes, I felt very uncomfortable, and my instinctive reaction was to stop. Dr. Trish assured us that this was normal and to push through.

After three cycles of 30 breaths, the last breath is released in the same fashion as the others before it, only this time you are instructed to hold your breath as long as you can. "At first your body is going to try to get you to breathe," Dr. Trish said. "That's just your autonomic nervous system doing its job. It has no basis on the actual oxygen levels in your cells right now. Once you let that initial instinct pass, you'll find that you'll be able to hold your breath much longer than you ever expected."

True to form, my autonomic nervous system was doing its job. Within moments of holding my breath, I felt like I needed to breathe, but as I remembered Trish's instructions, and let my body relax into the floor. I felt a sudden calm. The calm that came over my body was almost euphoric. "Thirty seconds," she said. This had already seemed like a long time considering we weren't working with a full breath and had already exhaled.

"One minute. Good job." Trish announced.

Shortly thereafter, I started experiencing some physical symptoms that my body would not be opposed to a breath of air, but I knew that I had to be close to 90 seconds.

I remembered a trick that my mom had taught me from her days in the Olympic development swimming program. When holding your breath, you can buy some extra time by slowly exhaling and releasing some of the acidic CO_2 in your lungs.

My mom's "biohack" bought me the extra time I needed to pass the 90-second mark. When the time came when we needed to inhale, I took a deep breath and held this new breath of fresh air for another 15 to 20 seconds. This allowed my body to partition the fresh oxygen to my thirsty, oxygen-depleted cells. Thinking back, I'm not sure if I had ever held my breath for 90 seconds before, let alone that long after exhaling.

Moreover, I noticed changes in my body, I felt clear headed and focused. A calm, relaxed energy came over me, and it was akin to what one might experience right after a meditation session.

Aidan, a 38 year old software engineer who owns a programming company, practices this method 4 to 6 times per week because it helps with his mental clarity, and morning grogginess.

The morning routine we put together for Aidan, which includes Wim Hof, has now replaced his morning cup of coffee.

As with anything, practice makes permanent. To improve your breathing, and subsequently, your body's energy production through more efficient and effective oxygen intake and utilization, requires practice. Some other strategies and biohacks to consider to improve your breathing and oxygen status are:

- Pranayama Yoga
- Art of Living classes
- The Expand-a-Lung Breathing Fitness Exerciser
- The Powerlung and Powerlung Sport Breathing Trainer
- The Elevation High Altitude Training Mask 2.0
- Meditation
- *Deep Belly Breathing:* Slowly bring a deep breath into your body. Try to count to 7 as you breathe in using your belly. Then push breath out with another 7 count using your belly to completely empty the lungs. Each breath should take around 14 seconds. Expand your lungs each time until you cannot take in any more

air, but not to the point where you are uncomfortable and unable to enjoy the practice. I recommend breathing in and out through the nose, if possible.

- *"Relaxation Revolution: The Science and Genetics of Mind Body Healing"* by Herbert Benson, William Proctor
- Exercising for more than 20 minutes in your target heart rate zone as described in the "Movement" section of this guide.
- *Hypoxic (or Reduced Oxygen) Training:* Hypoxico offers commercial home altitude systems that simulate low-oxygen environments and stimulate beneficial adaptive responses in the body.
- Hyperbaric oxygen therapy (HBOT)
- Free-diving (PerformanceFreeDiving.com)
- Qigong
- The Buteyko Breathing Method
- Sota Ozonator (highest quality medical grade components) or A2Z Aqua 6 Water Ozonator.
- *Oreck RAIRP-B Professional Air Purifier*
- *Air Purifier:* According to the EPA, the air in your home may be up to 5 times more polluted than the air outside, and we spend approximately 90% of our time indoors.
- *Austin Air Purifier Health Mate Plus:* Cleans benzene, wood smoke, formaldehyde and other volatile organic compound

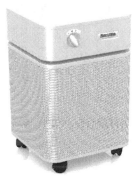
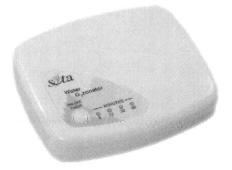

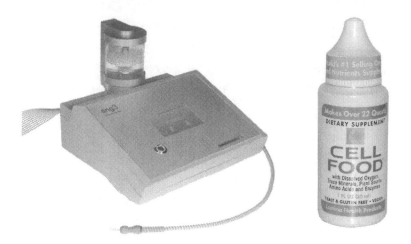

(VOCs) from the air. Capable of trapping 99.97% of all polluting particulates down to 0.3 microns (www.austinair.com).

– *NanoVi Bio-Identical Signaling Technology:* Designed to improve cellular activities, specifically by improving the body's response to oxidative stress (www.eng3corp.com).

– *Organic fulvic acid and humic acid (or humate substances):* Fulvic acid and humic acid contains approximately 45% oxygen that is highly bioavailable to all systems and cells in the body. Can be added to water. Because fulvic and humic acids carry both a negative and a positive charge, cells are energized, and can behave as an electron donor or acceptor, depending on the need. Newly energized cells in every system could have the potential to function at peak performance. Body weight balances naturally because fulvic and humic acids may correct chemical and hormonal imbalances, assisting in the proper metabolism of food, and diminishing mineral deficiency cravings.

– *CellFood:* Oxygen and nutrient supplement. Add 8 drops to 8 ounces of water up to three times daily. In a study conducted at the University of Pretoria, CELLFOOD was shown to increase oxygen uptake (VO2 Max), increase ferretin (iron storage), and decrease lactic acid accumulation (muscular fatigue). CELLFOOD's colloidal and ionic formula has a negative charge (as measured by Zeta potential testing). This negatively charged solution (like blood and lymph) allows for the rapid absorption and assimilation of nutrients. This process enables the body to more efficiently eliminate toxins and balance pH (www.cellfood.com).

– *Pulsed Electromagnetic Field Therapy (PEMF therapy):* Studies show PEMF therapy increases tissue and brain oxygenation.

– *Heal Respiratory Conditions and Sleep Apnea:* Take steps to heal any respiratory conditions like sleep apnea or nasal congestions, allergies, and other hidden infections that can restrict or prevent nasal breathing. There are a great deal of methodologies that you can use to combat this, ranging from supplements, to saline rinses, to anti-microbial sprays (both herbal and sometimes prescription). In some cases my clients and I even have to work towards recolonizing the nasal passageways with lactobacillus sakei bacteria.

– *Cyclic Variations in Adaptive Conditioning (CVAC) Pod:* Effort and workload are each varied and increased by using patterned sequential progression in amplitude of dynamic pressure changes to fresh air. Regular, rhythmic use of the CVAC Process 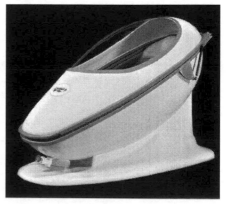 can elicit some of the same benefits gained through traditional aerobic and anaerobic exercise *(www.cvacsystems.com)*.

LIGHT

You've learned a bit about how late night exposure to light can disrupt our circadian rhythm, interfere with sleep, and has been implicated in many studies to have an association with heart disease, cancer, diabetes, and obesity.

When properly administered light therapy has been shown to:

- Reduce Pain
- Reduce Inflammation
- Increase Collagen Production
- Increase Blood Flow to Damaged Tissue
- Increase ATP production in the Body
- Help Heal Acne and Skin Conditions
- Boost the Immune System

We also know that exposure to light, or lack thereof, can have a profound impact on mood, cognition, and focus. That's why many people suffer from depression and fatigue in the low light winter months, a condition known as Seasonal Affective Disorder (SAD).

In this section, we will detail ways that you can utilize and manipulate light exposure to increase energy production, improve health, enhance brain function, decrease inflammation, and amplify focus.

You'll remember from the section on "Sleep" that blue light, which is the kind of light that's emitted from our computers, cell phones, televisions, and many compact bulbs in our homes, suppresses our body's endogenous production of the hormone melatonin for up to four hours. Lower melatonin levels can lead to compromised sleep, recovery, and elevated levels of the stress hormone cortisol (the hormones melatonin and cortisol oppose one another).

To counteract the unwanted suppression of melatonin and the spiking of cortisol that takes place as a result of your exposure to blue light, it's advised that you shut down all of your electronics at least one hour before bedtime.

It's also good for you to create a pitch black sleeping environment for yourself. You can do so by using blackout shades, a sleep mask, and either unplugging or putting tape over any LED-emitting electronics in your bedroom.

Some studies have shown that light, whether blue light or otherwise, is the most potent cue used by humans to synchronize our circadian rhythms (or internal clocks). The photoreceptors in our retina communicate with the hypothalamus in our brain, which is involved with the regulation of energy production, sleep, and multiple biological mechanisms.

You're probably familiar with The Pareto Principle which maintains that, in any situation, 20% of our efforts are responsible for 80% of our results. When it comes to light hacking, the simplest and most effective change you can make is immediately exposing your eyes to natural sunlight as close as possible to the time you wake up. I recommend that as soon as your alarm goes off, you open up the shades, look outside, and let the sun shine in.

At night, keep your house dark and minimize your exposure to blue light by using amber tinted glasses, low blue light bulbs, and candles for light.

NATURAL SUNLIGHT

Earth's most important energy source is the Sun.

Sunlight contains the entire electromagnetic color spectrum. And each color wavelength along the electromagnetic spectrum facilitates multiple vital biochemical processes within the body.

We are just starting to scratch the surface of the role natural light plays in energy production and peak performance.

The good news is, like electricity, you don't have to understand all the nuances to benefit from their existence. To benefit from electricity, you just have to flip the light switch and, voila, the room is illuminated. To reap the benefits of photobiomodulation, you just have to get outside and expose your eyes and skin to lots of natural sunlight. If you live somewhere that does not get consistent sunlight throughout the year, Dr. Jack Kruse suggests moving or taking frequent vacations. "Your zip code is a better determinant of health than your genetic code," says Kruse.

Not getting enough natural sunlight is just as harmful, if not more so, than getting too much. Many of us are doing far more harm than good by using dangerous sunscreens that contain toxins, petrochemicals, parabens, and lead. All of this is absorbed into the skin, and they block the natural sunlight that we need to produce the hormone vitamin D. What you have to understand is that vitamin D is almost totally absent from our food supply and many of us are deficient in it. This deficiency has been linked to depression, dementia, autism, cancer, and an increased risk of death.

Humans have adapted to sunlight and the 1,500 wavelengths that it contains to optimize our biological function. Light is very beneficial to us in many ways. Here are a few things that we know about how exposure to light can positively effect our health:

- *Blue light* has been used to treat bacterial infections, mood disorders, and skin conditions.
- *White light* has been shown to improve circulation, strengthen the immune system, increase antibody production, and dampen inflammation.
- *Red light* has been found to increase mitochondrial energy production, treat hypothyroidism, reverse cognitive issues after

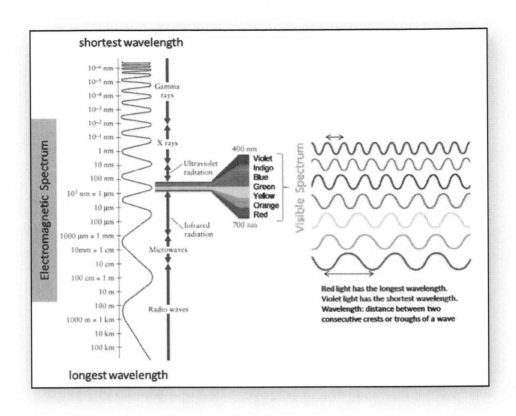

brain injuries, decrease cellulite, regrow hair, and decrease physical pain.

I have even used sunlight with some of my MS (multiple sclerosis) clients to facilitate a reduction in unwanted symptoms. A number of studies have shown that UVB light exposure also protects against melanoma, the most deadly form of skin cancer. New evidence confirms that exposure to the sun, in strategic amounts and specific time frames, has additional benefits beyond our body's production of vitamin D. A few of these include:

- Elevated release of endorphins, enhancing energy and mood
- Increased nitric oxide, which fights cancer, increases oxygenation,

kills pathogenic bacteria, and has cardioprotective effects in the body
- Regulation of melatonin via photoreceptors in the pineal gland
- Normalization of body temperature
- Synchronization of diurnal Biorhythms
- Even the elimination of body odors

Get at least 20 minutes of sunlight to your eyes and exposed skin per day, as close as possible to the time you first wake up. In climates where this is not possible, you'll still want to expose your eyes to natural sunlight as soon as you wake up.

Use sunscreen only as a last resort, after you have first sought out shade, shelter, and protective clothing to protect your skin from overexposure.

If you do use sunscreen, I highly recommend that you download the Environmental Working Group's (EWG's) sunscreen guide and their guide to sun safety as many contain potentially dangerous ingredients like oxybenzone.

Soap removes our skin's natural oils we need to absorb sunlight and synthesize vitamin D. This is why I see many clients who spend sufficient time in the sun with poor vitamin D status when we check their blood. Use soap only on your most important parts to avoid washing off these natural oils.

We all need sunlight, but the amount we need varies based on our geographic locations, genetics, and heritage. Here are some of the reasons why we need sunlight:

- *Vitamin D:* As you know, exposure to sunlight helps our bodies to produce vitamin D. Deficiencies in this vitamin have been linked to conditions such as over 17 different types of cancer, along with

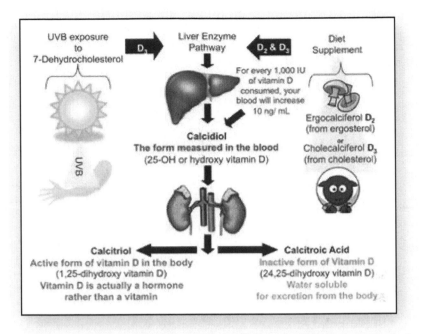

Diabetes, auto-immune diseases, birth defects, chronic fatigue, heart disease, and hypertension.

– *Blood Pressure:* A number of studies have shown ultraviolet light to reduce blood pressure. This includes both UV light from the sun and lamp sources. The blood pressure lowering effect of sunlight is also tied to the aforementioned production of nitric oxide, which has a relaxing and vasodilation effect on our blood vessels. As you probably know, high blood pressure is one of the strongest correlating effects of cardiovascular disease and yet another reason why daily exposure to sunlight is so important.

– *Inflammation:* Studies have found a strong connection between the development of MS and the amount of sunlight a person might get within the location where they were born. Two other sunlight-related factors tied to MS are the geographical locations the patient lives in as an adult, in addition to the time of year. Interestingly, relapse rates for MS are highest in the wintertime.

- *Longevity:* In a fairly new study, researchers followed the sun exposure habits of 30,000 Swedish women. They found that those women who avoided the sun had a twofold higher risk of early mortality. Sunlight exposure has also been shown to boost mood and resistance to stress, as previously mentioned. This happens because sunlight increases the production of feel-good endorphins and neurotransmitters like serotonin. Higher levels of these have also been correlated with increased longevity and quality of life.

Scientifically, light is a nutrient for the body. Similar to the way plants need light to survive, human cells need light of various wavelengths for energy production and well-being. As technologies push forward and our modern lifestyle has us spending more and more time indoors, temptations arise to derive the benefits of sunlight and vitamin D through other means.

Most experts now recommend that we maintain vitamin D levels in the blood of 50 ng/mL for optimal health. However, there is a great deal of controversy surrounding these recommendations.

A prospective cohort study involving 1.2 million participants showed that the lowest risk of all-cause mortality and the lowest rates of cardiovascular disease were found in people with vitamin D levels between 20 to 36 ng/mL. To put things in perspective, the low end of the laboratory reference range of vitamin D levels in the U.S is 30 ng/ml. So this study involving over a million people found those with borderline vitamin D deficiency to have the greatest health status.

Now, why could this be? One potential reason may be that vitamin A and vitamin K2, which are two vitamins that are often missing, protect our bodies from vitamin D toxicity. We have a large cross-section of the population supplementing with vitamin D. However, many of these people are still deficient in vitamin A and vitamin K, and therefore, the vitamin D supplementation may be exposing them to an increased risk of vitamin D toxicity. Hence, there are higher levels of all-cause mortality and cardiovascular disease.

Another possible mechanism is tied to the fact that vitamin D and vitamin K2 play a role in calcium absorption. Vitamin K2 is found in a number of green plants, and a much higher concentration of it is found in organ meats. It can also be found in a very nasty, foul-smelling Japanese soy dish called Natto. These are not the most popular foods with many Americans, and so many of us possess vitamin K levels below our body's requirements.

When we combine elevated vitamin D levels due to supplementation with deficiencies in vitamin K2, it increases the rate of calcification in our arteries and increases our chances of experiencing cardiovascular troubles. Light is the missing ingredient in many of our lives, and the best place to get the light that we need is from the sun. Unfortunately, family responsibilities, career demands, weather, modern lifestyle, and other such factors can sometimes impede our ability to receive proper amounts of sunlight. This deficit, however, is one of the main problems contributing to chronic and inflammatory diseases, which are rising to epidemic levels.

The good news is we can use blue and infrared light technology to safely deliver light energy throughout the body. This can help to:

- Increase energy levels
- Raise vitality
- Improve sleep
- Elevate mood
- Expand mental clarity

Another major benefit to all of this is that it can contribute to younger-looking skin as a result of raised collagen levels. Participants in light therapy are also likely to have:

- More optimal ATP levels
- Improved blood flow
- Enhanced oxygen and nutrient deliverability
- Improved recovery
- Cellular repair and regeneration

Already, there are many light-hacking technologies available to you. The ones that I utilize and recommend to clients are:

- *Sunlighten mPULSE CONQUER Infrared Sauna:* One of the most beneficial detoxification strategies. Aim for 45 minutes

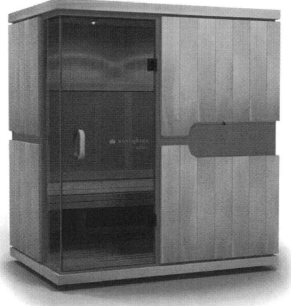

Sunlighten Infrared Sauna

around 140+ degrees. The more you sweat, the more toxins will be eliminated. Wipe the skin frequently to remove heavy metals, chemicals, and prevent reabsorption. You can find more info on the units I'm using now at www.BiohackingSecrets.com/sauna.

- *Pro Biomat 7000MX (infrared)*
- *TDP Far Infrared Heat Lamp*
- *Philips HF3520 sunrise simulation wake up light*
- *Beurer IL50 Infrared heat lamp*
- *VieLIGHT 655 Prime Intranasal Light Therapy Device* (circulation, inflammation, and pathogens)
- Sperti Vitamin D Lamp, model D/UV-F
- Sperti Fiji Sun Lamp
- *VieLIGHT 810 Intranasal Light Therapy Device* (brain and cognitive)

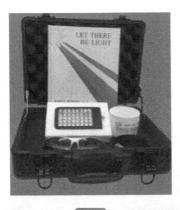

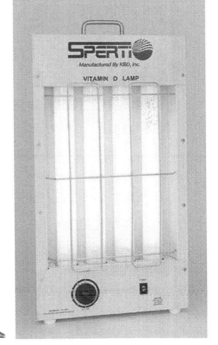

- *Naturebright SuntouchPlus Blue Light*
- *Anne Marie Gianni's Organic Cosmedic and Skin Care Line* (www.annmariegianni.com)
- *In Light Wellness Systems 6-Port* (www.BiohackingSecrets.com/ILWS)
- *Theralumen Light Therapy Device:* Designed to promote and improve energy and immune function via gentle infusion of specific wavelengths into the blood through the sub-lingual capillary system (www.millennialhealthsystems.com).
- *MHS SpectraMite* (www.millennialhealthsystems.com): To save $50 on the Spectramite and $100 on the Theralumen call Millennial Health Systems by phone at 405-478-4351 and use discount code "biohacks".
- *Low blue light night lights*
- *F.lux:* Blue light blocking software for laptops and computers (www.justgetflux.com).
- *Gunnar blue-light blocking glasses*
- *The Mercola Vitality Elite Tanning Bed:* Contains UVA, UVB, infrared, red, and blue light (www.mercola.com)
- *DreamSpa:* Biophoton system to upregulate mitochondrial function and ATP/energy production, reduce stress, and improve sleep. Many clients report feeling more well-rested and refreshed when using the DreamSpa during their treatment sessions (www.BioHackingSecrets.com/DreamSpa)
- *Photonic Health Pro Light Kit:* (www.BioHackingSecrets.com/photonichealth)
- *Advanced Photonic Laser Therapy McLaren Torch:* Photonic therapy is an advanced form of traditional complementary medicine using light to stimulate recognized acupuncture points. It involves safe, low frequency red light (not laser) which supports

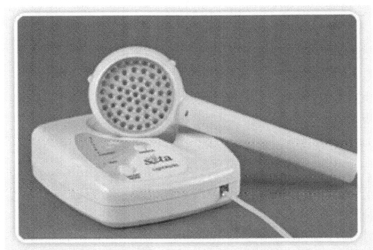

Sota LightWorks can direct Red or Near Infrared light anywhere on the body.

the healing of conditions and injuries. Dr. Brian McLaren, a clinical scientist and veterinary surgeon, is a veterinary acupuncturist in Australia with postgraduate qualifications in veterinary and human acupuncture. He developed the original photonic torch which many others have since attempted to replicate (www. advancedphotonictherapy.com).

– *Sota LightWorks:* The LightWorks by SOTA offers the benefits of LED light combined with healthy frequencies. These frequencies gently stimulate the body electric for more energy, health and well-being. Either Red or Near Infrared (NIR) light can be readily applied by placing the Paddle anywhere on the body. A built-in timer automatically cycles through healthy frequencies or individual settings can be chosen (www.Sota.com).

Just to clarify, I recommend that my clients use these in conjunction with natural sunlight exposure and only by themselves in the absence of opportunities for natural light exposure.

I use both the Biomat and the infrared heat lamp. I have the heat lamp next to my bed, in fact. It feels great when it's over your ankles and feet. Additionally, I have the Beurer infrared heat lamp (www.BioHackingSecrets.com/infraredlight). I use it when I'm standing at the sink, getting ready for my day. I sometimes will put it on the floor in front of me when I sit and meditate.

HOW TO HACK LIGHT AND TEMPERATURE

When I wake up in the morning, the first thing I do is drop my shades and let a bunch of natural sunlight in. There are a number of reasons that you'd want to do this. For one, it causes the photoreceptors in your retinas to react. It also helps to wake you up. Probably most importantly, however, is the fact that it helps to regulate your circadian rhythm. Plus, the sunlight coming in causes the room to heat up. We know that as temperature rises in the morning, the blood flow to the brain is increased. So, this helps us to get moving too.

From there, I will usually jump into a hot shower with my Natural Action Technologies structured water shower head. While I am waiting, I'll normally do things like brush my teeth and shave. I have a Beurer infrared light on the counter running while I get ready. I use a dry skin brush to remove dead skin, stimulate the lymphatic system, and increase blood flow to the surface of the skin.

If I have some extra time, I will throw two cups of Epsom salt, a cup of baking soda, a cup of food grade 35% hydrogen peroxide, and some lavender oil into the tub.

Most mornings I stick with a hot shower.

All showers end with the water on cold and some deep, oxygenating breathing.

After I take a bath and/or shower, I'll turn the Beurer infrared light back on, along with a 24-inch light that emits both UVA and UVB, while I finish getting ready. I don't towel off. Instead I air dry so that the water can help my skin absorb even more light.

The next thing I generally do is head into the living room and meditate. There are a number of different ways in which I integrate light into my meditation. Sometimes I'll use the David Delight Pro, which combines cranial electrical stimulation (CES) with a pair of glasses that emit visual light and audio frequencies for brain entrainment. They help to more quickly bring the brain out of a beta state and into a more relaxed alpha brain wave state. If I don't want the cranial electrical stimulation, I'll use the DAVID Smart device instead.

There are also times when I'll use my VieLight (www. BiohackingSecrets.com/vielight). This is an intranasal light therapy device. You see, the inside of our nose contains the highest concentration of capillaries in our body, and there's a tremendous amount of blood flow through that area. That's part of the reason why a person bleeds

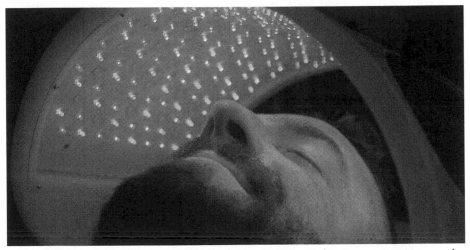

Specific light frequencies have been shown in scientific studies to generate increased collagen production, resulting in a more youthful appearance and skin.

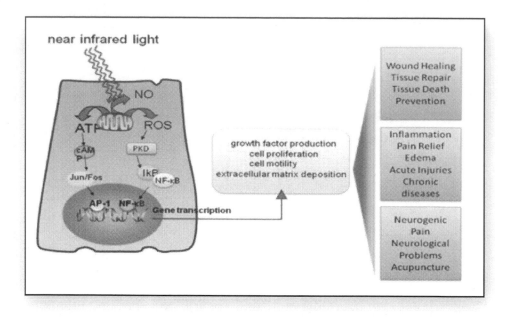

so much when they break their nose. It's also blood that's in close proximity to the brain, and these near infrared therapy devices have been shown to mimic many of the benefits of blood irradiation therapy.

This type of technology has been used to a much greater degree overseas, such as in Russia, Brazil, and China. They have been found to have a number of beneficial properties. For instance, this type of therapy has been known to improve mitochondrial efficiency. Also, they increase the activity of Cytochrome c Oxidase. This is an enzyme that accepts photon light energy, and in turn, becomes activated by that light when operating at suboptimal levels. All of these things have been shown to increase energy and ATP production.

This near infrared light has also been known to cause a low-level increase in oxidative stress, which stimulates our body's responses, resulting in positive and beneficial adaptations in the body. Among those adaptations, we see improved circulation and vasodilation as well as increased nitric oxide levels throughout the body. A number of the studies that have been conducted in Russia, China, and Brazil have shown that blood irradiation therapy, and this type of technology, have resulted in improved physical performance.

In one particular study, scientists found that after just 10 days of blood irradiation therapy, the participating athletes experienced a 20% boost in exercise capacity and this improvement lasted for a full 16 weeks after they stopped treatment.

So these infrared lights and blood irradiation therapies create adaptive changes within the body that increase oxygen utilization, increase ATP production, and mitochondrial efficiency. These adaptive changes continue beyond the cessation of treatment in many cases. When I use the VieLight, I simply put it in one of my nostrils, turn it on, and let it do its thing. I haven't been using it for very long, but within the first treatment or two, I had already noticed improvements. I felt like my circulation was better, and I felt less inflamed. In particular, my feet and ankles felt healthier and like they were receiving better blood flow.

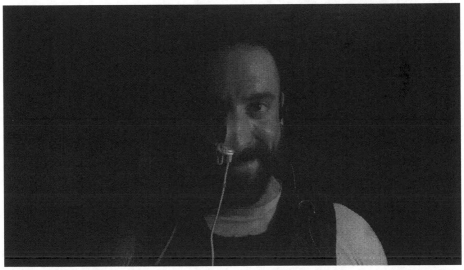

The nose is one of the most capilary dense areas in the body, making it a perfect location to expose large quantities of blood to beneficial wavelengths of red and infrared light.

To save 10% on the Vielight Neuro, 810, and 655 devices use discount code "biohacks" at www.vielight.com.

To get more natural sunlight, in the summertime, I'll throw on my shoes and take a jog around the lake. I don't run at a pace that's particularly stressful, just one that's going to oxygenate the cells, get my body moving, and up-regulate my production of BDNF (Brain-derived neurotrophic factor).

I use a Garmin Forerunner 220 heart rate monitor. Once I'm in my aerobic training zone, I'll jog for 20 to 30 minutes.

The things that are important for you to do in order to enhance energy, focus, and your performance overall are the things that you want to do every single day and make part of your routine.

This is part of the reason why I put a cap on how long I take a run and stop before I even feel like I want to. Doing so also minimizes the risk for injuries; it gives your body the chance to receive those hormetic stressors and stimulates your body's healing response, which results in improved cardiovascular strength. Nitric oxide production, blood flow to the brain, and other such things are also positively impacted.

Make sure that when the weather allows, you get outside and take advantage of the natural sunlight. There is no substitute for the physical and psychological benefits that come from exposure to full spectrum sunlight.

In the winter, I still run, but I'll do it on a Woodway treadmill. These are my favorite types of treadmills because they're made from a wood that's easy on the joints and feels like a more natural running surface.

If it's the winter time and I've gotten my run in, but I haven't had much exposure to sunlight, occasionally I'll use my SunTouchPlus device, by NatureBright. This is a blue light box. I keep it next to the standing desk, and I usually turn it on about 2 pm, while I work. I'll have it on for about 20 to 60 minutes. Blue lights such as these have been shown to combat some of the predispositions that some of us have to low mood, low energy, and seasonal affective disorder.

THE DREAMSPA

Scientifically, light is a nutrient for the body. Just as plants need sunlight to thrive, humans need light to maintain health and wellbeing. Human cells are activated by particular frequencies and wavelengths of light absorbed as photons.

Albert Einstein received the Nobel Prize and changed the course of physics for his incredible discovery on how photons, fundamental particles of light, interact with matter, the Photo-Electric Effect.

His discovery laid the groundwork for our understanding of the vital role light plays in our biology.

Human cells are activated by fundamental particles of light called photons.

At the cellular level, photons influence mitochondria to produce energy.

The photons produced by the DreamSpa are absorbed by the body through the skin and acupuncture points. The fiber optic properties of connective tissue conduct the light throughout the body.

Cells in the human body go through approximately 100,000 chemical reactions per second. These are not random events, but "a highly controlled process in

which the light acts as the communicator that makes the reactions happen at the right moment and in the right place."

In contrast to the chaotic light produced, for example, by an electric light bulb, biophotonic waves are "coherent" which allows them to be modulated and act as information carriers.

The DreamSpa's ™ unique programs deliver bio-active light directly to the cells promoting and stimulating:

- ATP (energy) production
- Increased blood flow
- Enhanced oxygen and nutrient delivery
- Cellular repair and regeneration
- Collagen production leading to wrinkle reduction

The DreamSpa stimulates cellular repair and regeneration, recharging the body like a battery and rebooting the brain.

The DreamSpa system is a comprehensive and natural solution to the effects of aging and stress: low energy, fatigue, poor sleep, stress, moodiness, brain fog, aches & pain, as well as the physical signs of aging: fine lines, wrinkles & hair loss.

It is based on over 30 years of research by NASA, NIH, universities and researchers around the world in the fields of Biophotonics, Bioenergetics, Tissue Optics, Cellular Communication, Phototherapy, Stress Management and Anti-Aging.

I use my DreamSpa 3-4 times a week, typically while meditating.

Save 10% on the DreamSpa by entering discount code "biohacks" at www.lighthealthresearch.com during checkout.

THE TRUTH ABOUT TANNING BEDS

Also in the wintertime, I will often use a natural tanning bed once or twice a week. When it comes to the actual science linking use of tanning beds and cancer, there's a lot of smoke and little fire.

The most commonly referenced statistic is that tanning bed use increases melanoma risk by 75%. This statistic is based on data pooled from a number of studies, the strongest of which followed 100,000 women over 8 years.

So what does a 75% increase really mean? The study "found that less than three-tenths of 1 percent who tanned frequently developed melanoma while less than two-tenths of 1 percent who didn't tan developed melanoma."

We are talking about 1/10th of a percentage difference between the tanning group and the non-tanning group.

Even still that's only a 55% increase. To get the figure up to the 75%, commonly referenced in the mainstream media, the reporters pooled the data from that study with a number of others. They pooled with studies that were conducted in different labs, by different scientists, using different methodologies, sample sizes, and durations. Lumping all of the studies together and referring only to the percentage difference is not only deceptive, it's bad science.

A number of other studies have suggested the overall health benefit of improved vitamin D status may be more important than the marginally (one tenth of one percent) increased risk of skin cancer.

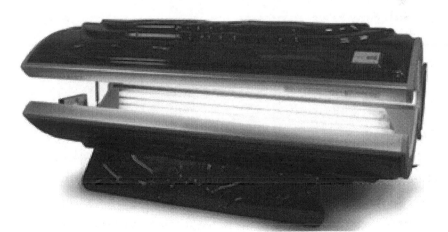

When using a tanning bed, look for one with:

- Greater than 5% UVB
- Low pressure bulbs (if they don't have low pressure bulbs high pressure is acceptable)
- Proactive bulb replacement program (newer bulbs replaced based on hours, not when they burn out)

UVLRX ULTRAVIOLET BLOOD IRRADIATION

"This is either going to be made illegal and seen in a similar light to blood doping, or it's going to be used by every professional sports team, endurance athlete, and Olympian within the next 20 years," I said to Dr. Jack Dybis at the IVME Hydration Clinic in Chicago.

I was experimenting with a new intravenous light therapy device called the UVLrx.

Reclined in a white, leather chair, I had a patented IV needle emitting ultraviolet light directly into the largest vein in my right forearm.

Blood irradiation therapy has been used in clinical settings since 1981. Most of the research surrounding its benefits has been conducted in Germany, Russia, and China.

It's a procedure in which the blood is exposed to low-level red (often laser) light for therapeutic purposes, most often to help clients with cardiovascular abnormalities.

More recent research has shown blood irradiation therapy to have wide-ranging therapeutic benefits including increased oxygen uptake and improved oxygen utilization in the cells.

This also provides a cleansing of the blood through the elimination of bacterial, viral, mold, fungal and other pathogenic organisms. Blood pathogens are five times more sensitive to photonic light than human cells. So we are able to expose a blood sample to UV light, removing many of these harmful organisms, without any detrimental impact to our own cells. Benefits of blood irradiation include, but are not limited to, the following:

- Increased oxygen uptake
- Improved oxygen utilization
  Cleansing of the blood
- Decreased inflammation
- Improved immune response
- Upgraded metabolism or uric acid, cholesterol, and glucose
- Increased ATP production
- Reduced oxidative stress
- Accelerated recovery from injuries
- Improved circulation
- Elevated production of red blood cells

The list above points out that blood irradiation therapy reduces inflammation. In addition to that, post-blood irradiation therapy patients exhibit lower levels of inflammation like CRP (C-reactive protein), Interleukin-6 (IL-6), and other inflammatory cytokines. UV light upregulates ATP production. Cytochrome C-oxidase (CCO) is an enzyme in our mitochondria, which utilizes light photons to increase ATP energy production and reduce oxidative stress in our bodies. By exposing our blood to UV light, a cascade of mitochondria and intracellular effects are triggered. This includes increased levels of cytochrome c-oxidase which leads to improved tissue repair and lower levels of oxidation.

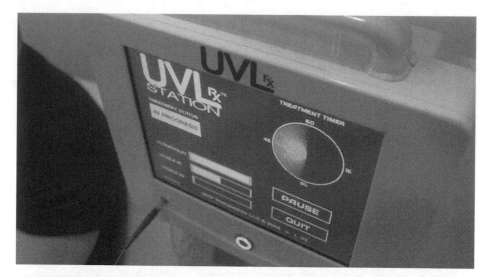

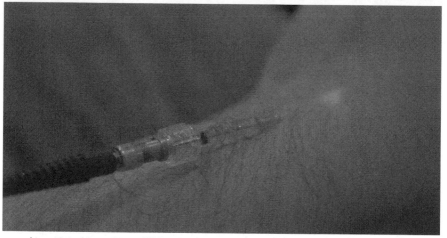

Associated benefits of UVLrx Ultraviolet Blood Irradiation include decreased inflammation, improved circulation and increased immune response.

A number of studies have shown that irradiation of the blood has resulted in improvements in lipids, cholesterol levels, and blood sugar levels as well as reduced platelet aggregation (a term for undesirable "stickiness" of the blood). In sports medicine, it has been shown to increase exercise times and capacity along with delayed onset of fatigue and improvements in post-exercise biomarkers, including creatine kinase and lactic acid.

A German study, published in 2008, found that athletes were able to increase exercise performance by over 20% in a number of different categories from just 10 days of blood irradiation. What's really cool is that the results lasted for 16 weeks after the cessation of treatment.

I've utilized this technology as part of an advanced program with a number of sports and performance-based clients. In doing so, we are often able to produce results comparable to 4 to 6 months of rigorous training in less than 30 days.

More specifically, global studies are underway to investigate the UVLrx's efficacy in treating the following conditions:

- Dengue Fever
- Tuberculosis
- Sepsis
- Renal Disease
- Post-Surgical Recovery
- Non-Healing Wounds
- Sports-Related Injuries
- Auto Immune Disorders
- Lyme Disease
- Adjunctive Care for Cancer
- HIV and Hepatitis C
- Nosocomial Infections
- Epstein-Barr Virus
- General Inflammation

Blood irradiation therapy has been used to help athletes heal faster from acute injuries and help my clients overcome nagging, treatment resistant aches and pains.

Recently, a Chicago Cubs player, who I was asked not to name, incurred a serious injury during one of their games. He was concerned that he would be out for 6 to 8 weeks. He used the UVLrx machine on the same day as his injury in order to reduce inflammation and to upgrade his body's ability to repair damaged tissues. The next day, he woke up with a markedly improved functional range of motion and said that he "felt 10 years younger."

The anecdotal evidence supporting the efficacy of the UVLrx machine and the blood irradiation therapy for a broad range of health issues and performance enhancement is abundant. While I talked with Dr. Jack Dybis, the Chicago trauma surgeon who runs the clinic, and his director of nursing, Gina, they shared story after story of how this technology was changing people's lives and helping them to overcome conditions which were previously unresponsive to other therapeutic interventions.

Blood irradiation therapy as a treatment modality was limited until very recently. This was because a byproduct of the red laser light was heat. This forced practitioners to first remove the blood from the body, one quart at a time, expose it to the ultraviolet light, and then inject that quart of blood back into the body. It was a long, tedious process with many redundancies. The UVlrx intravascular light therapy system has changed the game in this regard. It is the first medical device that allows us to administer light therapy intravenously without producing the heat which can damage surrounding tissues.

Early adopters of the UVlrx have been individuals who suffered from Lyme disease and related coinfections. We are now starting to see an explosion in its use as a healing tool and performance enhancer for professional athletes and weekend warriors. Healthy individuals using the UVlrx report increased energy, a decrease in aches and pains, and elevated cognitive functions.

As my forearm radiated a soft, iridescent red glow, I listened as Dr. Dybis shared stories about how the machine had helped them and dozens of other patients. Most recently, both had incurred injuries that they couldn't seem to shake within 1-2 treatments on the UVLrx, Dr. Dybis' knee was no longer bothering him, and Gina's thumb felt good as new. As an added bonus, Gina noticed that during her running workouts was much easier. She was admittedly a bad runner, but after her treatment, she noticed that rather than breathing heavy and feeling achy from the very beginning of her workout, her run felt easier and her breathing more effortless.

They told me stories about patients with chronic Lyme disease who, after several treatments with the UVLrx, suddenly displayed the stereotypical bullseye rash years after being bit by the tick. One patient was a woman who had spent the last 21 years suffering from chronic fatigue, achy muscles and joints, brain fog, digestive issues, depression, and a host of other debilitating health issues. Nine years ago, her son was born, and he came into the world covered with bullseye rashes. Then recently, after 21 years of experiencing a consistent and debilitating degradation in her health, she finally went to see Dr. Dietrich Klinghardt, and this was one last act in desperation to reclaim her life.

Klin Med (Mosk). 2009;87(6):22-5.

[Effect of intravenous laser blood irradiation on endothelial dysfunction in patients with hypertensive disease].

[Article in Russian]
Burduli NM, Aleksandrova OM.

Abstract
The aim of this work was to study effect of intravenous laser blood irradiation (ILBI) on endothelial dysfunction in 120 patients (mean age 53.4 +/- 1.3 yr) with grade I-II hypertensive disease (HD) allocated to 2 groups. Traditional drug therapy given to patients of control group was supplemented by ILBI using a Mulat laser therapy device in the study group. Endothelial function was evaluated from the total plasma concentration of stable NO_x metabolites, nitrates (NO_3-), nitrites (NO_2-), and Willebrand's factor. HD patients were found to have elevated activity of the Willebrand factor and show 3 types of response of the NO generating system: (1) decreased NO synthesis, (2) lack of its changes, and (3) increased NO synthesis. NO production in HD patients negatively correlated with systolic ($r = -0.59$) and diastolic ($r = -0.64$) arterial pressure (AP) which suggests the relationship between decreased NO production and elevated AP. Inclusion of ILBI in the therapy of HD resulted in a significant decrease of Willebrand's factor activity and normalization of the NO level regardless of its initial value.

This woman began treatment with Dr. Klinghardt in the state of Washington. She then returned back to Chicago and set up 3 weeks of one-hour daily treatments with the UVLrx. After her sixth or seventh consecutive session, she too developed a bullseye rash in the exact location she remembered being bitten by a tick 21 years earlier. With the help of a comprehensive Lyme protocol over the following months, she was able to get her life back.

They continued on with more stories. Some were about professional athletes, high-level executives, and entrepreneurs who were leveraging this technology to gain an advantage over their competition and optimize performance. As I listened, I noticed something strange was happening. At first it was subtle, but then it quickly became undeniable that I was becoming lightheaded and a little spacey.

The first half-hour of the treatment, I felt like my mental clarity was perceptively improving. Yet, at this moment, minutes after the light had changed to a different wavelength (which occurs around the 30 minute mark), I found myself having a little trouble concentrating. It was almost like what you experience at a high altitude or when you hyperventilate. "Is that normal?" I asked Gina. She said that this was a very common response. It happened to her and the doctor as well. It's suspected that this has to do with increased oxygen uptake and improved oxygen utilization in the body. Symptomatically, this has many commonalities with the feelings we experience when we over-breathe.

After my treatment, I scheduled an appointment for the same time the following week. Later on, the mild lightheadedness dispelled, and the feeling was replaced with a discernible improvement in word recall and verbal fluency along with a surprising amount of energy, regardless of my being up since 5 a.m. and having only slept a few hours. I stayed up working that night until 12 a.m. This made for an uncharacteristically long day, given my sleep deficit. Even more noticeable was that seemingly, my cognition and mental clarity were more resilient to my lack of adequate sleep, and I felt smarter.

There are literally dozens of these types of advanced biohacks that can be used in strategic combinations to produce unparalleled advancements in energy, focus, and performance. The limiting factor is often our own resistance to change. Dr. Dybis shared with me a story about a Dr. Erich Muhe. He was the first German physician to perform the laparoscopic cholecystectomy. This is a minimally invasive surgical procedure for removing the gallbladder.

For years, Muhe was ridiculed, criticized, and ostracized by the German surgical community. Despite nearly 100 successful surgeries and overwhelming anecdotal support, his article about the first laparoscopic cholecystectomy was rejected by the American Journal of Surgery in 1990. It wasn't until six years later that Muhe's work was recognized as one of the greatest original achievements of German medicine in recent history. He received the German Surgical Society Congress Anniversary Award.

Most people are resistant to change, even when confronted with overwhelming evidence against the status quo. It took six years for one of the greatest medical achievements in recent history to be recognized and accepted by other medical doctors. That timeline is commonly 5-10 times longer when it comes to acceptance and adoption by the general public. A number of the strategies in this guide fall into that category. Together we represent the leading edge in the advancement of our human potential. Stay curious, keep experimenting, and embrace intelligent change.

HYDRATION, OXYGENATION, & LIGHT BIOHACKS

This is not an all-inclusive summary from this section but will help you get started until you are able to explore in more detail.

The One Thing for Hydration is: Install a reverse osmosis water filtration system and then drink 70% of your current body weight in ounces of water away from meals (to prevent diluting stomach acids and digestive enzymes). Add back important trace minerals removed via RO.

The One Thing for Oxygen is: Practice deep, diaphragmatic breathing through the nose until this becomes your default breathing pattern. Suggested times to practice are during your morning steady state jog and meditation.

The One Thing for Light is: Get at least 20 minutes of sunlight per day. Expose both your eyes and your skin - eyes being the most important. Do this as close to the time you first wake up as possible.

Biohack #1: Commercial water filters do not remove fluoride. This includes many of the most popular brands, like Brita, PUR, and

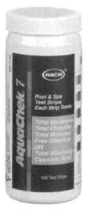

Culligan. The same is true for filtered bottled water, and we now know that filtered bottled water also exposes us to a number of chemical toxins beyond the widely recognized Bisphenol A (BPA). Get a reverse osmosis water filter or structured water system.

Other strategies to consider to improve your water quality and hydration:

– Check your water quality using *AquaCheck test strips*

- *Reverse Osmosis Water Filter*
- *ConcenTrace Trace Mineral Drops* (or Good State-Liquid Ionic Trace Minerals) for Water filtered via reverse osmosis
- *Rainshowr Bath-3000 KDR Crystal Water Filter Ball*
- *Shower Filter*
- *Natural Action Technologies Shower Head:* (www.naturalactiontechnologies.com)
- *Berkey KDSF*
- *Rainshower CQ-1000-MS Shower Filter*
- *Deluxe Showerwise Shower Filtration System*
- *Kangen SD501 Water Machine:* (www.biohackingsecrets.com/kangen)
- Find a local spring likely to have structured water: (www.findaspring.com)
- *Waterwise 9000 Countertop Distiller:* Be sure to add back beneficial trace minerals.
- *Berkey BK4X2-BB Big Berkey Drinking Water Filtration System*
- *Dr. Patrick Flanagan's MegaHydrate:* Dr. Patrick Flanagan holds advanced degrees in chemistry, nanotechnology, biosciences and medicine, and was named Scientist of the Year in 1997 by the International Association for New Science. MegaHydrate was created as a way to boost cellular hydration by reducing the surface tension of water within the body, essentially making the water in and between our cells easier to absorb. The idea is that with optimal hydration and surface tension of water we are able to more efficiently eliminate toxins and metabolic by-products on the most basic level. Add to this a potential increase in the delivery of important nutrients and you have a recipe for healthier cells and a healthier body. In a state of dehydration, body cells cannot assimilate nutrients and remove waste and relief pain from conditions like arthritis or fibromyalgia.

- *Book: "The Hidden Messages in Water"* by Masaru Emoto
- *Book: "The Fourth Phase of Water"* by Gerald Pollack
- *Vitabath Vita-c-bath Effervescent Vitamin C Dechlorination, 1000 mg, 100 Tablets*
- *Crystal Springs "Purified" Water Delivery:* Reverse osmosis, distilled, or both (www.crystalspringswaterslo.com)
- *Mountain Valley Spring Water:* Available in glass bottles and bubblers delivered to your home. (www.mountainvalleyspring.com)
- *Vitalizer Plus Hexagonal Oxygen Water Maker:* (www.vitalizerplus.com)
- Another high quality spring water is *Palomar:* (www.palomarwater.com).
- *Vinturi Essential Wine Aerator* (for structuring water via vortexing, also adds oxygen)

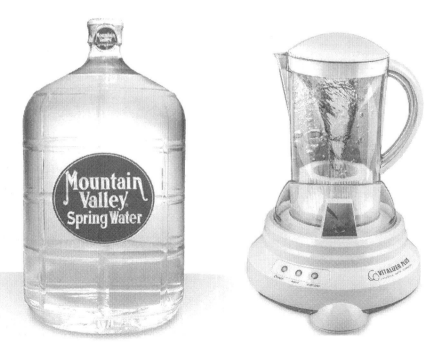

- *Natural Action Technologies Portable Structured Water Device* (www.naturalactiontechnologies.com)
- *Minerals and Electrolytes:* Healthy electrolyte status is associated with improved nerve signaling, muscle firing, and energy production in the body. Bioelectricity was first discovered in 1789 when Italian physicist Luigi Galvani used a charged metal scalpel to induce muscle contraction in the leg of a dead frog leg by touching the sciatic nerve. The muscle fired as if the frog were still alive. Electricity is a driving force behind many biological systems in the body and initiates muscle movement. Maintain healthy electrolyte status by adding pink Himalayan salt to your meals (this is different than iodized table salt which is associated with health risks). If you are prone to heavy sweating, physically active, or dealing with certain health issues it may be wise to supplement

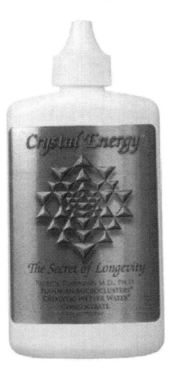

with buffered electrolyte salts, Schuessler cell salts, Crystal Energy (product invented by Dr. Patrick Flanagan after studying the energizing and longevity properties of Hunza water), magnesium, potassium, and/or add trace minerals to your drinking water.

- *The Original Dr. Hayashi Hydrogen Rich Water Stick:* Dr. H. Hayashi, a Cardiovascular Surgeon from Japan, developed a hydrogen-producing mineral stick, more commonly referred to as the Hydrogen Rich Water Stick. The Hydrogen Rich Water Sticks are backed by 25 years of clinical research and increase the antioxidant potential of your water offering superior hydration and energy.

- *Collagen Generators (BioSil, Great Lakes Gelatin, bone broth from grass-fed cows, Neocel Super Collagen + C Type 1 & 3, CellFood Essential Silica):* Collagen is the most commonly found protein in our skin, muscles and tendons. It works synergistically with water, especially structured water, to transmit electrical signals and nerve impulses throughout the body. Starting at age 21, collagen diminishes 1% per year. By age 30, the signs become visible and often felt. Replenishing collagen via supplementation and diet can improve the body's energetic systems and cellular communication. Many chronic infections can also sequester collagen for their own uses. For example, Lyme disease feeds on collagen thus accelerating this biological decline. That's another reason it is important to address any infections that will interfere with optimal energy production and cellular signaling.

Biohack #2: Practice the Wim Hof Method and deep diaphragmic breathing through the nose. Other strategies and biohacks to consider to improve your breathing and oxygen status, along with those listed earlier in this section, are:

- *Hyperbaric oxygen therapy (HBOT):* the medical use of oxygen at a level higher than atmospheric pressure. The equipment required consists of a pressure chamber, which may be of rigid or flexible construction, and a means of delivering 100% oxygen.
- *Pulse Oxometer:* Determine your SpO2 (blood oxygen saturation levels) and pulse rate in seconds.
- *Alcohol-Free ChlorOxygen:* Builds red blood cells. Increases hemoglobins capacity to capture oxygen in the lungs and distribute it throughout the body. Helpful in high altitude situations.

Supports pregnancy by maintaining healthy hemotocrit levels. Acts as an intestinal deodorizer and offers liver protection.

- *Floradix Floravital Yeast Free Iron and Herbs:* Iron deficiency is the leading cause of fatigue among women between the time of menstruation and menopause (it is estimated that up to 26% of reproductive aged women are iron deficient). Iron is an essential element for the body. It combines with copper and protein to make hemoglobin, a major component of red blood cells which transports oxygen from the lungs to all the tissues of the body. Iron is also needed throughout the body for adenosine triphosphate production (ATP). ATP is required for cellular energy and proper cell function. When iron is low, ATP production drops and energy levels decrease as a result. Most iron supplements can cause GI distress and constipation. I use Floradix with my clients, when appropriate, and it works without these unwanted side effects.

- *World Organics Chlorophyll Supplement:* Helps increase the amount of oxygen available to cells. It supports the production of red blood cells and their blood-oxygen carrying capacity.

- *Chlorophyllin:* Chlorophyllin, a water-soluble derivative of chlorophyll, has antioxidant properties that protect our DNA and improve tissue oxygenation. It also protects our mitochondria by reducing oxidative stress. And for the folks who put MCTs in their coffee, and fear mycotoxic molds, Chlorophyllin may also minimize the effects of dietary exposure to aflatoxin (a naturally occurring mycotoxin), by reducing its bioavailability.

Biohack #3: Get as much natural sunlight to your eyes and exposed skin daily as you can. If you live in an area with cold winters or low levels of sunlight, take frequent vacations to sunny places and consider moving. I'm looking at places in Santa Monica, Malibu, San Diego, and Miami for our future biohacking HQ.

Biohack #4: Light-hacking technologies I utilize and recommend to clients are:

- Expose your eyes to a few minutes of natural sunlight as soon as you wake up.
- Spend time throughout the day without glasses, contacts, or sunglasses to allow your intrinsically photosensitive retinal ganglion cells to absorb all the important wavelengths of natural light and optimize your circadian rhythms.
- Practice *dry skin brushing* before you shower or bathe and a loofah in the bath to remove dead skin cells and prep your body's largest solar panel to absorb photonic light.
- Use a *natural coconut-based soap or black african soap* as opposed to products with chemicals, fragrances, and unnatural additives that can interfere with these processes. Only wash the "important" areas to prevent removing your skin's natural oils

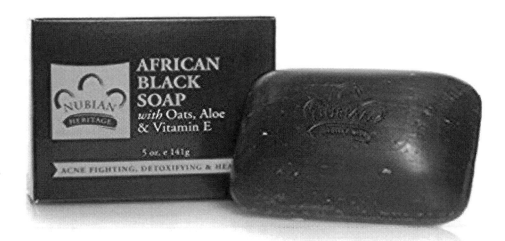

which are necessary to absorb and synthesize vitamin D. Many clients and physicians rave about Ann Marie Gianni's edible organic cosmetic line available at www.annmariegianni.com

- *Look towards the sun* (about 15-20 degrees off as to not stare directly at it) for 5-30 minutes at least once daily. You can do this during your outdoor exercise or any other activity you can integrate.
- Watch the sunrise and sunset whenever you can.
- Turn off electronics 1-3 hours before bed
- *Dim your lights at night.* Use candles as opposed to electric lights to illuminate your home.
- If you live in an area away from the equator with cooler winters and sub-optimal sunlight, take frequent vacations, use natural tanning beds with UVB greater than 5%, and consider relocation.
- *Use full spectrum infrared saunas often.* I recommend at least once a week for healthy clients in areas with lower levels of natural sunlight and more frequently for clients with compromised energy or health-related challenges.
- *Pro Biomat 7000MX (infrared)*
- *TDP Far Infrared Heat Lamp*
- *Philips HF3520 sunrise simulation wake up light*
- *Beurer IL50 Infrared heat lamp*
- *Sunlighten mPULSE cONQUER Infrared Sauna*
- *VieLIGHT 655 Prime Intranasal Light Therapy Device*
- *Valkee Human Charger*
- *Naturebright SuntouchPlus Blue Light*
- *Low blue light nightlights*
- *F.lux* (blue light blocking software for laptops and computers)
- *Gunnar blue-light blocking glasses*
- *The Mercola Vitality Elite Tanning Bed* (contains UVA, UVB, infrared, red, and blue light)

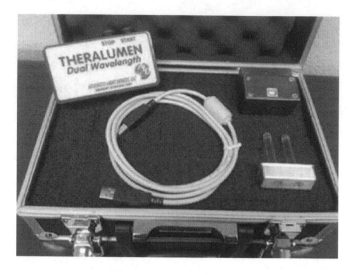

- *Philips 415836 Heat Lamp 250-Watt R40 Flood Infrared Light Bulb:* These are an inexpensive way to get infrared light and increase your bioelectric conductivity. Especially beneficial during low light winter months. I have two and use them when I'm working, getting out of the shower, meditating, or doing PEMF therapy.
- *Theralumen Immune Laser:*
  (www.biohackingsecrets.com/theralumen)
- *SpectraMite Light Therapy Device:* This system utilizes multiple frequency and color combinations to improve immune function and encourage healing mechanisms in the body. Based on NASA research over the past 20 years.
- *The Quantlet:* The QUANTLET, which looks much like a large watch, is worn around the wrist. It uses applied science and engineering to harness light and cold to improve human performance, which are both safe and effective mechanisms with no known side effects. In recent studies, photobiomodulation and thermoregulation have both demonstrated increases in exercise

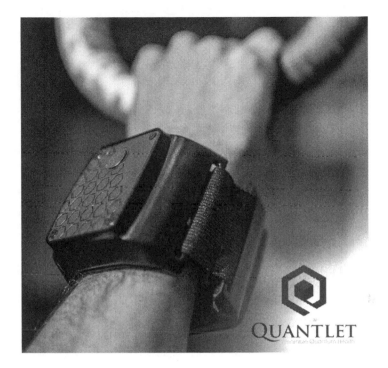

capacity, as well as improved cellular metabolism and, in some cases, even reduced levels of inflammation (www.thequantlet.com/biohacks)

– *GDV (Gas Discharge Visualization) Bio-Well Camera:* Developed by Gas Dr. Konstantin Korotkov, this camera provides a rapid method of assessment for monitoring the functional state of the organism during treatment and rehabilitation, for preventing the side effects of various therapies, for determining additional indications for allopathic, non-drug, and homeopathic treatment methods, and providing a more objective assessment of their effects (www.gdvcamera.com).

– *Book: "Life on the Edge"* by John Joe McFadden and Jim Al-Khalili

– *Book: "Light in Shaping Life"* by Roeland Van Wijk

– *Website:* www.MyLightTherapy.com

MINDSET & HABITS

"You will never change your life until you change something you do daily."

- John C. Maxwell

One of my clients Jill was a consultant. She worked 70 to 80 hours a week for close to a decade. Jill had become so unhappy at work that she would sneak off into empty conference rooms five or six times a day to cry. Obviously, someone can't be miserable for 70 to 80+ hours a week and be healthy.

Finally, Jill's body gave her no choice but to reevaluate her situation. She hit a wall and her body shut down. She was exhausted and burnt out. Jill and I started with the foundational elements she needed to reclaim her energy and wellness. But to only address the physical would be neglecting perhaps the biggest culprit responsible for Jill's current state of health. We had to address her psychology and patterns of thinking.

Growing up, Jill was an only child. Her parents taught her that play only got in the way of more worthy and admirable intellectual pursuits. They gave her attention and praise when she got good grades and did good schoolwork. So Jill was taught that by doing work she would get love and connection. By frowning upon games and leisure, her parents reinforced play as a juvenile and unproductive use of one's time.

My job was to help Jill relearn how to play. It's a skill we all have. Many of us have just repressed it for so long that it takes a little more effort to resurrect. I encouraged Jill and her husband Chris to play together. Make love. Give each other massages. Play pranks and joke around.

I told her she was not allowed to listen to books or podcasts about business, marketing, or anything non-fiction; especially, if it was related to personal development. She could, however, watch funny movies, stand up comedy, and listen to fiction audiobooks for enjoyment. We had to structurally reintegrate play into her daily life.

At first Jill had a hard time letting go. She was so focused on productivity, achievement, and progress that she was suffocating her inner child. Ironically, her mentality was the very thing holding her back. Activity cannot be confused with progress.

After about a month, I started seeing a shift. Her and Chris were going out together again. She messaged me ecstatic one Friday night after they were headed home from Sky High Sports in Niles, IL. "Trampolining was *awesome!!* I could go there everyday." They'd had the time of their lives at one of those places where the entire floor is one giant trampoline. She even wore her heart rate monitor.

A few days later, I sent her one of my favorite quotes from Dr. Wayne Dyer, "One of the most responsible things you can do as an adult is to become more of a child."

She responded, "Yes :) I'm going to incorporate at least one child-like thing today :)"

To which I replied, "Just don't go poopin' your pants and blaming it on me :)"

A few hours later, I received another message from Jill, "I definitely just colored this :)"

It was accompanied by the picture she'd colored of a red puppy, flowers, and butterflies. She was finally getting it.

DAILY ROUTINES TO UPGRADE YOUR LIFE

We can't think our way into new actions. We have to act our way into new thinking.

If you wait to take action based on the way you are feeling, you may be waiting for a really long time. Regardless of what's going on in your head, or what you feel like doing, you want to have smart feet, that just know what direction to walk in no matter what.

Dr. BJ Fogg, a PhD from Stanford University, has found that designing for behavioral change is a systematic process. It's not guesswork. Fogg has created a universal method for this, which involves three steps:

1. *Get Specific:* You have to decide what behavior you want by translating your desired goal or outcome into a specific behavior.

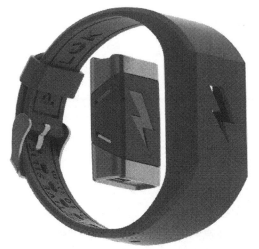

The Pavlok gives you a mild zap when you engage in an unwanted habit, training your brain to stop liking, and therefore engaging in, the habit.

2. *Make It Easy:* Think about how you can make the behavior easy to do because if it takes too long, or it's too complicated, you're not going to follow through long-term. Simplicity changes behavior.

3. *Trigger the Behavior:* You want to link the desired behavioral change to another action event or time.

The Pavlok gives you a mild zap when you engage in an unwanted habit, training your brain to stop liking, and therefore engaging in, the habit. Thousands of people have used it to quit smoking, nail-biting, and kick unhealthy eating to the curb.

One of the ways that I challenge my clients (www.BioHackingSecrets.com/coaching) to integrate more movement into their routine is to have a chin-up bar in their bathroom doorway. Each time they brush their teeth, they do one pull-up. I do have clients who can't do a pull-up, so they do a push-up or a bodyweight squat. The only rule is that they have to do at least one. They can do more, but they have to do at least one pull-up, push-up, or bodyweight squat, and in some cases, I have them do all three.

Another option is to set a recurring alarm on your Smartphone. When that alarm goes off, it's time for you to drop everything you're doing and take action on the linked behavior. So, if you need to be in bed by 11 pm, you might set a recurring alarm that goes off every day at 10 pm. When that alarm goes off, you know that you need to shutdown your computer and electronics in order to start winding down for bed.

The point is to get clear about what will prompt your desired behavior. Some of these triggers are natural and some you will have to design. No new behavior is going to occur consistently without a trigger.

I recommend creating a Daily Action Plan (DAP) where you have the list of daily habits, in chronological orders, that will help you achieve

24 HOUR DAILY ACTION PLAN (DAP)

	Hours	I Plan To...
MORNING	5 AM	
	6 AM	
	7 AM	
	8 AM	
	9 AM	
NOON	10 AM	
	11 AM	
	12 PM	
	1 PM	
AFTERNOON	2 PM	
	3 PM	
	4 PM	
	5 PM	
EVENING	6 PM	
	7 PM	
	8 PM	
	9 PM	
NIGHT	10 PM	
	11 PM	
	12 AM	
	1 AM	
	2 AM	
	3 AM	
	4 AM	

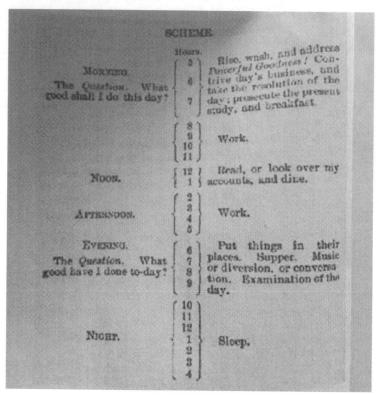

Example of Benjamin Franklin's ideal daily routine

your goals. Write it down. Keep it somewhere you can access it anytime and modify it easily.

On Tuesday, November 10, 2015, I wrote down some of the specific things I did that day. Feel free to write down any of these that would be relevant or helpful in your routine...

At 6:00 am, I woke up. One of the things I have been working on is not hitting snooze as much when my alarm clock goes off.

I make sure that I leave my phone set to airplane mode so that I'm not tempted to check texts or emails until the important stuff is done. Putting your phone in airplane mode while you sleep exposes you to less electrosmog (EMFs) during the night. I also stay away from my computer.

I opened up my windows to let some sun in, and I made my bed.

I went into the kitchen and filled one 12-ounce glass with my favorite spring water that I have delivered every week. I ran the spring water through a device to make the water particles smaller and lower the water's surface tension, so it could be more easily absorbed. If you've ever drank water and felt it uncomfortably sloshing around in your belly, this is a common unwanted side effect of low-quality, clustered water. Sometimes, when traveling, I'll substitute a bottle of Penta Ultra Purified Bottled Water. Penta water is purified in a 13-step, 11-hour process that provides advanced hydration. Penta's process involves spinning the water under high speed and pressure (cavitation) to produce smaller, more readily absorbed water droplets.

I drank that glass of water and repeated the process above, filling up a second 12-ounce glass. I then ozonated this structured spring water, for 5 to 15 minutes, to add oxygen. I let my ozonator run while I got

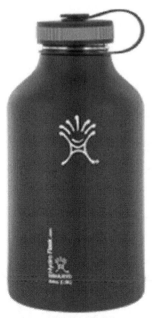

Hydro Flask

ready. Many ozonators use low grade materials made from chemicals which then leech into your water. I recommend investing in a quality ozonator. Pathogens and cancers are anaerobic (living without air). O3 aids their elimination by oxidation and speeds detoxification. Consuming O3 water flushes pathogens, wastes and toxins from your system. When using a pulse oxometer, you can literally watch your blood oxygen saturation levels rise in the minutes following the consumption of ozonated water. I use the Sota Water Ozonator available at www.Sota.com.

Next, I went into the bathroom to fill up my Hydro Flask, 64-Oz water bottle with clean, 9.5 pH, structured, ionized water from my Kangen machine. I then added some trace minerals, electrolytes, and other hydration and oxygenation cofactors to the water. This sounds fancy and complicated but it literally takes a matter of seconds.

At this point in my morning routine, I will sometimes check biomarkers like body temperature, blood pressure, fasting glucose, heart rate, blood oxygenation, etc. Today I only checked blood oxygen saturation with my pulse oxometer. It registered at 99%.

I then did a couple of pull-ups and pushups as I walked into the bathroom to brush my teeth and get ready.

I turned on my Beurer infrared light and took all of my empty-stomach vitamins. There have been several studies linking oral hygiene to increased longevity, so I've been using a tongue cleaner, flossing with floss picks, and brushing my teeth with an electronic toothbrush.

Sometimes when I'm getting ready, I'll also put on some good music to get me fired up and moving. I don't get to listen to music as much as I'd like during the day, so it's fun to check out some of the new music that's been released that week while I get ready. I also have playlists that I can count on to get me emotionally juiced if it's a slow morning.

I dry brushed my skin to remove dead skin cells, improve circulation, and stimulate lymphatic drainage. This improves the appearance of skin, enhances detoxification, and increases absorption of light.

Then, I jumped in the shower. I started with the water really hot to loosen up. Some days I also do some light stretching. This helps to get the body oxygenated.

I finished my shower turning the water as cold as it can go. I'm kind of a baby about the cold - especially in Chicago winters, but I do it anyway. I still have to get myself psyched up every single time. The greatest habit is doing the things you know you should, even when you don't feel like it. I usually time it by doing one cycle of Wim Hof for 35 deep breaths. If I'm feeling good, I'll exhale after my last breath and do a static breath hold as long as I can. For longer bouts of cold thermogenesis (CT) I'll add cold showers at the gym after the sauna, ice baths at the Chicago Recovery Room (or my bathtub), cryotherapy at the Chicago Cryo Spa, or a cold plunge in Lake Michigan when the water is cold (40-55 degrees Fahrenheit) but the air is tolerable.

After my shower, I let myself air dry (I do this on days when I'm not pressed for time). While I got ready, I turned on a couple infrared heating lamps and a high output fluorescent bulb that emits UVB rays. Our bodies produce vitamin D when ultraviolet B (UVB) rays interact with 7-dehydrocholesterol (7-DHC) present in the skin.

I'll then sometimes use the Heart Math emWave2 to get into coherence. Coherence is a state of synchronization between your heart, brain, and autonomic nervous system which has been proven to have numerous mental, emotional and physical benefits. I didn't on this particular day because I was a little short on time.

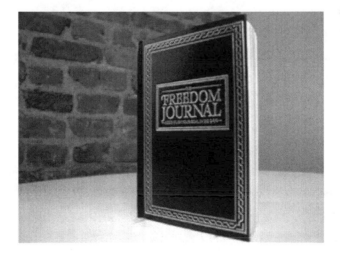

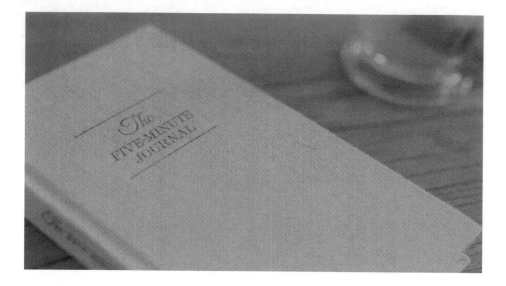

I used The Five Minute Journal. It only takes me two or three minutes to make an entry.

After that, I got to work on my most important task (MIT), which on this day was to work on this very guide. While I did this, I turned on my SunTouch Plus blue light for 20 minutes while I was working.

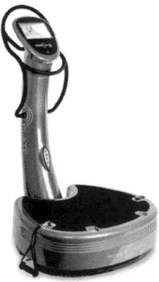

At noon, I jogged to the gym for a fast workout. While I did, I used the Power Plate Pro machine, which is a whole-body vibration machine.

At the gym, I did a dumbbell sequence with 50-pound dumbbells. During this workout, I incorporated overhead presses, deadlifts, squats, pushups, planks, and then I went for a 30-minute run, keeping my heart rate within my target heart rate zone. That would be 75% to 85% of my max heart rate.

After I finished that, I went for a 20-minute sauna in which I meditated. I also thought about some of my goals and spent some of my time visualizing and trying to feel those good feelings. I mentally planned the rest of my day by feeling and visualizing how I wanted the events to unfold.

After I got out of the sauna, I took another cold shower; but longer this time (2 full rounds of Wim Hof with the static breath hold). When I was through with that, it was around 1:00 or 1:30 and I still hadn't eaten. I usually fast until I feel hungry. That's, in part, for the epigenetic beneficial gene expression and, in part, a product of a busy schedule. My mind feels more sharp on an empty stomach. Sometimes, during my fast, I'll throw in one of my keto cocktails. This serves a few different functions. It's made up of a combination of exogenous ketones, pure Caprylic acid C-8 MCT oil, branched-chain amino acids, and a number of other things that increase the production of ketone bodies. Among other things, this helps me to fast longer without being too hungry or uncomfortable.

On this particular day, I didn't consume the cocktail. Instead, I had a huge salad with mixed organic greens, extra virgin olive oil, apple cider vinegar, Himalayan sea salt seasoning, some organic sprouted pumpkin seeds, and then I made a shake with a few different types of vegan protein powder. I also had some organic baby spinach, some organic frozen berries, and I threw in a bunch of other boosters for energy, detoxification, and overall health.

After eating, I took my vitamins that are supposed to be taken with food. These usually vary because there are some supplements that I take all of the time and some that I rotate in based on my goals, my workload, and my lifestyle. I will also adjust them based upon how I am responding to a supplement, either increasing or decreasing the dosage as needed.

Next, I went back to work. I worked for a few hours, and when I needed a break, I lay down on my biomat and did a guided meditation, listening to Brain.fm. Sometimes I use the Tooks headband. Not only does this headband have embedded headphones, but you can also put them over your eyes. So, it doubles as an eye mask.

For dinner, I had some wild-caught salmon, two big bunches of asparagus cooked in extra virgin olive oil with Himalayan sea salt, a couple of Dorot frozen garlic cubes, sweet potato, and an organic green apple. After dinner I got back to work. I'm always running Flux on my computer to block blue light, and then when it starts getting later, I'll throw on my Gunner intercept glasses. On this day it was especially important because I was on a tight deadline, so I wasn't always observing the "one hour before bedtime rule." Sometimes I was working right up until I had to go to bed. I am trying to get better at making sure that I'm allocating at least 7 ½ hours of time in bed.

When I'm getting ready to lie down in bed, I'll usually do "The Five Minute Journal" nighttime entry. I will take my empty-stomach vitamins, and I will open up a window to let my room cool off and facilitate the onset of sleep. Then, I use my David Delight Pro and put it in sleep mode, and I was finally in bed right around 11 pm.

This is just a glimpse of one of my typical days, except that on this particular day, I was able to do more things. Some days I do a lot less, and some days I'll do even more. It all depends on how much work I have to do and what I'm able to squeeze in.

Two of my mentors, Tony Robbins and Tim Ferriss, also adhere to regimented, daily routines. Some of the things that Tony includes in his morning routine are practices such as using the NuCalm device to manage his energy and stress, and he also relies on daily exercise, an ageless attitude, and blood tests. Let's look at some of the ways he integrates these things into his day...

Tony's exercise routine comes from Stu Mittleman's book, *"Slow Burn."* It's essentially a steady-state cardio workout. Stu recommends jogging within your target heart rate zone, which you can calculate by subtracting your age from 180. Robbins does not consume alcohol, caffeine, nicotine or any other recreational drugs. His diet consists of mostly green vegetables and wild-caught fish, and he makes slight adjustments to his diet based upon the results of his blood tests.

Robbins also prepares himself for a high energy day by doing three-minutes of a breathing exercise, followed by three minutes of gratitude, and three minutes of wishing good things for other people (blessings). When he's home, he also immerses himself in a cold plunge pool or his full-body cryotherapy tank.

Tim Ferriss recently did a podcast where he talked about the five things that he tries to do most mornings to set himself up and make the day a win. Those are:

- Make his bed
- Hanging
- Meditates
- Journal
- Makes tea

Tim either uses his Teeter gravity boots or Teeter inversion table to hang upside down. You can hook gravity boots up to a bathroom door-mounted pull-up bar if you would like to try this for yourself. Tim uses the The Five Minute Journal for his journaling, and, in some instances, he uses Morning Pages, which is an exercise that's used frequently by writers.

Some activities should be done every day, but some are impractical to do each day. The former pertains largely to certain workouts. When you're constructing your weekly workout schedule, it's important to keep in mind that you need to work all three energy systems and find a balance between strength, endurance, cardiovascular conditioning, and mobility.

Some of the specific areas you'll want to integrate into your weekly physical activity include:

- Strength/Resistance Training
- The Body by Science Method by Doug McGuff
- Occam's protocol from Tim Ferriss' book, *"Four Hour Body"*
- ARX Fit Omni machine (www.arxfit.com)
- The StrongLifts 5X5 program
- *PEMF Therapy:* I was introduced to a 49-year-old power lifter, with a 600 lb bench (in competition), who was able to add 100 lbs to his bench press in 3 weeks. Training in his basement, he

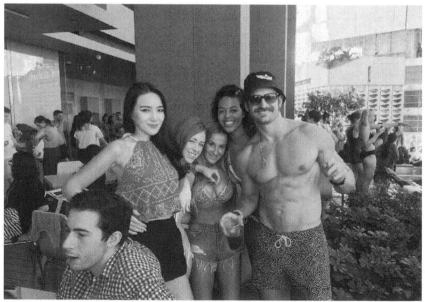

My client Cary poolside with some friends.

was repping 450 lbs "out of chains" for that 600 lbs lift. After 3 weeks of PEMF therapy, he was repping 550 lbs out of chains for the same number of reps. Many clients and professional athletes have achieved similar improvements in strength, endurance, and recoverability using our customized, performance-based protocols including PEMF (www.biohackingsecrets.com/coaching).

Mobility, breathing, soft tissue work:

- Deep tissue massage (aim for 30-60 minutes every week or every other week)
- Joe DeFranco's "Limber 11" (you can find this video on YouTube)
- TriggerPoint Roller or Rumble Roller
- LaCrosse ball or a TriggerPoint ball
- The Elevation Training Mask 2.0
- Boss Rutten 02 Trainer
- Vibrant Breathing
- The Wim Hof Method
- Bounding or Rebounding either on the floor, grass, or mini trampoline (rebounder)

Yoga & Flexibility:

- Budokon: Flow and Flexibility yoga DVD
- Stretching in the shower

Steady State Cardio (oxidative energy system, exercises > 2 minutes in duration):

- 20-30 minute outdoor jog in your target heart rate zone, verified by target heart rate monitor

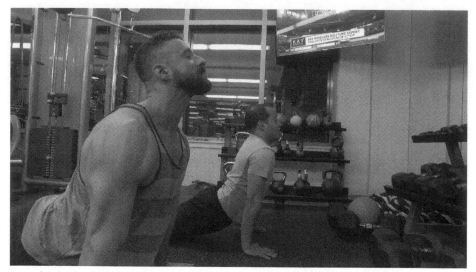

Apply the 80/20 rule to your physical activity, with 80% focused on building a bigger aerobic engine and improving mobility, flexibility and biomechanics.

- Garmin Forerunner 220
- Any Polar device
- StairMaster treadmill, Woodway treadmill
- Row machine, Concept 2
- Airdyne bike, Assault AirBike

Anaerobic System (glycolytic energy system, exercises ranging from 30-120 seconds):

- Make about 20% of your conditioning, high-intensity exercise
- Power Speed ENDURANCE by Brian Mackenzie
- Warrior Cardio by Martin Rooney
- Crossfit: Grace, Fran, Murph, Filthy Fifty, The Seven, 300 FY, OPT repeatability test, Annie, Angie, Fight Gone Bad, Helen, Cindy
- The extreme care about cardio 1&2 DVDs

- The Creatine Phosphate System (phosphagen system < 30 seconds in duration)
- Barbell powerlifting, squats, deadlifts, rows, snatch
- Bench press, overhead press, clean and press
- Floor to clavicle upright rows
- Weighted pull-ups
- Maximum-effort sprints (10-30 seconds in duration)

In a moment, I'll be providing you with a sample of how you might put together some of these different types of workouts and movement patterns into a weekly workout schedule. First, understand that we try to take every important area and apply the 80/20 rule the same way. With nutrition, for example, 80% of the food that you take into your body should be plants, and most of those plants should be vegetables, especially starting out. And you want most of those vegetables to be green.

Once you improve your insulin sensitivity, restore endocrine balance, and increase your metabolic rate, you can strategically incorporate more variety in your plant sources. For instance, you can start consuming things like starchy tubers (yams, squash, white potatoes), organic fruits, and for some individuals, organic grains. You're also going to want to apply this 80/20 rule to your physical activity.

You will get the greatest improvement in energy production and mental clarity by putting forth 80% of your efforts towards activities that build a bigger aerobic engine such as:

- Morning outdoor steady state cardio
- Vinyasa yoga
- Budokon yoga
- Martial arts
- Swimming

- Rowing
- Airdyne biking
- Stair climbing

These cardiovascular activities should be performed using a heart rate monitor to ensure that you are within 65% to 85% of your max heart rate. Healthy individuals should be 75% to 85% of their max heart rate. Individuals who are older, out of shape, or dealing with health issues can start at the lower end of the spectrum. The other 20% of your efforts should focus on building strength, muscular endurance, mobility, and bringing up any weak parts of your game.

Here's one of the biggest secrets to making movement a lasting part of your lifestyle: *Do what you love.* Clients ask me all of the time what the most efficient workout is or the best way to burn the most belly fat in the least amount of time. This mentality sets us up for failure.

On a long enough timeline, the things that we stick with and continue to do are the things that we enjoy and love. If you spend too much time thinking about something, you'll never get anything done. Don't confuse internet research with taking action. 80% of my workouts now consist of jogging and yoga. That's it. The other 20% is focused on building relative strength, increasing my mobility, and maintaining (or improving) absolute strength as well as muscular endurance.

I used to train like a body builder with a focus on absolute strength. The term "absolute strength" refers to the maximum amount of force someone can produce, independent of body size or weight. So, when someone asks you how much you can bench or how much you can squat, they are referring to absolute strength. When I got sick, for the first time in my life, I began integrating more yoga and body weight relative strength exercises into my regiment. Relative strength is the amount of strength someone can produce in relation to their body weight or size.

In terms of real-world application and functional relevance, developing a mastery over your own body weight and increasing your relative strength will produce a much higher ROI than bodybuilder-style training focused on increasing absolute strength. There's also the added benefit that improvements in relative strength and bodyweight training do not require a gym. These types of exercises can be done anywhere because your body is your gym.

For most male clients (www.BioHackingSecrets.com/coaching), developing absolute strength beyond 225 pounds in any major lift produces diminishing returns, and these diminishing returns often come at the expense of flexibility, mobility, muscular endurance, and the maintenance and development of their aerobic engine. Here is a sample week of how you could integrate all of these different movement patterns and workout types into your exercise routine.

Monday - Friday

In the a.m., do 20-30 minute outdoor jog with lots of skin exposed to direct sunlight. Make sure that you are in your target heart rate zone. If you hate jogging or are physically unable to jog, you can also use the Assault AirBike or Airdyne Bike, the Concept 2 Row Machine, StairMaster treadmill or Woodway treadmill, or the Stairmaster.

Find your target heart rate by subtracting your age from 220. You want to work 65% to 85% of that. A shortcut for this is to subtract your age from 180. For a 40 year old man, this would be 140 beats per minute. Then, subtract 10 from that to get your lower threshold. You would jog for 20 to 30 minutes, keeping your heart rate between 130 and 140 beats per minute. This should be verified by a heart rate monitor with a chest strap.

Tuesday & Thursday

On Tuesdays and Thursdays, you can do a similar workout, but in order to prevent injury, after you've warmed up, you would then do 4-6 minutes of active-time, maximum-effort sprints. These sprints can vary in length from 20 seconds all the way up to 2 minutes and 30 seconds. Some sprint patterns that work well starting out are:

- 30 seconds on and 30 seconds off
- 20 seconds on and 10 seconds off
- 45 seconds on and 75 seconds off

After you've performed 4 to 6 minutes of sprinting (not total time, but the actual time you spent sprinting) you would go into your steady state cardiovascular workout. If you're a beginner, and you're too exhausted after your sprints to jog, you can also substitute incline walking on a treadmill. You would want the incline to be set around 8.0 and the speed to be around 3.2. For an added challenge, this can also be performed with a 20-50 pound weight vest. I use a short MIR weighted vest.

If you're unable to jog because of pains, aches, tightness, and stiffness, this is fixable. It's your body's way of giving feedback that something is out of balance, and is almost always partially derived from the food that we are eating. This is something that I've helped many clients with. We will touch on some of these in a later section that focuses on eliminating pain. Since there can be many compounding factors that cause such a state, and if this is something that you'd like more individual help with, we have an executive coaching program available for that.

If you're unable to jog because you're overweight, start doing what you are capable of when it comes to physical activity, and in the meantime, focus on getting the weight off. Use the recommendations in this book to get your energy up. You should also consider hiring an expert to help you with any problems you may be having.

If you feel like you can't run because you don't like to run, then do it anyway. You are an adult, and adults sometimes have to do things that are good for us, and improve our quality of life. You cannot achieve optimal health and performance by just sitting on the couch eating chips. So, you're going to have to switch your focus from short-term gratification to long-term satisfaction. That means sometimes doing things that you don't want to do.

Just to reiterate, make sure that you are using a heart rate monitor. You shouldn't guess when it comes to this stuff. Monday through Friday, do your fractionalized workouts. This is something that should be done every day, and you should make it part of your morning routine.

One thing that you can do, which will help you exercise more regularly, is to put a pull-up bar in your bathroom doorway. You can also do pushups and bodyweight squats as soon as you wake up and put your feet down on the floor. There are endless ways to incorporate

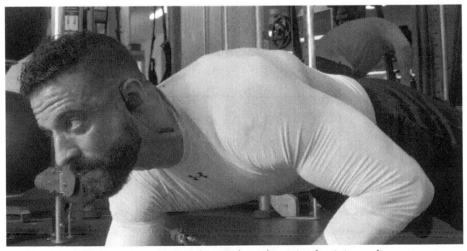

Do some form of stretching, rebounding, steady-state cardio or body-weight exercise within the first hour of your day.

fractioned workouts into your routine. Some of the most popular exercises for fractionalized workouts are:

– Pull-ups
– Pushups
– Chin-ups
– Planks
– Prisoner Squats
– Dips
– Lunges
– Jumping jacks

Wednesday

Incorporate 15 minutes of whole body vibration training either by using a Power Plate Pro machine or a rebounder.

I recommend using a whole body vibration machine like the Power Plate Pro. In the 1960's, during the Cold War, the democratic United States and the communist Soviet Union battled for space flight supremacy. This was a competition that came to be referred to as The Space Race. One of the biggest limiting factors back then with space travel were muscle wasting and bone loss. These problems would come about when people spent a significant amount of time in zero gravity space. To counteract this muscular atrophy and compromised bone density, the Soviets discovered a technology that they referred to as "vibrational training."

This discovery allowed Soviet astronauts to last an average of 400 days in space at one time, whereas US astronauts could only last an average of about 130 days. This technology was later refined and quickly incorporated into the training regimens of Olympic athletes and professional sports teams.

The two simplest ways to incorporate vibration training into your fitness regimen are by using the Power Plate Pro whole body vibration machine or a mini trampoline, which is also known as a rebounder. A lower cost alternative to the Power Plate Pro is the Bulletproof Vibe. Personally, I have most of my clients go barefoot, get out on some grass in contact with the earth, and do 100 gentle bounds as if they were jumping on a trampoline.

The advantage of the Power Plate is that it's able to create 25 to 50 vibrations per second. This forces the body's kinetic chain and muscular skeletal system to respond each time, improving balance, stabilization, coordination, strength, and endurance.

Healthcare professionals are now using the Power Plate whole body vibration technology in the management of:

- Idiopathic peripheral neuropathy
- Osteoporosis
- Multiple sclerosis, Parkinson's disease
- Cerebral palsy
- Rheumatoid arthritis

If you don't have access to a gym with Power Plate machines, you can also use a rebounder. Some of these "mini trampolines" are better than others. One of the best ones that I have found is the JumpSport Fitness Trampoline model 250. A mini trampoline subjects your body to gravitational pulls ranging from zero, at the top, to 2 or even 3 times the force of gravity at the bottom, depending on the height of your jump.

Whole body vibration training has been shown to improve:

- Strength
- Tone

- Flexibility
- Fitness
- Bone density
- Range of motion

The best part of all this is that these changes can begin to take place with as little as 15 minutes of exercise on the trampoline. This technology is being used by athletes and celebrities, including: The NFL Broncos, olympian Rebecca Romero, Rafael McDowell, and Serena Williams.

I recommend many clients (www.BioHackingSecrets.com/coaching) perform dumbbell circuits on the Power Plate, but these benefits can also be achieved by stretching, holding isometric yoga postures, or simply standing on the machine. Whole body vibration training also increases energy, stimulates circulation, and helps the body eliminate toxins by increasing lymphatic drainage. The lymph system is a network of organs, lymph ducts, lymph organs, and lymph vessels, which helps to rid the body of toxins.

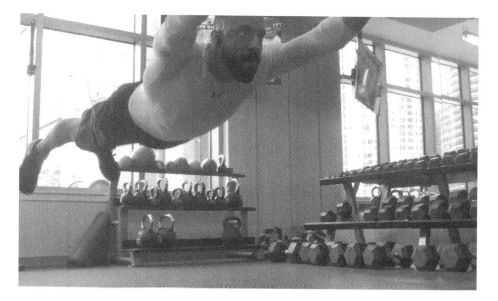

Friday

I recommend doing a high-intensity glycolytic workout. Some simple ways to do this include:

- The Extreme Cardio 1 & 2 DVDs
- *Crossfit WODs:* Grace, Fran, Murph, Filthy Fifty, The Seven, OPT repeatability test, 300 FY, Annie, Angie, Fight Gone Bad, Helen, Cindy
- *100 Burpee Challenge:* Do 100 burpees in the least amount of time possible. For an added benefit, you can incorporate jumping. The most advanced athletes can include jumping push-up burpees. My most well-conditioned clients are able to perform the 100 Burpee Challenge doing jumping Burpee pushups, in the 4-7 minute range. You can also use and follow the Insanity Fast and Furious DVD. This is an intense glycolytically-demanding workout that's just 20 minutes long.

Saturday

Saturday is for strength. This is when I recommend that you work your anaerobic and creatine phosphate systems. You should also go outside and workout, if at all possible. This is a great time to follow *"Body by Science"* by Doug McGuff and *"Power of 10"* by Adam Zickerman and Bill Schley. You might also use the ARX Fit machine (www.arxfit.com), or you could go for an outdoor trail run or hike.

Sunday

Sundays should be used for yoga, flexibility, and mobility. Hot yoga is best for detoxification. I am in Miami at the moment, finishing up this chapter, and I got to start my day by dropping in on a hot yoga class at a small studio around the corner from where I've been staying. I used to teach yoga, by the way. It was mostly because it kind of force me into doing yoga. However, I eventually got too busy with coaching, so I had to hang up the yoga instructor hat. When that happened, I found my own yoga practice occurring less and less frequently.

After three days of shenanigans in Miami, I pretty much got my butt kicked by a 115 pound female yoga instructor. She had a good laugh watching me pour sweat all over my mat. I'm not going to lie. About 45 minutes into the class, I was looking at the door and considering how rude it would be to pick up my mat and make a run for it. In spite of being a little worn out this week, I have to admit that it's pretty normal for me to start losing patience about 40-60 minutes into a yoga class. I did stick with it today though, and I felt incredible by the time we were done.

There is a bit of a learning curve when it comes to yoga. A lot of guys, especially, miss out on its benefits because they don't give themselves the opportunity to get used to it. Many men feel like they aren't any good in the beginning. It's true that a large majority of guys aren't good at yoga starting out. However, it's been my experience that if a guy will do it once or twice a week, within the first seven or eight sessions, they will start seeing massive improvements in their flexibility and focus as well as huge reductions in their stress levels.

Another one of my favorite products is the Budokon: Flow and Flexibility DVD. It incorporates some martial arts and bursts of higher-intensity movements. It's a great way to improve flexibility, relative strength, and also burn body fat. If you don't do hot yoga, Sundays are a great time to incorporate 20-30 minute saunas, post workout. The way I like to do this is to spend 20-30 minutes in the sauna, followed by a 2-minute cold shower. Two cycles will give you the greatest benefit.

You could also do soft tissue and trigger point work in the sauna using a foam roller or a lacrosse ball. If you've already incorporated soft tissue work and flexibility work into your weekly routine, and you don't

WEEKLY HABITS

MONDAY	
TUESDAY	
WEDNESDAY	
THURSDAY	
FRIDAY	
SATURDAY	
SUNDAY	

have any injuries, this is also a great chance to meditate. Some other great ways to include flexibility, mobility, and range of motion include:

- Active release technique (ART)
- Deep tissue massage
- Rolfing
- Muscle activation technique
- Advanced muscle integrated therapy
- Graston technique
- Trigger point therapy
- Lacrosse ball, golf ball, or trigger point ball
- The stick
- The orb
- Cranial sacral therapy
- The theracane
- Foam roller
- The Trigger Point Roller, Rumble Roller, PVC pipe

As mentioned previously, you can use a lacrosse ball, a golf ball, or a trigger point ball to release knots and trigger points. The Stick is also a tool that one can use to relieve muscle pain and soreness as well as to improve muscle strength. It also accelerates recovery time and helps with endurance.

The Orb is another such tool which provides a focused massage and contributes to flexibility.

The Theracane is also a massaging device which can be used to ease your body's aches and pains. The Trigger Point Roller, Rumble Roller, PVC pipe can also be used in this way, or you can just turn your 64-Oz Hydro Flask on its side and use that to IT band (Iliotibial band), quads, and glutes.

MINDSET

"You are not your job, you're not how much money you have in the bank. You are not the car you drive. You're not the contents of your wallet. You are not your fucking khakis."

- Tyler Durden, Fight Club

Our energy is a reflection of our physical health, our emotional state, and where we focus our attention. The two greatest skills we can develop to achieve this are:

- *Where We Focus Our Attention:* Every person, situation, and circumstance has aspects that make us feel good and aspects that make us not feel good. Which particular aspects we focus our attention on determines the meaning that we attribute to that person, situation, and circumstance. Energy and good feelings come from intentionally focusing our attention on the aspects of any situation that make us feel good.
- *The Ability to Get Ourselves in a Peak State:* Our state is the psychological and emotional patterns and moods we go to most frequently. Many times people passively allow their state to be dictated by their circumstances. However, our state is something that we can control.

The fastest way to change your state, is to change your physiology:

- Change the way you carry yourself, the way you move your body.
- Stand tall and proud.
- Pull your shoulders back and walk with purpose.
- Cultivate an external focus by helping others to experience the feelings and emotions you want for your own life.

- Cultivate feelings of gratitude and appreciation for all of the good things that are already in your life and the good things that are still on their way.
- Visualize your future, both in the short and long-term, and see things unfolding in your favor. Plan ahead in your mind by briefly rehearsing the way you want the next part of your day to unfold. This practice is called Segment Intending.

The simplest tool I have found to help direct thoughts and emotions in a more positive manner is The Five Minute Journal.

What makes this particular journal so effective is that it only takes 2 minutes in the morning and 2-3 minutes at night.

Each day you are given a quote, and each of these quotes are from some of the greatest thinkers in history. This is a great way to immediately focus our attention in an empowering direction. You then write down three things you are grateful for, followed by three things that will make the day great. This helps you to generate feelings of gratitude and helps you to start visualizing right away.

The morning journal entry concludes with affirmations. You finish the sentence, starting with "I am" and include characteristics and traits that you want to reinforce or cultivate in your life. Writing out affirmations is a powerful way to rewire your limiting beliefs and strengthen beliefs that bring about positive thoughts and actions.

During your nighttime entry, you'll write down three amazing things that happened during your day. You also reflect on anything that you could have done to make the day better. Obviously, there's nothing revolutionary about this practice, except that the simple act of doing these exercises causes you to direct your attention towards more positive outlooks, amplifies your state, identifies and changes limiting beliefs, and makes small incremental improvements by consciously reflecting on the events of your life.

WHY SO SERIOUS?

"The most wasted of all days is one without laughter."

- E. E. Cummings

After a stressful trip to cold-war Russia in 1964, Saturday Review (a weekly U.S. magazine publication) editor Norman Cousins developed a debilitating illness which left him bedridden.

After hospitalization and a battery of tests, he was diagnosed with an arthritic disease known as ankylosing spondylitis. His condition continued to deteriorate and prognosis was not good.

Cousins noticed that the depressing routine of hospital life, and poor quality of food, tended to produce side effects that made his condition worse. With his doctor's blessing, he checked out of the hospital and into a a more comfortable, and less expensive hotel where the food was better and he could watch funny movies while he medicated himself with high doses of Vitamin C.

He started to improve and was convinced that his results were a byproduct of his individualized methods and taking charge of his healing protocol. His approach has since come to be known as "Laughter Therapy."

Cousins recounted his own self-treatment with humor in an article in the New England Journal of Medicine in 1976.

Ed Diener, a professor of psychology at the University of Illinois, began studying happiness in 1981. "Many of us have material things and our basic needs met, so we are looking for what comes after that. Materialism isn't bad. It's only bad if we use it to replace other things in life like meaningful work, a good marriage, kids and friends. People are recognizing that those who make money more important than love have lower levels of life satisfaction."

Studies have revealed that laughter reduces pain, decreases stress, improves hormonal health, and strengthens the immune system. Many hospitals now offer laughter therapy programs. I recommend a healthy dose of daily laughter and comedy to all my clients, not just folks faced with a life threatening illness.

Second by second, we lose the opportunity to become the person that we want to be. Where most of us drop the ball is with consistency.

Most of the time we're initially motivated by pain. The problem is, eventually, the pain dissipates and we lose our motivation.

Most of us fail to create lasting, long-term change because we operate based on *push motivation* (the desire to move away from pain), but *pull motivation* is far stronger when it comes to building habits that foster and support long-term change. Here are some recommendations to put pull motivation to work for you:

- Write down clear, specific goals and reinforce them daily.
- According to research, less than 3% of Americans have written goals and less than 1% review and write their goals down on a daily basis. High performance expert Brian Tracy refers to written goal setting and daily reinforcement as "the single most important skill that you can learn and perfect." It's a process that allows you to control the direction of change in your favor.

CREATE ENJOYMENT & PLEASURE IN THE PROCESS

Most of us have heard the advice that we should take the stairs instead of the escalator, but few people actually do this. Researchers in Sweden went to the Odenplan Metro Station in Stockholm to perform an experiment. The passengers who were exiting the train had both an escalator and a staircase to choose from at this station. Both led up to the city streets. They installed cameras to track how many people took the stairs compared to the escalators.

The researches then installed piano keys and lights on the stairs. These would emit and play lights as people stepped on them. There was an immediate shift. By making the experience of walking up the stairs fun, the researchers observed a 66% increase in people taking the stairs over the escalator. Humans are playful creatures. On a long enough timeline, the behaviors that we continue to follow through with are those that we enjoy and find to be fun. This is a concept that has come to be known as "Fun Theory."

If you want any change to last long-term, you have to find ways to create fun and enjoyment in the behaviors that support your desired outcome. Now, this doesn't mean that you have to find the behavior itself fun. For example, you may not be crazy about jogging, but for many of my clients, their morning jog is the time that they get to listen to an audio book, podcast, or their favorite music. These are activities that they normally don't have time for in their busy schedules.

By layering in these other aspects of their training, it makes their daily jog more fun and enjoyable.

In addition to adding fun to your tasks, there are a number of neuro-linguistic programming (NLP) strategies and exercises you can use to bulletproof your mind and create lasting change.

OVERCOMING LIMITING BELIEFS

Before we can overcome our limiting beliefs, we have to first identify what those limiting beliefs are.

There are three types of limiting beliefs:

- Beliefs about cause
- Beliefs about meaning
- Beliefs about identity

All three types of beliefs influence our perspective of the world, which aspects of reality we observe, and which get ignored. When we have a belief about someone or something, we look for evidence in our world that supports that belief. So, it's vital that we overcome limiting beliefs because our beliefs ultimately determine the experiences we will have in life. All situations are neither good or bad. It is our thinking and the meaning that we attribute to these situations that determine whether our beliefs are positive or negative. All negative beliefs are limiting.

Our tendency to notice evidence that supports our beliefs is a byproduct of the reticular activating system (RAS). The RAS is a set of connected nuclei in the brains of vertebrates that are responsible for wakefulness and sleep-wake transitions. Beliefs are simply thoughts that we think over and over again. These beliefs, in turn, stimulate the reticular activating system, which then consciously scans our environment for real-world evidence to support those beliefs. This is why reframing situations, overcoming limiting beliefs, and consciously creating beliefs that empower us are vital skills in creating a positive outlook and optimal performance.

Here's an example. If you just got out of a really bad relationship, you might start thinking that all women, or men, are the same. This limiting belief will ultimately only sabotage your ability to have loving, meaningful relationships.

There are three strategies that you can use to overcome limiting beliefs. They are:

- *Activate your RAS:* Once you've identified the limiting belief that's holding you back, you then need to create a new empowering belief in that area. As mentioned, a belief is simply a thought that we think over and over again. Therefore, we have the ability to reinforce this new empowering belief by using our RAS to look for evidence that supports it in our environment.
- *Spend five minutes a day affirming your new belief:* To do this, you'll want to think, say, and feel the emotions behind that new belief. Amplify the intensity of your new belief with movement and physical activity. Visualize that belief, having already occurred. Tools that you can use for this are The Five Minute Journal and The 6 Phase Meditation read by Vishen Lakhiani, the founder of Mindvalley. I also recommend using the Omvana smartphone app.
- *Write down the new belief that you are going to adopt 20 times per day, by hand:* As you write, don't just think about the words on the page. You want to feel them and connect with the emotions you will experience when that belief becomes a reality in your life. Visualize and see that belief coming true in your mind's eye.

ANCHORING

Anchors are triggers that bring about a specific emotional state or thought. Anchoring is a process in which we apply a touch, gesture, movement or sound when we are in a peak state. With repetition, we would eventually be able to trigger our desired states simply by initiating that same movement, sound, touch, or gesture.

The most famous example of anchoring is Pavlov's Dog (theory). If you've never heard of this before, Ivan Pavlov was a Russian scientist who lived in the 1800's. He did an experiment where he rang a dinner bell and then gave his dog food directly afterwards. He repeated this process over and over again for many days in a row, and after some time had passed, every time the dog heard the bell it would start to salivate and get excited.

The dog associated the sound of the bell with food. So essentially, Pavlov was able to trigger this response just by ringing the bell.

This experiment led to a big progression in understanding how our brains work. You can use anchoring to initiate a desired state as well. Here's how:

1. Identify your desired state (e.g. excitement, energy, happiness, focus, courage).
2. Do whatever you need to do to get yourself into that state. The best way to do this is to think of someone who possesses your desired state and characteristics, and then adopt their physiology by mirroring their body language.
3. When you are completely in the state you wish to be in, clap your hands and say "yes." Continue clapping and saying "yes" for 20 to 30 seconds more, then stop, and think of something totally unrelated to the emotion that you felt.
4. After a couple of minutes, clap and say "yes" the same way that you did the first time. Try to bring yourself back into that desired state. Some clients of mine will incorporate a specific song that helps them activate that state (www.BioHackingSecrets.com/coaching).
5. Practice bringing yourself in and out of states. Through repetition you will strengthen the effectiveness of your anchor and your ability to quickly initiate that state.

One of the most effective biohacks for anchoring a state of peak performance is Tony Robbins' Unleashing the Power Within (UPW) event. Over three days, he uses specific movement, music, and other strategies from neuro-linguistic programming to bring you into a peak state and then anchor that state so that you have the ability to trigger it on your own.

REFRAMING

All the meaning that you attach to things depends on your point of view and your attitude. So, the meaning of any event is determined by the frame of reference, or lens, through which we see the world. When we change the frame, along with our state, we change the meaning of the events in our lives. In turn, our responses and behaviors are changed as well.

In 2008, I was working on the 94th floor of the Sears Tower (now the Willis Tower). I had been hired by a Belgian bank called Dexia to work in their commercial mortgage backed securities (CMBS) division. For three years prior to taking on this position, I had worked in commercial banking. This whole time, I had been doing health and fitness training on the side because I loved it.

I was not a banker. Every morning I was overcome with dread at the thought of putting on my suit and tie and spending the next 10 hours in a cubicle crunching Excel spreadsheets and underwriting loan documents. I felt trapped, and I was terrified by the thought that I would have to spend the next 40+ years doing something that was sucking the life out of me.

At Dexia, things were much better. I worked for a man named Steve Kemph, who had been a rock star over at JP Morgan and was hired by Dexia to build a flourishing CMBS department. Steve was only a few years older than me, and he had played college football at Minnesota. We got along great and worked well together. In fact, over that next year, we became really good friends. In 2008, the CMBS market tanked, and without warning, our office was shut down, and I lost my job.

I was making well over six figures, which was a good amount of money for someone my age. When we got news that our office was being shut down, I was devastated. Not only had my source of income come to a screeching halt, but I had lost what I thought to be the only job I could tolerate in the finance industry. As Steve broke the news, I remember being filled with a sense of dread. What was I going to do? How could I replace my income? The entire mortgage industry was in a tailspin, and I knew I couldn't possibly find anything in the same industry. If I had to start over I was looking at an entry level salary and bonus... there was no way I could possibly make ends meet. For the first time in my life I was truly worried about just paying my bills.

As I walked out of the Sears Tower that afternoon, suddenly a different feeling swept over me. It was like the dread and horror of my situation stopped following me when I hit the doorway, and within seconds I felt free, like I was throwing shackles and chains from my body.

What if all of this had happened so that I could pursue my life's true purpose? What if our office was shut down because some higher power knew that I was too scared to take that leap myself? Maybe I needed that extra nudge. I decided at that point that I would reframe that setback and look at it as an opportunity to pursue my entrepreneurial dream in health and fitness. This set me on a path that would lead me to eventually help tens of thousands of people. I've been able to help people lose weight, overcome health challenges, and dramatically increase their quality of life.

Anytime we have an experience that we don't like, what we really don't like is our response to that experience. One way of changing the way that you're likely to respond is to understand that the response itself is not based on the actual experience. It's based on the meaning that we give to that experience. At any moment, we have three choices. We can choose:

- What action we take
- What we focus on
- What meaning we give to our circumstances

So much about winning this game comes down to our attitude. Consciously choose to focus your attention and attribute meaning to situations and circumstances that help you feel good.

COMMUNICATION & RAPPORT

The four simplest hacks you can employ to become a better communicator and more rapidly build rapport with other people are:

- Talk less.
- Listen more.
- Develop a genuine interest and curiosity in the person you're communicating with.
- Practice making eye contact with everyone you pass and communicate with until it no longer feels awkward.

Making eye contact with people that I either didn't know or hardly knew was a huge sticking point for me for a long time. If it's not something that you are currently doing, I can almost guarantee that you are short-changing your personal and professional success. We communicate using our body language, tone of voice, and of course, our words. There are literally thousands of courses and books on how to improve each of these areas, but you don't need them. The information you need to get better in each of these areas is all around you. Become a student of life.

Pay attention to how other people communicate verbally and non-verbally. Notice how others react. Find people who are good in these areas and deconstruct what they do that makes them good, and then practice applying what you've learned. All of this comes down to practice. If your motivation is some destination end point, your results will always be temporary.

The secret of high performers is that their training never stops. Their motivation is not six-pack abs or a higher IQ. These may be added benefits, but what truly drives top performers is the desire to be the best version of themselves they can possibly be. Here are some additional strategies you can use to become a better verbal and nonverbal communicator:

- Improvisation classes
- Public speaking courses (Toastmasters, or Stand and Deliver by Dale Carnegie)

Jerry Seinfeld once joked that according to most studies, people's number #1 fear is public speaking, and #2 is death. However scary it may be, learning to communicate more effectively can really open up the world to you and allow you to build stronger relationships. To be a communicator, you need to work on your non-verbal communication, too, as studies have shown that this is more what people pay attention to than the words you actually say. For help with this, you might try:

- Taking dance classes (Salsa, Hip Hop)
- Dance Floor Arsenal (course by Nick Taylor)
- Mixed martial arts (Brazilian jiu-jitsu, Capoeira)

Capoeira is a mixed martial art that combines elements of dance and acrobatics. All three are good ways to develop your ability to communicate non-verbally. The movement practitioner Ido Portal also has some awesome videos on YouTube. You can learn more about his program, Movement Culture, at www.IdoPortal.com. Another recommended natural human movement program is Erwan Le Corre's MoveNat (www.MoveNat.com).

FEED YOUR MIND

One of the best ways for you to go about feeding your mind is to read a little bit each day. I recommend that you do so in the morning. We live in one of the greatest times in human history, and part of that is because we can choose just about anything we like from the massive amount of information within reach. Rather than reading that article your friend posted on Facebook, why not start with some of the greatest books of all time? Here are some of my personal favorites:

- *"Striking Thoughts"* by Bruce Lee
- *"Tao Te Ching"* by Lao-Tzu
- *"Letters from a Stoic"* by Seneca
- *"How to Win Friends and Influence People"* by Dale Carnegie
- *"Think and Grow Rich"* by Napoleon Hill
- *"The Compound Effect"* by Darren Hardy
- *"Meditations"* by Marcus Aurelius
- *"Influence"* by Robert Cialdini
- *"The Slight Edge"* by Jeff Olson

Consciously cultivate all of the inputs in your life, from the books you read, to the movies you watch, to the podcasts you listen to. This also includes the people you surround yourself with. Only allow seeds into your garden you want to grow.

MINDSET & HABITS BIOHACKS

This is not an all-inclusive summary from this section but will help you get started until you are able to explore in more detail.

The One Thing: Invest in The Five Minute Journal (available on Amazon) and use it each morning and every night.

Biohack #1: One of the most beneficial tools that you can use is a daily action plan. Get it down on paper so that you have a roadmap to follow and you can modify and correct course along the way.

Biohack #2: Here are some of the practices, tools, and resources I recommend to help build new habits and cultivate a bulletproof mind:

- Set a recurring alarm on your Smartphone. When that alarm goes off, it's time for you to drop everything you're doing and take action on the linked behavior.
- Once you take action, celebrate victory. As soon as you do it, tell yourself that you're awesome. Literally, say the words, "I'm awesome."
- The Five Minute Journal. It only takes me two or three minutes to make an entry.

Biohack #3: Fractionalized workouts you might work into your daily routine are: Pull-ups, Pushups, Chin-ups, Planks, Prisoner Squats, Dips, Lunges, and Jumping Jacks.

Biohack #4: The fastest way to change your emotional state is to change your physiology:

- Change the way you carry yourself, the way you move your body.
- Stand tall and proud.
- Pull your shoulders back and walk with purpose and strength.
- Apply the meta habits we discussed in the previous section.
- Cultivate an external focus by helping others to experience the feelings and emotions you want for your own life.
- Cultivate feelings of gratitude and appreciation for all of the good things that are already in your life and the good things that arc still on their way.
- Visualize your future, both in the short and long-term, and see things unfolding in your favor.

Biohack #5: Integrate some of the specific training modalities discussed in this section into your weekly movement training.

TROUBLESHOOTING

THE MOST OVERLOOKED ENERGY VAMPIRES THAT KEEP US PHYSICALLY & MENTALLY FATIGUED...

1. Gut Dysfunction
INCLUDES DIGESTIVE ISSUES AND INTESTINAL PERMEABILITY (LEAKY GUT).

2. Nutrient Imbalances
LIFESTYLE AND ENVIRONMENTAL FACTORS HAVE RESULTED IN EPIDEMIC LEVELS OF NUTRIENT IMBALANCES IN OUR CULTURE.

3. Toxic Overload
OUR BODIES ARE CONSTANTLY BOMBARDED WITH ENVIRONMENTAL TOXINS IN OUR FOOD, WATER, AIR, AND MORE.

4. Low Testosterone
& Human Growth Hormone (HGH)
THERE ARE SEVEN PRIMARY REASONS WHY WE MAY EXPERIENCE LOW TESTOSTERONE AND HGH.

5. Adrenal Fatigue
HPA Axis or Cortisol Dysregulation
THIS MAY BE A FACTOR IF YOU WAKE UP TIRED, DESPITE GETTING ADEQUATE SLEEP.

6. Hypothyroidism

60% OF PEOPLE WITH THYROID PROBLEMS MAY BE
UNAWARE THEY HAVE A HORMONAL IMBALANCE.

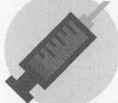

7. Blood Sugar
& Metabolic Issues

THESE ARE SOME OF THE MOST COMMON CAUSES
OF COMPROMISED ENERGY PRODUCTION.

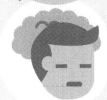

8. Neurotransmitter Imbalances

LEARN WHAT FACTORS CAN EXACERBATE THESE.

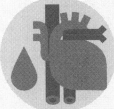

9. Chronic Infections

THE UNNATURAL ALTERATIONS WE'VE MADE TO OUR
ENVIRONMENT ARE THREATENING OUR HEALTH.

10. Brain Inflammation
(Neuroinflammation)

THE GUT-BRAIN AXIS IS AN OFTEN OVERLOOKED
FACTOR IN ENERGY PRODUCTION AND MENTAL CLARITY.

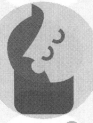
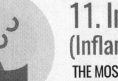

11. Immune Dysregulation
(Inflammatory Imbalance)

THE MOST COMMON TRIGGER FOR THESE AUTOIMMUNE
REACTIONS ARE THE FOODS WE EAT EVERY DAY.

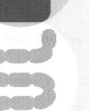

12. Impaired Methylation
(and genetic polymorphisms)

OFTEN CONTRIBUTES TO ENERGY FLUCTUATIONS,
SYMPTOMS OF CHRONIC ILLNESS, AND OTHER PROBLEMS.

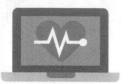

13. Mitochondrial Dysfunction

MITOCHONDRIA ARE THE TINY, BACTERIA-LIKE ENERGY PRODUCTION CENTERS OF OUR CELLS.

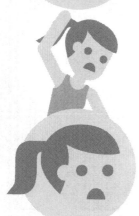

14. Circulation and Oxygen Deliverability

AS WE GET OLDER, WE LOSE THE ABILITY TO UTILIZE OXYGEN.

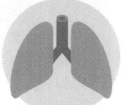

15. Movement Patterns & Biomechanics

USE IT OR LOSE IT. THAT'S THE WAY IT GOES WITH THE HUMAN BODY.

16. Estrogen Dominance, Elevated Androgens, and PCOS

FATIGUE AND BRAIN FOG MAY BE SYMPTOMS.

Read on to pinpoint the factors that may be contributing to suboptimal energy and focus & recommendations to help turn them around...

TROUBLESHOOTING

Let's assume you've already put The Foundational pieces into place.

In this Troubleshooting section, we will help you identify and eliminate some of the most overlooked energy vampires that can keep us physically and mentally fatigued.

Each section contains functional diagnostic questions that will help you assess your situation and pinpoint the factors that may be contributing to suboptimal energy and focus.

TROUBLESHOOTING #1: GUT DYSFUNCTION

Please circle "Yes" or "No" for each statement below:

1. I've experienced abdominal pain or discomfort multiple times in the past year. *(Yes or No)*
2. I occasionally have irregular bowel movements, including diarrhea and/or constipation. *(Yes or No)*
3. I feel better after having a bowel movement. *(Yes or No)*
4. I sometimes go two or more days without a bowel movement. *(Yes or No)*

5. My poop is occasionally very hard or soft and watery. *(Yes or No)*
6. My digestive symptoms interfere with my daily life. *(Yes or No)*
7. I experience digestive problems after eating certain foods. *(Yes or No)*
8. Sometimes it hurts to go poop. *(Yes or No)*
9. I have had blood or mucus in my stool in the past six months. *(Yes or No)*
10. I have unintentionally lost weight in the past 12 months. *(Yes or No)*
11. I burp and fart more frequently than what feels normal. *(Yes or No)*
12. I experience heartburn two or more times a week. *(Yes or No)*
13. I sometimes have difficulty swallowing. *(Yes or No)*
14. I frequently wake up with a sore throat in the morning. *(Yes or No)*
15. Sometimes heartburn wakes me up in the middle of the night. *(Yes or No)*
16. I take antacids or acid reducers such as Tums, Rolaids, or Pepcid more than once a week for heartburn symptoms. *(Yes or No)*
17. I have a family history of irritable bowels, Crone's disease, colitis, heartburn and/or digestive problems. *(Yes or No)*

Gut dysfunction includes digestive issues and intestinal permeability (leaky gut). You do not have to have gut symptoms to have a leaky gut. Any of the following conditions may also be indicative of gut dysfunction:

- Arthritis
- Depression
- Anxiety
- Obesity
- Diabetes
- Chronic fatigue
- Parkinson's

- Heart disease and cardiovascular problems
- Inflammatory Bowel Syndrome (IBS)
- Hashimoto's
- Autism
- Mental illness
- Arthritis
- Pains, Aches, Tightness, and Stiffness
- Autoimmunity
- Thyroid issues
- Acne, Eczema, Psoriasis, and Skin conditions

Over 2,000 years ago, Greek Physician Hippocrates observed, "All disease begins in the gut." Medical advances made over the past 20 years have shown just how right he was. We now know our gut to play a central role in our immune health (the gut is home to 70-80% of the body's immune cells), mood (close to 90% of the body's feel-good neurotransmitter, serotonin, is produced in the gut), energy production, and mental clarity.

Our gut is home to approximately 100 trillion microorganisms. The human gut contains 10 times more bacteria than all of the human cells in our entire body. So, technically, humans are more bacterial than we are human. There are two primary components to gut health:

- The intestinal microbiome (the quantity and diversity of bacterial species in gut).
- The gut barrier (the structural integrity of the single layer of cells lining our intestines).

A disruption in either of these components can initiate a wide range of health issues that erode our energy and focus. It's important to note that not all individuals with compromised intestinal integrity or suboptimal gut health exhibit physical symptoms. We now know that gut dysfunction results when a genetic predisposition intersects with an environmental trigger (often grains and/or gluten).

There's much debate around the percentage of the population who are affected by sensitivities to grains and gluten, but the real question we should be focusing on is whether or not *you* are sensitive to these environmental triggers. You must determine whether or not they are interfering with your optimal energy production and mental clarity. I have yet to encounter a client who has not experienced an improvement in vitality, strength, body composition, and brain function by reducing or eliminating their consumption of most grains and gluten.

In November of 2015, tennis star Novak Djokovic surpassed American tennis legend John McEnroe by spending 171 weeks in the #1 ranked position, according to the Emirates ATP Rankings. Djokovic has been called the greatest tennis player of all time. However, it was not always a steady and easy rise to fame. Even as an elite athlete at the highest level, it wasn't until Djokovic embarked on a gluten free diet that he saw his asthma, allergies, and chronic fatigue disappear.

When many people argue that they are not sensitive to gluten, what they are saying is that they have not consciously noticed. They have not consciously made the connection between the consumption of gluten-containing foods and suboptimal health. As you know, there is a vast difference between the absence of disease and optimized physical and mental performance.

Along with grains and gluten, there are several modern lifestyle factors that can contribute to gut dysfunction, such as:

– Consumption of commercial dairy and its derivatives
– Antibiotics and certain other prescription and over-the-counter medications

- Diets high in processed foods, sugars, and refined carbohydrates
- Diets low in plants and fermentable fibers (food for the good bacteria in our gut)
- Other dietary toxins like vegetable oils (canola, soy bean, corn, and wheat)
- Consumption of genetically modified organisms (the three biggest being corn, soy, canola oil, and their derivatives).
- Chronic infections like SIBO (small intestine bacterial overgrowth), candida, parasites, and H. pylori.
- Hypochloridia (low stomach acid production)
- Fluoride, chlorine, and other chemicals in our water
- Inadequate consumption of living plant foods (organic plants contain enzymes our body needs to effectively digest, assimilate, and absorb nutrients from our food).

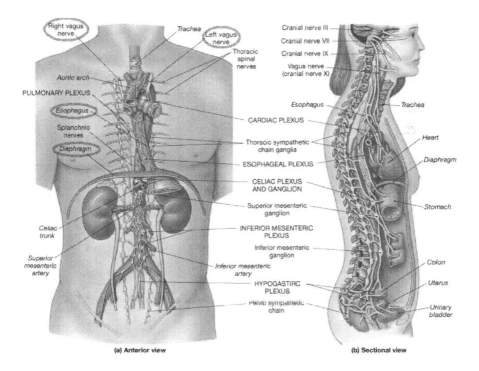

(a) Anterior view   (b) Sectional view

When a patient comes to me with skin problems like eczema, rosacea, psoriasis, or autoimmune conditions like Hashimoto's, or even just stubborn body fat, joint or back pain (including rheumatoid arthritis), anxiety, depression, and/or chronic fatigue, one of the first places we focus our attention is healing the gut.

While we can't change an individual's genetic blueprint, we can influence whether or not certain genes express themselves. The most effective way to positively affect gene expression, as it pertains to the gut, is to remove environmental triggers from the diet.

For many of us, consumption of grains and gluten damages nerve cells in our digestive tract, which compromises motility (our ability to

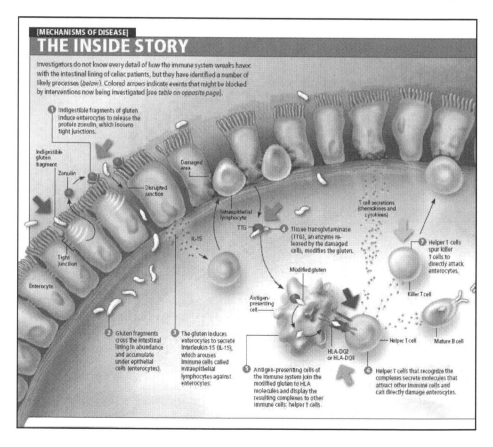

effectively eliminate toxins through the evacuation of our bowels). This also causes an over expression of a protein called zonulin, which results in increased intestinal permeability. You can look at our intestines as a 15 to 20 foot tube that's lined with a single layer of cells. These cells function like doors, and in a healthy individual, these doors are closed. However, when we consume foods that initiate an immunogenic or an allergenic response, we see an increase in the protein zonulin, which in turn causes these doors to open.

When these doors are open, undigested food particles and other compounds are able to enter the bloodstream where they are not recognized by our body's immune system. Our body then mounts an attack, which causes inflammation, pain, and fatigue. Researchers have now found that most autoimmune diseases, including Type 1 diabetes, multiple sclerosis, arthritis, inflammatory bowel syndrome, and celiac disease, are associated with abnormally high levels of zonulin and leaky gut.

Besides eliminating or reducing environmental triggers like grains, gluten, dairy, vegetable oils, sugar, processed foods, and alcohol, what else can you do to improve gut function? Here are some other solutions:

- Aim to get about 80% of your nutrition from local organic plants (most of those plants being vegetables, most of those vegetables being green) which still contain their natural water content. If you experience gas, bloating, or digestive symptoms, try lightly cooking your vegetables to aid in the digestive process.
- Aim for at least 32 grams of fiber daily, coming from these organic plant sources. This is very different from the fiber found in processed, refined foods, including many supplements and "health bars."

- Take a high-quality broad-spectrum probiotic daily. Unfortunately, many probiotics are ineffective. There are only four on the market that I use with my clients. The best probiotic for you depends largely on the current bacterial composition of your gut and your health status.

- Consider supplemental stomach acid as Betaine HCL, digestive enzymes, digestive bitters, and/or ox bile to more effectively digest, assimilate, and absorb food. Stomach acid will also reduce risk of pathogens getting a foothold in the gut.

- Treat hidden infections. If you have small intestinal bacterial overgrowth, parasites, candida, H. pylori, or other gut-related infections, these are going to hinder any chance at optimal performance.

- Until you've re-established a healthy gut microbiome consider minimizing exposure to foods that can be problematic for individuals with sensitivities to histamines, tyramines, and arginine.

- Stimulate the vagal/vagus nerve: The vagal nerve is the longest nerve in the body. It originates in the brain and then travels down the neck and wraps around the digestive system, liver, spleen, pancreas, heart and lungs. In people with gut problems, a sluggish vagus nerve is almost always involved. It plays an indispensable role in regulating the parasympathetic nervous system, responsible for rest and digestion. A latent vagal nerve has been implicated in a variety of conditions including epilepsy, rheumatoid arthritis, and inflammatory bowel syndrome (IBS). You can stimulate the vagus nerve by humming, gargling, meditating, singing, projecting your voice when speaking, and slow rhythmic diaphramic breathing.

Signs of Low Stomach Acid (*courtesy of www.thealternativedaily. com*): *If you feel poorly when you eat meat or protein-rich foods, low stomach acid may be to blame. Many people take nausea or sluggishness after eating meat as a sign that they should become vegetarian. While this may be true for some people at some life stages, it is a good idea to test for hypochlorhydria. Eating sustainable, healthy and humane sources of animal protein is critical for lasting health for most people.*

Along a similar vein, those who have previously chosen to eat a vegetarian or vegan diet may have decreased hydrochloric acid production, because it is naturally downregulated by the body when little animal protein is consumed. If you choose to reintroduce animal foods, this must be done gradually so that acid production can resume accordingly.

Other digestive discomforts can also result from inadequate stomach acid production. Acid reflux and GERD, or heartburn, seem to be related to overproduction of acid but are actually caused by acid escaping from the stomach into the soft, sensitive tissues of the esophagus. This uncomfortable condition results from pressure in the stomach due to low stomach acid.

In addition, burping, gas, bloating or heaviness after eating are clear indicators that the digestive process is not happening as it should. It is likely that the excessive growth of bacteria (left unchecked due to low stomach acid) results in fermentation of the food you eat, with gas as a by-product. The smelly burps that many people have are a sign that food is sitting in the stomach for too long, when it should already have moved into the small intestine. When pH levels are too low in the stomach, the signal that should move food onward into the intestine never happens, and food is left to provide a feast for unhealthy bacteria. Bacterial infections such as H. pylori can result.

This incomplete digestion can also contribute to constant hunger, because nutrients cannot be absorbed when food is left whole by inadequate stomach acid. The body believes it is undernourished and continues to trigger hunger signals.

Digestive illness such as inflammatory bowel disease, celiac symptoms, Crohn's disease or ulcerative colitis that just won't get better even after numerous diet and lifestyle changes could be a sign of low stomach acid.

Since a lack of strong stomach acid can let bacteria grow beyond optimal levels, bad breath can result. If you have persistent bad breath, it may not be coming from your teeth, tongue or gums, but rather from deeper down. When food sits in the gut, bacteria breeds and lets off foul gases that can come out of your mouth.

Another "cosmetic" side effect of hypochlorhydria is weak and peeling fingernails. This results from deficiencies in proteins and essential fatty acids that are missed out on when food is not properly digested.

Case Study: Nick P

Nick is a well-known expert in the health and weight loss industry. He's had a few best selling programs and helped thousands of men and women discover the truth about nutrition for fat loss.

Over the years, Nick has referred many of his hardest cases to me because he knows that diet-resistant, hard-to-lose weight is often accompanied by issues that go beyond diet and exercise. When one of his clients isn't getting results, he sends them to me.

This was a unique case because it was Nick who was in need of help. He'd spent almost two years sleeping less than 4 hours a night. Although his nutrition had been almost perfect, chronic stress and poor sleep habits had burned out his HPA axis and he was experiencing a number of unwanted symptoms including constipation, low energy, muscle aches and tension, acne, and brain fog.

After some functional testing, I put together a program that started by addressing Nick's gut microbiome and detoxification pathways.

We utilized supplements to restore intestinal integrity and support Phase I and II detoxification.

In less than 3 weeks, Nick was well on his way to feeling superhuman. He felt more energized,, the tension in his back and neck were down significantly, and he had less acne on his face than ever before. Nick told me he could literally feel himself getting healthier. He joked that I was "turning him into a superhuman, one day at a time."

SIBO (Small Intestinal Bacterial Overgrowth)

Small Intestinal Bacterial Overgrowth is one of the more common challenges I see in clients (www.BioHackingSecrets.com/coaching) struggling with gut dysfunction. I typically start them on an herbal protocol which includes Biotics Research FC Cidal and Biotics Research Dysbiocide at a dose of two caps, two times a day, for four weeks, of each formula. I then incorporate one of the four probiotic formulas in order to repopulate the gut, based on the individual's symptoms, as well as a prebiotic as additional food for the bacteria in the gut (like Klaire Labs Biotagen). I also supplement enzymes and Betaine HCL as an individualized dosage that I help the patient to determine.

Occasionally, we will incorporate low-dose Naltrexone (LDN) to improve intestinal motility, which may have been caused by nerve damage. Also, when warranted, nutrients are added to the mix as well as natural prescription medication to support the thyroid. The thyroid, by the way, can often be compromised in autoimmune conditions like Hashimoto's. This herbal protocol is based on the John Hopkins study, which found it to be as effective as prescription medications. So, this is where we usually start.

If the herbal protocol doesn't work, we then move on to a combination of four prescription medications in order to strategically eradicate the pathogenic bacteria and yeast. This protocol is like hitting the reset button on your metabolism. You start with a clean slate. That protocol includes Rifaximin (Xifaxan at 1600 mg a day for 10 days) plus neomycin (1,000 mg a day for 10 days). We then follow up with two antifungals. These are Nystatin and Diflucan. I recommend a dosage of two tablets 3-5 times a day for 30 days when it comes to the Nystatin, and for the Diflucan, I recommend 200 mg a day for 30 days.

Some physicians balk at Diflucan because some studies have shown an association with liver damage. However, this usually occurs only with long-term use and the elevated liver enzymes return to normal promptly after the discontinuation of use. A common mistake often made when treating SIBO and other bacterial infections in the gut is going on a low FODMAP diet. This results in a reduction in symptoms, but also sends the bacteria into survival mode. It also reduces the efficacy of the herbal and prescription antibiotics. Happy bacteria that are being well fed are more easily killed by antibiotics, herbal or otherwise.

Whether you are dealing with dysfunction of the gut, thyroid issues, or weight-related challenges, I recommend most clients begin by addressing the gut microbiome. Healing the gut can be a complicated symphony of nutritional, lifestyle, and supplemental interventions. If I had to start with just one recommendation, it would be to put out the fire. In other words, find out what foods you may be sensitive to and cut them out entirely. Aim for no less than 28 days.

Once you have eliminated the triggers, then I recommend adding colostrum. There is only one kind of colostrum I use and recommend to clients. It is a 100% pure bovine colostrum collected within the first 16 hours after birthing. This colostrum is a natural whole-food that provides a rich source of IgG and PRPs (Proline-Rich Polypeptides).

It also supplies protein, immune factors, growth factors, vitamins and minerals to support gut health and vitality naturally. Restoring energy and focus by healing the gut can be complicated and take time. I have seen clients with severe gut dysfunction continue to experience improvements for as much as 3 to 4 years.

Other supplements and herbs that I have used with patients in order to correct gut dysfunction include:

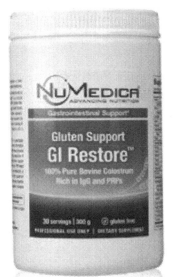

- Non starch polysaccharides (inulin, FOS, and arabinogalactan)
- Resistant starch (cold potatoes)
- Prebiotics (Klaire Labs Biotagen)
- Prebiotin, Prebiogen
- Acacia fiber
- Psyllium husk
- Glucomannan
- Digestive enzymes
- Protease
- Lipase: Plant enzyme supplement that aids in the digestion of fats
- Amylase
- Ox Bile: Important supplement for individuals with gallbladder issues or who have had their gallbladder removed.
- Papaya
- Pancreatin
- Bromelain
- Papain cellulose pepsin
- Berberine HCL
- Oregano oil
- Undecylenic acid

- Magnesium glycinate
- Coconut activated charcoal
- Mastic gum
- Garlic
- Cinnamon
- Artemisinin
- Potato starch
- Plantain flour
- Dehydrated green plantains
- Green banana flour
- Extra virgin cod liver oil: High in the anti-inflammatory omega-3s, EVCLO also contains bioavailable, fat-soluble vitamins A & D which help build the immune system and fight inflammation in the gut.
- Biocidin gut cleanse formulas
- Metagenics candibactin-AR
- Metagenics candibactin-BR
- L-glutamine powder
- Deglycyrrhizinated licorice (DGL)
- Aloe Vera
- Slippery Elm
- Marshmallow root
- Cat's claw
- Quercetin
- Methylsulfonylmethane (MSM)
- Loratadine
- Saccharomyces boulardii
- Caprylic acid
- Wormwood extract
- Olive leaf extract

- Lauricidain (Monolaurin Supplement)
- Black walnut extract
- Pau d'arco
- Organically soaked and sprouted legumes that have been cooked for at least 20 minutes to reduce anti-nutrient content.
- Bone broth from grass-fed cows or free-range poultry (can be purchased online at www.GrasslandBeef.com, www.BoneBroths.com, or www.AZGrassRaisedBeef.com).

Also, an article about a recent study examining 21 people with Crohn's Disease said, "Half were given cigarettes without cannabinoids and the other half were given joints to smoke. The joints contained 23% THC and .5% CBD. 45% of the people given joints every day for eight weeks experienced complete remission of their Chron's disease."

Parasites can be a challenge to get rid of as well. I usually start clients out on an herbal protocol, which combines therapeutic dosages of cloves, black walnut, wormwood, milk thistle, chanca piedra extract, protease, amylase, cellulase, and lipase for 30 days. If this doesn't work, we then move on to multi-drug treatment protocol that was developed by the Center for Digestive Diseases in Sydney. This protocol typically includes 400 mg of secnidazole (30 capsules, three times a day), 500 mg of diloxinide furoate (30 capsules, three times a day), and Septrin DS (20 capsules, two times a day).

Other antiparasitic medications I have had clients use are Ivermectin, Albendazole, Metronidazole, Tinidazole, Doxycycline, Minocycline, Alinia, and Pyrantel Pamoate (available over the counter). Albendazole and Alinia both cross the blood brain barrier.

Additional anti-parasite interventions include rectal artemisinin and garlic via suppository, elimination of dietary grains and sugar, and rectal and oral MMS.

Some of the most important tests you can use to determine if you have gut dysfunction are:

- Doctor's Data Comprehensive Stool Analysis
- Biohealth 401 Culture-Based Stool Method
- SIBO Breath Testing by Genova
- Urinary Organic Acids Profile from Genova
- Cedars Sinai Irritable Bowel syndrome (IBS) blood test developed by Mark Pimentel, MD

In many cases, when the patient is open-minded, we also incorporate coffee enemas, probiotic enemas, and bentonite enemas to improve detoxification and reintroduce beneficial bacteria to the gut. Coffee enemas are not some new health fad, nor are they a practiced reserved solely for health nuts. I'll admit, the idea of putting coffee in our "out hole" is not the most appealing of propositions, but once we move past our psychological reservations, the benefits are immense.

When I first started doing coffee enemas in 2013, I immediately dropped 8-10 pounds and saw a visible increase in definition around

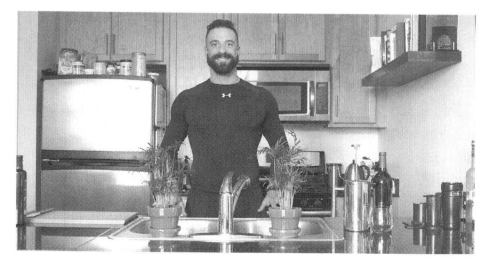

my midsection. The enemas allowed me to flush layers of body fat that had been resistant to diet, exercise, and supplements. Our body stores toxins in fat tissue as a protective mechanism to keep them away from our cells and vital organs.

When we improve our body's ability to detoxify, through coffee enemas and other means, we enable our body to remove these fat stores and achieve greater levels of leanness and improved body composition. Furthermore, this brings about substantial increases in energy, focus, and mental clarity. Again, this is nothing new:

- Ancient cultures in Africa, Greece, Babylonia, India, and China all used enemas.
- American Indians also performed enemas.
- Louis XIV had almost 2,000 enemas in his lifetime, and he was known to exhibit robust health.
- American actress, singer, and sex symbol, May West, started every day with a morning enema.

Did you know that Princess Diana was one of the first vocal advocates for colon hydrotherapy? The Globe quoted her saying, "For years, I've been trying to bury my troubles under mountains of food, but after I binge, I worry about my figure and I make myself throw up. It's a terrible, vicious compulsion, but now that I'm getting regular colonics, I don't worry so much about what I eat. I know all the excess food will be washed away, along with the poisons that cause my terrible headaches. My migraines are caused by my food allergies, and I haven't had one since I started the treatments."

Oprah Winfrey dedicated an entire episode of her show to colon cleansing enemas and its benefits. She is one among a number of celebrities who believe in this form of treatment. Madonna, Leonardo

DiCaprio, Britney Spears, Usher, Gwyneth Paltrow, John Lennon, Damon Wayans, Janet Jackson, and many others have all used enemas to maintain their health, energy, and youthful appearance.

TROUBLESHOOTING #2: NUTRIENT IMBALANCES

Please circle "Yes" or "No" for each statement below:

Vitamin A

1. I have dry skin or have to use large amounts of lotion to stay moisturized. *(Yes or No)*
2. I have difficulty seeing at night. *(Yes or No)*
3. My eyes often feel dry. *(Yes or No)*
4. I have issues with my nails and my hair is dry. *(Yes or No)*
5. I deal with unwanted acne. *(Yes or No)*
6. I get small bumps on my arms, face, or legs. *(Yes or No)*
7. I have an autoimmune condition like Crohn's, Hashimoto's, rheumatoid arthritis, etc. *(Yes or No)*
8. I think organ meats like liver, hearts, and kidneys are gross, and I do not eat them regularly. *(Yes or No)*
9. I have recently been restricting my dietary fats. *(Yes or No)*
10. When eating meat, I usually go with whatever is offered at the grocery store or restaurant (I do not seek out grass-fed meats nor do I eat them regularly). *(Yes or No)*
11. My diet includes foods that I could not find anywhere on earth 10,000 years ago (processed and refined foods; products that come in a box, a bag, a wrapper, a can, a tube, or a jar). *(Yes or No)*

TROUBLESHOOTING

Vitamin D

1. Most of my time is spent indoors. *(Yes or No)*
2. I get less than an hour of direct sunlight to exposed skin per week. *(Yes or No)*
3. When in the sun, I wear sunscreen or cover my skin with clothing. *(Yes or No)*
4. I do not take a vitamin D3 supplement. *(Yes or No)*
5. I have Crohn's, colitis, IBS, celiac disease, or other GI disorder. *(Yes or No)*
6. I am very overweight or obese. *(Yes or No)*
7. I have high blood sugar, diabetes, a slow metabolism, and/or high blood pressure. *(Yes or No)*
8. I have asthma. *(Yes or No)*
9. I have an autoimmune condition. *(Yes or No)*
10. I have been diagnosed with depression, anxiety, or experience a low mood more often than normal. *(Yes or No)*
11. I currently have, or have had, cancer. *(Yes or No)*
12. I have osteoporosis. *(Yes or No)*
13. I do not like fish and I eat less than two servings of cold water fatty fish per week. *(Yes or No)*

Magnesium

1. I often feel tight, stiff, and inflexible. *(Yes or No)*
2. I get muscle cramps on a regular basis, especially during physical activity. *(Yes or No)*
3. I often feel anxious or stressed. *(Yes or No)*
4. I'm often tired and sometimes experience low mood or depression. *(Yes or No)*
5. I have asthma or difficulty breathing. *(Yes or No)*
6. I do not sleep well. *(Yes or No)*

7. I am often constipated. *(Yes or No)*

8. I suffer from frequent headaches or migraines. *(Yes or No)*

9. I have been diagnosed with or suspect that I may have fibromyalgia or chronic fatigue syndrome. *(Yes or No)*

10. I have high blood sugar, diabetes, high blood pressure, or cardiovascular problems. *(Yes or No)*

11. I have osteoporosis. *(Yes or No)*

12. I am more than 25 pounds overweight. *(Yes or No)*

13. I'm on a prescription medication for high blood pressure or a diuretic. *(Yes or No)*

14. My diet includes foods that I could not find anywhere on earth 10,000 years ago (processed and refined foods; products that come in a box, a bag, a wrapper, a can, a tube, or a jar). *(Yes or No)*

15. I do not eat green vegetables every day. *(Yes or No)*

16. I do not eat many plants, nuts, or seeds. *(Yes or No)*

A variety of lifestyle and environmental factors have converged, resulting in epidemic levels of nutrient imbalances in our culture. We have more and more people blindly taking supplements in the wrong forms, incorrect quantities, and without essential cofactors to facilitate their absorption and prevent toxicity. One popular example of this is vitamin D, which can be toxic without adequate levels of bioactive vitamin A supplemented with vitamin D2. Supplementing with vitamin D in the absence of vitamin K2 is also problematic as it does not prevent the calcification of the arteries and may even contribute to the problem further.

There are literally dozens of examples like this. When a client comes to me on a self-prescribed supplement protocol, there are often multiple high-risk nutraceuticals in the mix. These nutrient excesses can be just as deleterious as some deficiencies are, and a growing body of research has found them to contribute to everything from heart disease to cancer and early mortality. On the other end of the spectrum, we have the far more common nutrient deficiencies. These can result from:

– Our modern calorie dense, nutrient poor diet, compromised digestion due to gut dysfunction or inflammation
– Ingestion of compounds that bind to nutrients and prevent the body from absorbing them (insoluble fiber in many processed foods)
– Decreased nutrient content in our soil, and therefore, our food

Many vegan and vegetarian diets also lack nutrients vital to optimal physiological function. Some of the most common nutrient deficiencies include:

– All of the B Vitamins (particularly folate, B12, B6, and B2)
– Magnesium
– Iron
– Vitamin D3
– Vitamin K2
– Selenium
– Iodine
– Vitamin A
– Lithium
– Essential fatty acids (EPA, DHA)

Here are some of the most effective ways to improve nutrient imbalances:

1. Eat a whole food, plant-based diet with a focus on organic, local, and seasonal plants.

2. For protein, focus on wild-caught fish and, to a lesser degree, free range organic poultry, free range organic pork, grass-fed beef, wild game, and other animals raised on their natural diet. These are among some of the most nutrient-dense foods available. The problem is that many people eat these foods in excess (they should make up no more than 20% of your food intake), and they consume unhealthy versions of these foods (i.e. commercial meat and dairy not specified as "organic," "grass-fed," "wild-caught," "free range," or "pastured"). For more in-depth exploration of nutrient density, I recommend Mat Lalonde's "Nutrient Density: Sticking to the Essentials" presentation, which took place in the Ancestral Health Symposium back in 2012. The video for this is available on YouTube.

3. Remove dietary toxins that can damage the gut. These include grains, gluten, dairy, alcohol, genetically-modified foods, industrial seed oils, sugar, and refined carbohydrates.

4. Before meals, consume a high-quality digestive enzyme along with supplemental betaine HCL to assist in the digestion, absorption, and assimilation of nutrients from your food.

5. Address nutrient deficiencies. I build out a customized settlement protocol for each client to help them optimize energy, focus, and performance because everyone is unique. Some of the supplements that I use most commonly include: Sublingual B-12 (methylcobalamin and hydroxocobalamin forms), Extra Virgin Cod Liver Oil, Magnesium Glycinate, and Vitamin D3.

For some individuals, we used intramuscular B-12 injections (methylcobalamin form or hydroxocobalamin form) to circumvent possible absorption issues due to compromised joint health.

We also occasionally use other injectable nutrients, including:

- Vitamin C
- B-Complex vitamins
- Glutathione
- Magnesium

Myers cocktails (which contain B-complex vitamins, vitamin C, Magnesium,vitamin B-5, Calcium, and frequent additions including B12, B6, adrenal cortical extract, glycerol and glutathione) can be especially helpful.

If I suspect that a client may be dehydrated, I will recommend 1,000 ml of saline solution or Lactated Ringer's solution. Some of the most important tests for evaluating nutrient status include:

- The Genova NutrEval
- The Urine Amino Acids Test through Genova or Doctor's Data
- Quicksilver Scientific Heavy Metals Test
- Serum 25- Hydroxyvitamin D Test

TROUBLESHOOTING #3: TOXIC OVERLOAD

Signs that you are suffering from toxic overload include:

1. Gut problems:
   - Gas
   - Bloating
   - Belching
   - Constipation
   - Diarrhea

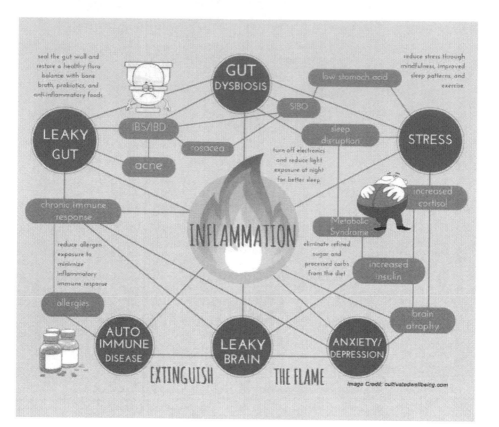

- Headaches
- Digestive problems
- Unexplained weight gain/weight loss
- Low energy
- Autoimmune conditions
- Difficulty sleeping
- Heartburn

2. Brain fog
3. Headaches/migraines
4. Unexplained weight gain/weight loss
5. Frequent urination

6. Stress or anxiety
7. Aches, pains, tightness, stiffness (including joints, lower back, and neck)
8. Skin problems
   - Acne
   - Psoriasis
   - Eczema
   - Rosacea
9. Blurry vision
10. Hemorrhoids
11. Weakened immune system
12. Fatigue/ low energy
13. Fungal or yeast infections
14. Swelling, bloating, or edema
15. Fluid retention
16. Chemical sensitivities:
    - Lotions
    - Perfumes
    - Cleaners
    - Cosmetics

How to Upgrade Your Energy & Focus by Reducing Your Body's Toxic Burden:

1. Avoid, or at least minimize, the most common dietary toxins: grains, dairy, alcohol, genetically modified foods, and anything containing corn, soy, canola oil, or any derivatives of these.

2. Eat a clean, plant-based, organic diet
   - 80% of your food should come from plants, most of those plants being vegetables, most of those vegetables being green.
   - Your primary protein source should be wild-caught fish

3. Drink filtered, structured water. Assuming a quality source and structure, aim for 70% of your bodyweight in ounces of water per day. I start with spring water from a bubbler then run it through my Kangen SD501 machine before structuring it via vortexing. You don't have to get all weird with it like I do, just get the toxins out (including fluoride if your municipality fluoridates).

4. Use enemas to assist your body's detoxification pathways
   - Use coffee enemas (daily, ideally two back-to-back for optimal results starting out). You can reduce your coffee enemas based on how you feel.
   - Bentonite enemas (once a week max)
   - Probiotic enemas

5. Take a high-quality, broad spectrum probiotic daily. Rotate type and dosage periodically.

6. Include probiotics in your coffee enemas

Our bodies are constantly being bombarded with environmental toxins in the food we eat, the water we drink, the air we breathe, the products that we put on our skin, and the chemicals we encounter. These environmental chemicals, especially when combined with a genetic predisposition, open the door for pathogens in the gut and compromised detoxification that further exacerbates our body's toxic burden.

Furthermore, we've seen an explosion in incidence of chronic inflammatory response syndrome (biotoxin illness), the most prominent trigger being exposure to mold in old or water-damaged buildings.

Some of the strategies that I use with clients (www.BioHackingSecrets. com/coaching) to lower the body's toxic burden include:

1. Chelation therapy to remove heavy metals (DMSA, EDTA, zeolite, bentonite, coconut activated charcoal, cilantro, cruciferous vegetables, etc).

2. Dry saunas (not steam rooms, which use tap water, and therefore, do the opposite of what we are after because they expose our body to higher levels of chlorine, fluoride, pharmaceutical drugs, and other chemicals that this water contains). In addition to activating the body's detoxification system, particularly through our largest organ, the skin, dry sauna treatment has been found to have a number of performance-enhancing benefits, including:

- Mimics the physiological effects of exercise, improving cardiovascular function and lowering heart rate
- Increases blood flow
- Increases oxygen transport and utilization
- Increases red blood cell count
- Improves insulin sensitivity
- Reduces the rate of glycogen depletion
- Enhances muscular and cardiovascular endurance

I try to go to Chicago Sweatlodge or Red Square at least once a week to use their dry saunas and cold plunge facilities. These bathhouses are popular in Eastern Europe and Russia, and they play a central role in the social landscape of these cultures. The sauna is a big room with multiple levels, which get hotter the higher up you go. The room is heated by a giant wood-burning oven. You can hang out in the sauna with friends and hit yourself with white oak or birch branches to further improve circulation. By the way, when you are using these saunas, you can enhance sweating by wearing a Kutting Weight suit or using a coconut oil-based Sweet Sweat on your skin.

Once you get hot, you leave the sauna and enter a cold plunge pool which is kept at a cool 41° F. In Eastern European and Russian cultures, men spend all day in these types of bath houses, socializing, drinking, eating, and connecting with friends. After a pretty late Saturday night with friends, watching the UFC 194 event, I hit the Chicago Sweatlodge with two of my buddies not too long ago, and after just a couple of hours, I felt like a new man.

Infrared saunas, like the Sunlighten mPulse cONQUER sauna, should be considered as well. Whereas traditional saunas heat the body from the outside in, infrared saunas heat the body from the inside out. Both kinds improve circulation and oxygenation of the tissues in addition to ramping up the body's detoxification channels.

3. A plant-based diet high in cruciferous vegetables. These are vegetables that contain large amounts of Indole-3-Carbinol and subsequently diindolylmethane (DIM) compounds. These are derived from cruciferous vegetables like:

- Broccoli
- Brussel sprouts
- Cabbage
- Kale
- Collard greens
- Sprouts

These help the body to eliminate toxins.

4. *Liquid meals*, which help the body's digestive burden. For many clients, I recommend starting the day with an energizing green smoothie that includes:

- 12-16 oz of water
- A vegan protein powder like Sunwarrior WARRIOR BLEND, Epic Protein, Vegan Shakeology, or Vega Sport
- One scoop of D-Ribose
- A big 6 oz bag of organic baby spinach or dark leafy greens
- A scoop of prebiotic
- A tablespoon of organic Chia seeds
- Possibly some organic berries as well (blueberries, raspberries, blackberries)

5. *Intermittent fasting*. Our body operates in two distinct phases. The first is "digestion and absorption," and the second is "elimination and detoxification." These processes are mutually exclusive. When we fast, our body initiates a cellular waste removal process called autophagy. This is where our body breaks down proteins and removes toxins that build up inside our cells over time.

Fasting is also a hormetic stressor that triggers beneficial adaptations in the body, and besides improved detoxification, fasting for periods of 18-36 hours has been shown to:

- Increase HGH levels by 2,000% in men and 1,300% in women.
- Improve body composition
- Result in more lean muscle, less body fat
- Increase insulin sensitivity
- Initiate therapeutic ketosis
- Increased levels of ketone bodies like beta-hydroxybutyrate and acetoacetate

Ketone Production by Liver During
Fasting Conditions (Ketosis)

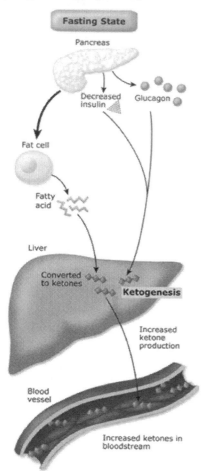

Fasting State

Pancreas

Decreased insulin   Glucagon

Fat cell

Fatty acid

Liver

Converted to ketones   **Ketogenesis**

Increased ketone production

Blood vessel

Increased ketones in bloodstream

– Protection against several diseases, including dementia, Alzheimer's, and many cancers

Intermittent fasting is not recommended for people with blood sugar and metabolic issues, at least not until those challenges have been corrected through diet and lifestyle interventions. I recommend starting out slowly by making dinner your last meal, and then simply skipping breakfast.

At first, aim for 12 to 14 hours between dinner and your first meal of the day. Then, as your body adapts, you can gradually increase your fasting window to the 18-24 hour range. This is the range in which many of the scientifically-reported benefits occur.

There are many ways to fast and they all have benefits:

– Skip breakfast
– Skip lunch
– Fast for 16 hours
– Fast for 36 hours

These are all valid strategies as long as you aren't dealing with adrenal or blood sugar issues. The best type of fast for you is the one you'll actually do.

Coldplay frontman, Chris Martin, prefers to eat 6 days a week and then stick to nothing but water for one day a week.

The truth of the matter is that simply eating less will help your body partition more faculties towards detoxification pathways.

Exogenous ketones and MCT oil can also be used to make fasting easier and increase the production of ketone bodies. When fasting, I will

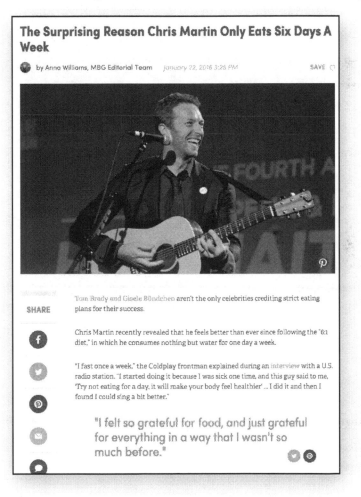

The Surprising Reason Chris Martin Only Eats Six Days A Week

by Anna Williams, MBG Editorial Team   January 22, 2016 3:25 PM   SAVE

SHARE

Tom Brady and Gisele Bündchen aren't the only celebrities crediting strict eating plans for their success.

Chris Martin recently revealed that he feels better than ever since following the "6:1 diet," in which he consumes nothing but water for one day a week.

"I fast once a week," the Coldplay frontman explained during an interview with a U.S. radio station. "I started doing it because I was sick one time, and this guy said to me, 'Try not eating for a day, it will make your body feel healthier' ... I did it and then I found I could sing a bit better."

"I felt so grateful for food, and just grateful for everything in a way that I wasn't so much before."

strategically use a tablespoon of Caprylic acid MCT oil (Bulletproof Brain Octane, Parrillo CapTri) along with exogenous ketones like Keto OS. I have been playing around with what I call a Keto Cocktail. This includes:

- 12 oz of filtered water
- One packet of Keto OS
- 1-1.5 tbsp of Pure Caprylic Acid MCT Oil
- One scoop of a color-, sweetener-, and flavor-free branched chain amino acids supplement.

Some of my more advanced clients have experimented with even longer 3-7 day fasts. These are not recommended for beginners, nor should they be done on your own without professional supervision. There is a pretty rough adaptation period, but then many clients report huge improvements in cognitive function and energy, along with a surprising lack of hunger.

The transition period can also be eased with the therapeutic use of exogenous ketones and C-8 MCT oil. To find out what exogenous ketones I'm currently using, go to www.BioHacks.Pruvitnow.com.

6. *Coffee Enemas.* Coffee enemas mechanically wash the colon, removing toxins, debris, bacteria, parasites, and yeast. The average human has 5-7 pounds of impacted fecal matter in their colon. Coffee enemas also increase Paracelsus of the colon, improving the body's ability to remove toxins through the elimination of feces. Compromised Paracelsus is a major contributor to toxic overload.

Elvis Presley's physician, Dr. George Nichopoulos ("Dr. Nick"), said that Elvis' autopsy revealed his colon was 5-6 inches in diameter, whereas a normal colon is just 2-3 inches. Also, instead of being the standard 4-5 feet long, his colon was 8-9 feet in length. Elvis did not talk about his struggles with constipation. He saw himself as a man's man, and admitting to and vocalizing these challenges would be a sign of weakness.

"Dr. Nick" hypothesized that much of Elvis' weight gain and bloated appearance was due in part to his severe constipation and toxic overload. Coffee also contains beneficial antioxidants which reduce oxidative damage, and the enema process allows us to access parts of the digestive tract that are otherwise difficult to get to. Coffee enemas have been a part of the Gerson therapy for cancer treatment for almost 100 years. The purpose of enemas in the Gerson therapy is to remove toxins in the liver and free radicals from the bloodstream.

In the 1920's, doctors at the University of Minnesota found that coffee which was administered rectally stimulates our body's primary antioxidant in the liver, glutathione S-transferase, by 600-700% above normal levels. Higher glutathione levels have been linked to greater energy, stronger immune function, and a slower aging process. Other benefits of coffee enemas include:

- Increased cellular energy production
- Improved circulation
- Higher glutathione levels
- Enhanced tissue health
- Stronger immunity and tissue repair
- Cellular regeneration
- Reduced body fat (greater leanness)
- An opening of the bile ducts which allows the liver to release both bile and toxins

It's important when doing coffee enemas to only use organic coffee. I recommend Purelife (www.PurelifeEnema.com) or the therapy roast coffee available at Cafe Mam (www.CafeMam.com). For more information on how to prepare your coffee and perform a coffee enema, I recommend checking out some of the free information at Gerson.org. Also, for maximum benefit you'll want to perform two coffee enemas back to back.

7. *Coconut Oil Detox*. Another beneficial detoxification strategy is a 1-3 day fast using raw, organic extra virgin, unfiltered coconut oil. During this fast, aim to drink 70% of your current body weight in ounces of filtered water per day. Ideally, this should be water from a reverse osmosis filter (the only effective way to eliminate fluoride). When you get hungry, have two tablespoons of raw, organic, extra virgin coconut oil. This can be repeated for up to 12 tablespoons per day. The fast can continue for up to three days.

8. *Bentonite Enemas*. Combine ½ cup of bentonite clay (I recommend Sonne's No. 7 Detoxificant) with 12-28 ounces of filtered water. Hold the enema for 10-30 minutes, and then release into the toilet. If performing a coffee enema and a bentonite enema in the same day, be sure to do the bentonite enema second as to not wash out the bentonite enema with the coffee enema. The benefits of the bentonite enema are that it is able to bind to toxins in the colon and assist the body in eliminating these compounds.

9. *The Biomat 7000MX*. This biomat utilizes infrared technology and, from a practical standpoint, has many benefits that a Far Infrared Sauna does not. Clients who have purchased Far Infrared Saunas for their home find that due to the amount of time it takes for the sauna to heat up, they don't end up using it as much as they would like. The Biomat 7000MX, however, quickly gets up to temperature and can be easily used daily during meditation or even at night during sleep.

10. Ionic Foot Baths using the IonCleanse machine (www. amajordifference.com)

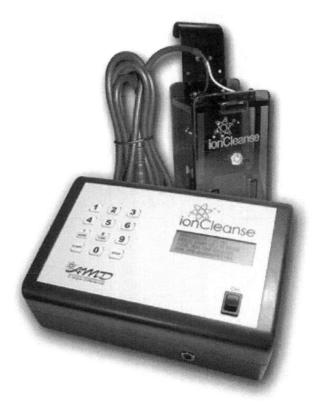

11. NanoVi: Stimulates cellular pathways associated with antioxidant support to combat oxidative stress from free radicals. This device offers a range of detoxification benefits for people interested in improving their health, slowing the aging process, and optimizing mental and physical performance. It is used in wellness centers, professional practices, and homes throughout North America and Europe. I only recommend their two higher end units that operate using 15-minute and 30-minute treatment sessions.

If you're interested I suggest speaking with Rowena. She's an expert in the technology and can help with your questions. We've arranged a discount for our readers if you decide you'd like to invest in a unit for your home or practice (www.eng3corp.com).

12. *Dynamic Neural Retraining System DVD Series* (www. dnrsystem.com) - Limbic System Rehabilitation for:

– Multiple Chemical Sensitivities
– Chronic Fatigue Syndrome
– Fibromyalgia
– Electric Hypersensitivity Syndrome
– Chronic Pain
– Gulf War Syndrome
– Anxiety
– Food Sensitivities
– Postural Orthostatic
– Tachycardia Syndrome

Here are some other tips for reducing exposure to environmental toxins and your body's toxic burden:

– Exercise. Particularly steady state cardiovascular exercise, where the body is sweating for 30 minutes.
– Ditch the plastic. Don't use plastic bottles or containers, even Tupperware, and never put these products in the microwave. This includes plastic bottled water.
– Open your windows. Let fresh air into your home. See Sick Building Syndrome (SBS).
– Walk around barefoot in your home.
– Replace carpets with hard wood floors or tile (not synthetic materials).

- Wash your hands.
- Keep leftovers in glass pyrex containers as food can absorb toxins from plastics.
- Install a reverse osmosis filter on your water faucets and change filters every three or four months. If you rent an apartment, take note that there are reverse osmosis countertop filters. Just add back minerals removed during the filtering process.
- If you run on a tight budget, at a minimum, get yourself a carbon countertop filter. These are selling for less than $30 on Amazon. They don't remove fluoride, but they are better than having nothing at all.
- Replace cleaners, household chemicals, soaps, and cosmetics with organic products. Ann Marie Gianni has a great line of skin cosmetic products so pure you could eat them if you wanted to (www.annmariegianni.com).
- If biotoxin illness is suspected, follow Richie Schumacher's 11-step protocol for Biotoxin Illness (for the detailed protocol visit SurvivingMold.com).
- Use Greenwave EMI (electromagnetic interference) filters in outlets to reduce electrosmog.

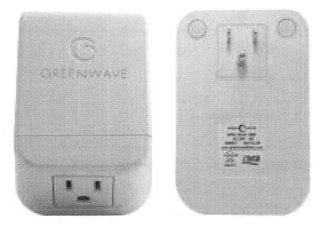

- Unplug electronics in the bedroom and put your cell phone in Airplane mode while you sleep. Or, even better, turn it off and leave it in another room.
- Get an EMP Protection device such as the Silver Retro SRT-3 Q-Link Pendant (www.BioHackingSecrets.com/emf). The Q-Link Clear devices can be placed on your cell phone and other high-EMF electronics to reduce your exposure.

Other supplements for detoxification include:

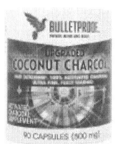

- Organic liquid chlorophyll
- Chlorophyllin
- Wasabi
- Curcumin/turmeric
- Organic chlorella
- Activated coconut charcoal
- Green tea (green tea helps regulate levels of a protein molecule HMGB1 responsible for controlling the signaling compounds known as cytokines that generate inflammation)
- Sulforaphane Glucosinolate (as found in broccoli extracts; can be especially beneficial in individuals with caffeine sensitivity and children with Autism Spectrum Disorders)
- Resveratrol
- Pterostilbene
- Alpha lipoic acid
- Watercress
- R-lipoic acid
- Ubiquinol form of CoQ10
- Vitamin C

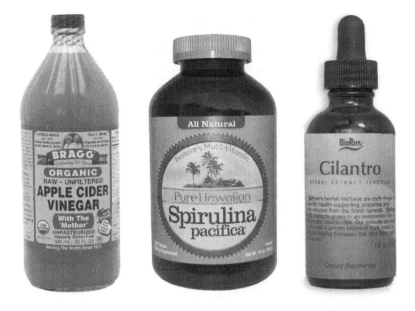

- Liposomal glutathione
- Selenium
- N-acetylcystine
- Melon pulp concentrate (providing superoxide dismutase)
- Natural form or Quali-C (not synthetic adsorbent acid which is often derived from genetically modified corn) broccoli extract
- Schisandra extract
- Milk thistle
- Calcium-d-glucarate
- DIM
- Cilantro can be juiced for additional heavy metal detoxification benefits. For convenience, or if you don't have a juicer, BioPure offers a high quality organic cilantro tincture. Take 10-30 drops up to twice daily.
- Bragg organic apple cider vinegar
- Organic spirulina pacifica

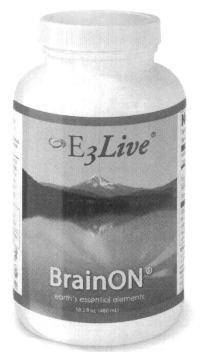

- E3Live BrainOn
- DMSO and ETDA chelating agents

TROUBLESHOOTING #4: LOW TESTOSTERONE & HUMAN GROWTH HORMONE (HGH)

Signs that you are suffering from low testosterone and/or HGH issues include:

- Low libido
- Erratic mood, cognitive function, difficulty concentrating
- Loss of muscle mass
- Sweating attacks in men

TROUBLESHOOTING

Please circle "Yes" or "No" for each statement below:

1. During sex it takes me a long time to climax. *(Yes or No)*
2. I carry excess fat in my belly. *(Yes or No)*
3. I have a low sex drive. *(Yes or No)*
4. I have thin arms and legs (usually along with a bigger belly or a potbelly). *(Yes or No)*
5. I have noticed decreased semen volume or have questioned whether I ejaculate as much as I used to. *(Yes or No)*
6. I shave less frequently than I did when I was younger. *(Yes or No)*
7. I have less hair on my body than I used to. *(Yes or No)*
8. My physician has told me that my testosterone levels are low or I found this to be true in a blood test. *(Yes or No)*

There are seven primary reasons why we may experience low testosterone and HGH. The first is biological aging.

As we get older the levels of various hormones start to decline more and more with each passing decade. Around age 30 we start seeing a decline in HGH, and around age 40 testosterone, estrogen, and progesterone. By age 50 we start seeing declines in DHEA and thyroid hormones. Then, around age 60 we start seeing lower levels of insulin and parathyroid hormone.

The other six, environmental and lifestyle, causes of low testosterone and/or HGH are:

- Gut dysbiosis
- Cortisol dysregulation (AKA hypothalamic, pituitary adrenal axis dysregulation)
- Insulin resistance
- Liver detoxification problems
- Methylation issues
- Fatty acid imbalance

Sleep. In the "Sleep" section of this book, a number of studies were referenced which associated the quantity and quality of sleep with healthy testosterone and healthy hormone levels. One of those studies, in fact, states that for every additional hour of sleep over four hours researchers observed a 15% increase in testosterone. Individuals that slept 8 hours had 60% higher testosterone levels than those who slept just 4 hours per night.

If you were to only do one thing to optimize your testosterone and HGH levels, it should be to spend at least 7 ½ hours in bed per night, aiming for at least 7 hours of deep restful sleep. A close second would be to reduce or even eliminate alcohol consumption. Multiple studies have linked alcohol consumption to substantially-reduced testosterone levels and increased estrogen levels. Alcohol also boosts aromatase activity, an enzyme which converts the male sex hormone, testosterone, into the female sex hormone, estrogen.

Alcohol metabolization also lowers coenzyme NAD+ (nicotinamide adenine dinucleotide), which plays an essential part in the production of testosterone and energy. Studies have shown that even just two drinks a day can lower your testosterone levels. For beer drinkers, the hops in beer are so estrogenic, they are now being studied to treat hot flashes in menopausal women. A pear-shaped body, characterized by a "beer belly" and skinny arms or skinny legs is now recognized as a physical manifestation of elevated estrogen levels in males.

Intermittent Fasting. Another strategy for optimizing testosterone and HGH levels is intermittent fasting. Let's say that you start out eating a normal diet and then you stop eating. The body mobilizes stored glycogen from the liver and muscles and then utilizes this glycogen for energy. Our central nervous system demands a steady fuel supply, and in the absence of dietary glucose, our body begins to deplete liver glycogen down to regulate insulin and assemble free fatty acids for fuel.

The problem is that long chain fatty acids do not cross the blood brain barrier efficiently. So, the body utilizes beta oxidation to break down these long chain fatty acids, which in turn start to form ketone bodies. These ketone bodies are more or less water soluble fat molecules that are able to be used as fuel by the muscles and brain. A number of studies have shown that the muscles and brain are able to run 70% more efficiently on ketones than glucose.

During fasting and this subsequent ketosis that occurs, blood levels of human growth hormone may increase by as much as five-fold, some studies have shown. Higher HGH levels meant greater fat burning and muscle gain, among other benefits such as greater energy levels and a more youthful appearance. A recent study at Intermountain Medical Heart Institute found that during 24-hour fasting periods, HGH increased an average of 1300% in women and nearly 2000% in men. In addition to the other hormonal benefits that have been spoken of, intermittent fasting may also:

- Increase the growth of neurons that protect the brain from damage
- Protect against neurogenic diseases like Alzheimer's, Parkinson's, and dementia
- Prevent cancer and reduce the side effects of chemotherapy
- Trigger autophagy, which removes waste from cells
- Improve numerous risk factors for blood pressure, cholesterol, triglycerides, and inflammatory markers
- Improve increased insulin sensitivity and lower blood sugar levels
- Burn fat and maintain lean muscle when in a calorie deficit
- Positively effect gene expression

Bioidentical Hormone Replacement Therapy (HRT). Wait, steroids? Sort of. But before we examine the important distinctions between anabolic steroids, as utilized by many professional bodybuilders for physique enhancement, and bioidentical hormone replacement therapy let's take a step back.

Steroids have got a bad rap. They destroy your liver, give you pizza face, shrink your man parts, and turn kind, gentle men into "roid raging" maniacs. Right?

Well, there's some truth to these statements. Steroids are, however, not so black and white. It's important to understand that all chemicals, even water and oxygen, are toxic to the human body if the dose is high enough. The dose makes the poison.

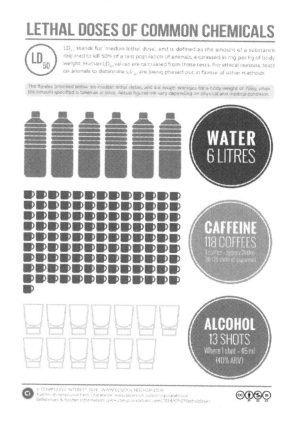

On one hand we have have 1/3 of the WrestleMania XI roster who have dropped dead from something other than old age (12 wrestlers at the time of this publication).

On the other hand, of the 44 football players who started for the Denver Broncos and 49ers in that year's Super Bowl, only one has passed away. And that was from diabetes and subsequent coronary complications.

You also have people like Sylvester Stallone and Arnold who have admitted to using large amounts of anabolic steroids, yet they are a picture of vibrant health and continue to build upon their successes at the 69 and 68 years of age, respectively.

But, rather than examining anecdotal cases in search of the truth, let's take a look at what the scientific literature tells us.

Here's an excerpt from Dunks, Doubles, and Doping: How Steroids are Killing American Athletics:

Enter HBO. *Real Sports with Bryant Gumbel* took the first significant step toward a mass-media outreach on the facts of steroids. In his specialized segment on steroids, Gumbel leads by saying, "As frequently evidenced by officials nationwide, Americans, when drugs are concerned, rarely choose logic when they can opt for hysteria. Case in point, the recent hoopla over steroids."

Furthermore, Americans don't necessarily jump to conclusions but are instead fed with hysteria. When the media pushes hysteria over logic, there is no going back. Gumbel's point is clearly made, and he continues by saying, "In light of the media excess, the public pronouncements and the wailing in Washington, one would assume that the scientific evidence establishing the health risks of steroids is overwhelming." He pauses for a moment, probably giving most viewers the opportunity to nod their heads. He continues, "But it's not. On the contrary, when it comes to steroid use among adult males, the evidence reveals virtually no fire despite all the smoke."

Before the program switches to the HBO feature on steroids, Gumbel leaves the viewer with, "The science of steroids, or the absence of it, suggests some conclusions that few people want to hear."

Not to defend steroids, or make an appeal against them, HBO and Gumbel use one very, very powerful fact in their presentation: evidence.

Whether hormones are beneficial or harmful depends on many factors. Not the least of which are the individual's age, gender, liver and kidney function, dosage, objectives, and the type of hormone administered.

However, before considering this route, it's imperative to first investigate and correct the six primary causes of low testosterone and HGH that are listed in the beginning of this section. If exogenous hormones are introduced to the body without correcting the root cause of hormonal imbalance, the resulting negative feedback loop could further exacerbate these imbalances, leading to more severe problems in the future. For most clients (www.BioHackingSecrets.com/coaching), I recommend getting as much out of your body's endogenous hormone production as you can before supplementing with bioidentical hormones.

Maintaining youthful hormone levels as we age is an essential tenet of optimal energy and focus. From a body composition standpoint, testosterone promotes lean body mass and a reduction in body fat. It does so by blocking the enzyme lipoprotein lipase (LPL), which is responsible for the uptake of body fat into fat cells. Testosterone also increases insulin sensitivity, enhances the growth of muscle tissue, and decreases fat deposits by signaling receptors on cell membranes to release stored fat.

Many placebo-controlled trials have demonstrated significant changes in body composition, including increases in lean body mass and decreases in body fat in men receiving bioidentical testosterone replacement therapy for 12 months or longer. Testosterone has also been shown to positively influence a number of inflammatory pathways. In a study involving 184 men with low testosterone levels, 18 weeks of bioidentical hormone replacement therapy lowered a number of inflammatory biomarkers, including C-reactive protein and tumor necrosis factor alpha (TNFα).

Low testosterone levels have also been associated with depression. This is further compounded by the reality that many antidepressant medications further suppress libido and adversely affect tumescence. Bio identical hormone replacement therapy is associated with elevated mood, positive outlook, and increased feelings of well-being.

Cognition and focus are also regulated in part by testosterone's effect on the central nervous system. Testosterone has neuroprotective qualities and has been shown to reduce oxidative stress along with beta amyloid accumulation. This is an important risk factor in the prevention of dementia and Alzheimer's disease. An association has been identified between low testosterone levels in men and a higher prevalence of neurodegenerative diseases.

For a long time it was assumed that since men had a higher incidence of heart attacks and cardiovascular disease it was all tied into testosterone. However, new research indicates that the opposite may be true. A growing body of scientific literature now shows a clear relationship between low testosterone levels and increased incidence of heart disease, cardiovascular incidents, and the mortality rates in men.

The bioidentical hormones for estrogen, testosterone, and progesterone are all approved by the FDA. Bioidentical hormones have the same molecular structure as the hormones naturally produced in the human body. The body cannot distinguish between them and the natural ones. As a result, these compounds are often free from the myriad of unwanted and dangerous side effects commonly anabolic and synthetic hormones.

Non-bioidentical hormones and synthetic anabolics have been associated with an increased risk in cancer, heart attack, and stroke. Bioidentical hormones are made from hormones extracted from soy or yams. When considering hormone replacement therapy, make sure:

- You only use bioidentical hormones
- Use the minimum effective dose (to prevent undesirable elevations in IGF1 (Insulin-Like Growth Factor 1) which can put you at an increased risk of cancer)
- Work with a physician who specializes in biological hormone replacement therapy who will monitor your blood work and adjust your hormone dosages accordingly
- A full blood panel is recommended no less frequently than every six months

For men, the standard dosage for testosterone injections is 200 mg every 1 to 4 weeks. Other forms of testosterone delivery include:

- Pellets inserted under the skin
- Patches
- Gels
- Pills

Included below is an image that compares the various forms of testosterone therapy:

Table 4. Testosterone Replacement Products

Formulation	Products Available	Dosing Ranges	Advantages	Disadvantages
Testosterone enanthate or cypionate	Delatestryl or Depo-Testosterone	100 mg/wk IM or 200 mg every 2 wk IM	Improves symptoms, inexpensive, longer intervals between dosing	Requires injection; fluctuations in serum testosterone levels
Topical gels	Testim and AndroGel	5-10 g (50-100 mg testosterone) applied daily	Corrects symptoms, flexible dosing, ease of application, good tolerability	Potential for secondary exposure
Transdermal patches[a]	Androderm	1-2 patches (5-10 mg) every 24 h	Ease of application, corrects symptoms, mimics diurnal rhythm, less erythrocytosis	Lower serum testosterone levels achieved, skin irritation likely
Buccal tablets	Striant	30-mg controlled-release tabs applied twice daily	Corrects symptoms	Gum and mouth irritation
Implantable pellets	Testopel	4-6 75-mg pellets implanted every 3-6 mo	Corrects symptoms, long duration of activity	Requires surgical implantation; pellet extrusions, infection

[a] Patches available in 2.5 and 5 mg.
Source: References 2, 7, 12.

Studies have shown bioidentical testosterone injections, in the range of 100 to 200 mg a week, do not increase growth factors and hormones that would cause cancer to grow and spread. In gums where people are taking more than 300 mg a week, there starts to be increases in systemic IGF 1 levels, which can lead to unwanted changes.

The one exception to this rule is that oxandrolone (Anavar) should be taken at a dosage of 10-50 mg per day. This oral testosterone has been used for decades as an intervention against cancer and HIV/AIDS-related muscle wasting, infections, severe burns, and major surgeries. It demonstrated itself to have an excellent safety profile and low toxicity levels. Oxandrolone is also popular among bodybuilders and physique competitors as a cutting agent, used to accelerate fat loss and increase muscle definition.

Cachexia is a form of muscle wasting and tissue atrophy that is common with cancer patients. Our risk of cancer increases with age, so there's frequently a perfect storm resulting in cachexia wherein four factors contribute to accelerated muscle and activity deterioration:

- The cancer itself
- Chemotherapy
- Inactivity/lack of mobility
- Age

Chemotherapy has been shown to increase muscle loss and fatigue, which in turn, results in less physical activity. Inactivity and lack of mobility further contribute to this problem. In individuals over the age of 40, it is common for sarcopenia (age-related muscle loss to also amplify these detrimental side effects.

The strategic use of anabolics can be instrumental in preventing cachexia and even sarcopenia. This is important because as people lose the ability to move, their mental health and physical health quickly deteriorate. This doesn't just apply to extreme cases like those related to cancer, HIV, and AIDS.

Both our energy production and our movement decrease as we age. This initiates a negative feedback loop where we move less and thereby experience a more rapid degradation of body composition as well as physical and mental health. Keeping people strong and mobile, even through the use of bioidentical hormones and low toxicity anabolics like oxandrolone, is of paramount importance for maintaining peak performance and a high quality of life.

Now, let's discuss HGH a little further. As previously stated, levels of HGH start to decrease around age 30. It is released during REM sleep, and while we hit REM sleep a number of times throughout the night, the greatest growth hormone release occurs within 90-110 minutes of going to bed. HGH plays an important role in growth, cellular reproduction, and tissue regeneration in addition to maintaining youthful energy levels, mood, and mental clarity. Symptoms of low growth hormone include:

- High levels of body fat, particularly around the midsection
- Low mood, depression, anxiety, and increased stress
- Decreased interest in sex
- Decreased sexual function
- Loss of motivation
- Fatigue
- Reductions in social connectedness
- Greater sensitivities to temperatures (cold and hot)
- Decreases in muscle strength and stamina
- Reduced bone density

Following the recommendations in this book, especially ensuring at least 7 ½ hours in bed every night, will maximize your natural production of HGH. Additionally, the presence of elevated insulin levels has been shown to interfere with growth hormone release. So, minimizing the consumption of sugar, carbohydrates, and insulin-spiking foods, within 3 hours of your bedtime, will further optimize endogenous growth hormone production.

Endogenous growth hormone injections have been used since the late 1950s to treat growth disorders in children, and they have been used for almost 35 years in body building competitions as an anabolic agent. In the past two decades use of HGH and performance enhancing drugs has exploded with celebrities, professional athletes, models, and business looking for a competitive edge. Hollywood trainer Happy Hill, who has helped Jake Gyllenhaal and Ryan Phillippe prepare for roles, estimates that around 20% of actors use performance enhancing drugs (PED) to help them bulk up and become more defined.

Actors like Sylvester Stallone and Arnold Schwarzenegger (as mentioned earlier) have been open about long-term anabolic PED use, as have Oliver Stone, Nick Nolte, Lance Armstrong, Marion Jones, and Alex Rodriguez. In 2008, the Albany Times Union reported that Timbaland, Mary J. Blige, 50 Cent, Tyler Perry, and Wyclef Jean were among thousands of celebrities who were receiving shipments of HDH and anabolic steroids.

For adults who have a growth hormone deficiency, or suboptimal levels of this youth hormone, HGH injections may provide increased strength and exercise capacity, greater bone density, increased muscle mass, lower body fat, greater motivation, and elevated mood. A number of my clients (www.BioHackingSecrets.com/coaching) use HGH injections to combat growth hormone deficiencies and reap these benefits. HGH is also approved to treat adults with short bowel syndrome or AIDS/HIV-related muscle wasting.

Before becoming illegal and being labeled as "the date rape drug," GHB (gamma-hydroxybutyric acid) was used to boost natural growth hormone production. A 1970 study from Japan found that by taking 6 grams of GHB, subjects experienced 600% higher levels of natural growth hormone production. It is important to note that subjects also experienced no change in insulin or glucose levels, which is important because growth hormone injections can cause insulin resistance and elevated blood glucose levels.

Another study found GHB doses ranging from 2.5 to 4.5 grams, administered at bedtime, increased durations of Stage 3 and Stage 4 sleep, which are thought to be the most restorative of sleep stages and the stages wherein our body actually produces growth hormone. Unfortunately, because GHB was used by some to take sexual advantage of others, it has since become a very tightly-controlled and regulated substance. Today, GHB is used solely as a treatment for narcolepsy and is available by prescription under the name XYREM. In order to get a prescription for XYREM, you must undergo an overnight sleep study which costs around $1,000 and be diagnosed with narcolepsy (at least in the state of Illinois).

Perhaps the biggest risk of human growth hormone injections is increased risk of cancer and accelerated cancer cell growth and replication. Cancer cells divide and replicate more rapidly in an environment of elevated IGF1, which is another reason blood tests 2-4 times a year are of paramount importance when utilizing these compounds. Here are some other strategies for maintaining healthy testosterone and HGH levels:

- Eat foods like wild-caught oysters, grass-fed beef, cruciferous vegetables (broccoli, kale, Brussel sprouts, cabbage), free-range eggs (including the yolks), garlic, wild-caught cold water fish
- Avoid excessive calorie restrictive diets, alcohol, soy, and caffeine (Several studies show that alcohol consumption significantly lowers testosterone levels).

- Avoid beer because it is one of the worst alcoholic beverages to consume if you are trying to maintain optimal test levels. It contains a strong form of estrogen called 8-Prenylnaringenin. It also contain xanthohumol, which is a polyphenol that has been shown to interfere with hormone signaling. Furthermore, most beers contain immunogenic and allergenic compounds like gluten, high fructose corn syrup, corn, genetically modified corn syrup, genetically modified dextrose, caramel coloring, yeast stabilizers, tannins, fish bladders, and/or anti-freeze, CLEP chemicals like propylene glycol.
- If you are going to drink, I recommend sticking to the minimum effective dose you need to achieve your desired affect, but no more, and have those drinks come from either a clear agave tequila or a potato- or grape-based vodka. Some individuals also do fine with low residual sugar red wines like Cabernet Sauvignon, Pinot Noir, and Merlot. However, you have to remember to listen to your body. If you don't feel good when drinking wine (i.e. you get tired, brain fogged, spacey, etc.), then don't drink anymore. Many wines contain allergens, such as pesticides from unwashed grapes, tannins, sulfites, preservatives, antihistamines, yeast, and egg whites (used as a fining agent).

When optimizing hormone levels, look first to the diet and lifestyle factors that could be interfering. Only after those potential issues have been addressed should you assess whether additional interventions should be made and weigh the pros and cons of exogenous bioidentical hormone replacement therapy. Even minute amounts of exogenous hormones can disrupt the body's endogenous production through negative feedback loops and complicated regulatory mechanisms.

We also have to decide for ourselves whether we are willing to improve mood, energy, motivation, body composition, and performance if the tradeoff is an increased risk of early mortality. I caution anyone considering these options to invest the resources necessary to work with an experienced expert who can help create a customized program that will maximize benefits while minimizing potential risks. There are also supplements you can take which are helpful in boosting HGH and/ or testosterone levels. You may consider taking this route prior to using any type of hormone therapy. They are:

- DHEA (dehydroepiandrosterone)
- Bioidentical testosterone cypionate and enanthate
- Melatonin
- Anavar (oxandrolone): When asked about using Anavar, I always recommend adding a few specific supplement formulas that include milk thistle (silymarin), chlorophyllin, a bioactive turmeric, broccoli extract, and a few other herbs that support liver detoxification and been shown to help maintain healthy liver enzyme levels.

Clin Endocrinol (Oxf). 1999 Nov;51(5):637-42.

The effect of melatonin administration on pituitary hormone secretion in man.

Forsling ML[1], Wheeler MJ, Williams AJ.

Author information

Abstract

OBJECTIVE: Evidence is accumulating that the nocturnal increase in melatonin may influence pituitary hormone secretion. The aim of this study was to determine the effect of exogenous melatonin, in concencetrations spanning the physiological range, on the release of pituitary hormones in man during daylight hours.

DESIGN: A double blind, randomized, crossover study.

SUBJECTS: Eight healthy male volunteers with a mean age of 21 +/- 0.5 years were studied on four occasions, observations being made after the adminstration of melatonin in doses of 0.05, 0.5 or 5.0 mg or placebo. They refrained from taking heavy exercise, alcohol and from smoking for 24 h prior to the study.

MEASUREMENTS: Serum cortisol, growth hormone, prolactin and plasma oxytocin, vasopressin, sodium, osmolality and packed cell volume were measured in samples taken at 30 minutes intervals for 150 minutes after the administration of melatonin.

RESULTS: Melatonin produced dose-dependent changes in circulating concentrations of oxytocin and vasopressin, the 0.5 mg dose being stimulatory, while 5.0 mg was inhibitory. These two doses stimulated growth hormone release, while there was no significant effect on prolactin or cortisol release.

CONCLUSIONS: These results confirm that the nocturnal increase in melatonin could contribute to the patterns of oxytocin, vasopressin and growth hormone release seen over 24 h.

- Bioidentical estrogen (for women)
- Progesterone
- Pregnenolone
- Vitamin D (Include vitamin A from an animal source like extra virgin cod liver oil to prevent vitamin D toxicity)
- Chrysin
- Muira Puama
- Tribulus Terrestris
- ZMA (Zinc Monomethionine Aspartate)
- Maca
- Moringa
- Calcium-D-Glucarate (to lower estrogen)
- DIM (Diindolylmethane, to metabolize estrogen)

TROUBLESHOOTING #5: ADRENAL FATIGUE (HPA AXIS DYSREGULATION, CORTISOL DYSREGULATION)

Please circle "Yes" or "No" for each statement below:

1. I get lightheaded, faint, or dizzy when I stand up. *(Yes or No)*
2. I have trouble falling asleep. *(Yes or No)*
3. I often wake up during the night. *(Yes or No)*
4. I'm very tired and groggy in the morning, and it is very difficult to get out of bed. *(Yes or No)*
5. I do not feel refreshed, even when I sleep eight or more hours. *(Yes or No)*
6. I have been diagnosed with hypoglycemia (low blood sugar) or know that I suffer from issues related to having low blood sugar. *(Yes or No)*

7. I get moody, anxious, or agitated when I miss a meal. *(Yes or No)*
8. I have seasonal allergies. *(Yes or No)*
9. My allergies have gotten worse in the past 12 months and/or I'm finding it more difficult to breathe through my nose. *(Yes or No)*
10. I get sick more often than other people. *(Yes or No)*
11. I have a below-average memory and would consider myself forgetful. *(Yes or No)*
12. I crave salt and salty foods. *(Yes or No)*
13. I have excess belly fat. *(Yes or No)*

When our bodies are exposed to chronic stress, the hypothalamic pituitary adrenal axis (HPA) is triggered. This results in a downstream release of various hormones, which ultimately result in increased levels of cortisol (the stress hormone). Chronic stress can come from poor diet, lack of sleep, psychological stress, chronic infections, overuse of caffeine and/or stimulants, overtraining (exercise that is too high in intensity or duration), and a wide variety of other factors.

The HPA axis, and more specifically our adrenals, are responsible for the body's fight or flight response. In healthy individuals, when stressors are removed, HPA axis returns to homeostasis. However, many of us are in a state of chronic stress, and on a long enough timeline, this can result in adrenal fatigue or full-blown adrenal burnout. Our bodies are constantly producing high levels of cortisol and our cells become less sensitive to its effects. This causes a condition known as cortisol resistance.

When this happens, more cortisol is required to produce the same effects, and eventually our body can't keep up. Cortisol levels then become too low and adrenal fatigue sets in. Symptoms of adrenal fatigue include:

– Waking up tired, despite adequate sleep
– Chronic fatigue throughout the day

- Decreased cognitive function or brain fog
- Low sex drive
- Food sensitivities
- Inability to effectively manage stress
- Low mood
- Low blood sugar
- Low blood pressure
- Feelings of dizziness or spaciness when standing up too quickly or getting out of bed
- Craving sweets or salty foods
- Feeling overwhelmed, irritable, tired, or wired
- Difficulty falling or staying asleep

The key to healing adrenal fatigue is to remove or reduce unhealthy stressors in your life and to develop more effective practices for managing stress and facilitating the body's ability to rest and recover. The most important ingredient is sleep. When we have adrenal fatigue, we need 8-9 hours of sleep per night. This would probably require you to spend 8 ½ - 9 ½ hours in bed per night. This can be very difficult for people with demanding jobs and family responsibilities. However, in many cases this still can be accomplished with careful planning.

In addition to a good night's sleep, 20-30 minute power naps taken in the afternoon can be instrumental in maintaining and restoring healthy cortisol rhythms. If you have difficulty falling asleep and staying asleep at night, follow the recommendations outlined in the sleep section of this guide. Other things that you can do are:

- Make your first meal of the day high in protein with carbs coming only from non-starchy green vegetables. I recommend a shake that contains:

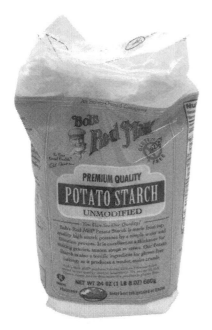

- 6-10 ounces of organic greens (baby spinach is most palatable)
- 10-16 ounces of water, coconut milk, or almond milk (make sure it does not contain carrageenan)
- 1 tbs of raw organic chia seeds (can substitute flax, sunflower, or hemp)
- 1-2 scoops organic vegan protein like SunWarrior Warrior Blend

  – *Additional resistant starch:* Bob's Red Mill potato starch unmodified, organic banana peel, Natural Stacks Prebiotic Plus, Klaire Labs Biotagen, Prebiotin

– Another all-in-one option is Dr. Alan Christiansen's Adrenal Reset Shake (http://store.drchristianson.com/)

– Limit or eliminate caffeine and stimulants which artificially induce the body's fight or flight response and worsen HPA axis dysregulation.

– Eat a complete protein with every meal, which would ideally come from a small serving of wild-caught fish. This would help to minimize hormonal fluctuations and support adrenal health.

– Eat every 2-3 hours

– Eliminate or reduce hidden infections like H. pylori, Lyme, herpes, parasites, Epstein-Barr, etc. (see the "Chronic Infections" section of this troubleshooting guide).

– Supplement wisely by taking one of the adaptogenic, herbal formulas recommended below along with nutrients to support adrenal health, a cortisol regulation.

Do not follow an intermittent fasting protocol or skip meals in cases such as this since these can be an additional sources of stress on the body. Be careful not to restrict your calorie intake too much either, as this can be an additional source of stress. You can better manage your stress by meditating daily, preferably in the morning, and practicing gentle yoga and getting frequent massages.

Depending on where a client of mine is at, I will often encourage some individuals to exercise and perform light steady state cardio in the morning. While some physicians do not recommend this, I've found that it depends on the individual. When we keep their heart rate around 65% of their max heart rate, this can have therapeutic benefits in re-establishing endocrine health.

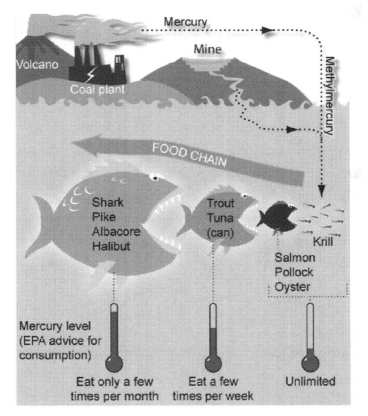

It also helps to lower inflammation by getting 80% of your nutrition from organic plants, most of those plants being vegetables, and most of those vegetables being green. Make wild-caught fish and oysters your primary source of protein and supplement with additional healthy fats like Udo's Choice Oil, 3.6.9 blend, extra virgin cod liver oil, and Yes Parent Essential Oils. There are a number of others that I use, which I choose from based on an individual's needs.

Again, you shouldn't overtrain. Any physical activity that you perform should result in increased energy afterwards. If you experience fatigue, decreased sex drive, increased aches and pains, or changes in mood, those are indications that you are pushing your body past its capacity to recover. Therefore, you should decrease the intensity or duration of your workouts and find a program that helps you to feel good as well as increase your quality of life. Furthermore, you should limit artificial light at night and get bright light during the day. (Be sure to also follow the recommendations outlined in the "Sleep" and "Light" sections of this guide).

A great resource is Dr. Alan Christiansen's *"Adrenal Reset Diet"* book. He categorizes adrenal dysfunction into three distinct categories: crashed, wired and tired, and stressed. By using his diagnostic test at www.AdrenalQuiz.com you can answer a few questions that will help you to determine which state of adrenal dysfunction most accurately reflects your situation. From there, he suggests specific nutrients, supplement packs, and adaptogens to bring your cortisol rhythms back into balance.

Use adaptogenic herbs to support the body's response to stress:

– Ashwagandha
– Rhodiola
– Siberian ginseng

- Eleutherococcus
- Phosphatidylserine
- Liposomal vitamin C
- Pantethine
- Adrenal glandular
- Natural vitamin C (Not ascorbic acid which can come from GMO corn)
- Licorice root to help increase circulating cortisol levels (not recommended for individuals with high blood pressure)

I have also used a number of broad spectrum adaptogenic formulas, based on individual situations. They include:

- Seriphos
- Adrenotone
- Gaia Adrenal Health
- Metagenics Adreset

You might also use hormones, such as:

- Pregnenolone
- DHEA

Be careful to avoid hydrocortisone, which has many unwanted side effects, including weight gain, immune suppression, cardiovascular problems, diabetes, insomnia, osteoporosis, and many others. Choosing the right brands and quality of supplements is of paramount importance. Avoid ascorbic acid, the popular choice for vitamin C supplements, as it is a synthetic compound usually made from genetically modified corn. It also kills the good bacteria in our digestive tract.

Many supplements also contain the filler magnesium stearate, which has been implicated in the formation of bile films. Some bile films can protect chronic infections from our immune system. I've also used the CT3M (Circadian T3method for low cortisol with a number of clients (www.BioHackingSecrets.com/coaching). The nuances of this approach are beyond the scope of this guide. However, I encourage you to do your own research and align with an expert who can help if this is something you would like to integrate into your treatment protocol.

TROUBLESHOOTING #6: HYPOTHYROIDISM

The three main hormones that control your metabolism and weight are cortisol, insulin, and thyroid. I've worked with many clients who have experienced symptoms of hypothyroidism despite taking prescription medications and having normal lab work. It is estimated that around 60% of the people who have thyroid problems are completely unaware that they are suffering from this hormonal imbalance. Symptoms of hypothyroidism include:

- Cold sensitivity
- Constipation
- Dry skin
- Diet resistant/hard to lose weight
- Fatigue
- Low mood or Depression
- Low sex drive
- Memory problems
- Brain Fog
- Cramping or Muscle weakness

- Excessive gas and bloating
- Water retention
- Inability to exercise
- Hair loss
- Brittle nails
- Hoarseness or losing one's voice easily
- Irregular menstrual cycles

Please circle "Yes" or "No" for each statement below:

1. I have an enlarged neck. *(Yes or No)*
2. I often feel tired or weak. *(Yes or No)*
3. I'm more sensitive to cold than other people, and I notice that my hands and feet are frequently cold to the touch. *(Yes or No)*
4. I've been told that I am anemic or been diagnosed with anemia. *(Yes or No)*
5. I have a slow pulse. *(Yes or No)*
6. My metabolism has grown slower as I've aged. *(Yes or No)*
7. I have delayed reflexes. *(Yes or No)*
8. I'm often constipated. *(Yes or No)*
9. I lose my voice more easily than other people or am often horse. *(Yes or No)*
10. I have been diagnosed with hypothyroidism or Hashimoto's disease. *(Yes or No)*
11. I often eat grains, flour, baked goods, or processed foods. *(Yes or No)*
12. I need to sleep more than other people. *(Yes or No)*
13. I have been unable to lose weight or feel like other people are able to lose weight much easier than me while putting forth the same effort. *(Yes or No)*

14. I frequently have hard poop, and it can be difficult to go to the bathroom. *(Yes or No)*
15. I often find it difficult to stay positive and struggle with low mood or depression. *(Yes or No)*
16. The outer part of my eyebrows are thinning. *(Yes or No)*
17. I have noticed my hair thinning, my hairline receding, and/or my hair falling out more than normal. *(Yes or No)*
18. I have dry skin. *(Yes or No)*
19. I have a dry scalp or dandruff. *(Yes or No)*
20. I have high cholesterol. *(Yes or No)*

Every cell in the body has receptors for thyroid hormone. Even people with normal thyroid levels experience improved energy, cognitive function, and mood when the levels of this hormone are functionally optimized. Here are a few of the ways that I have corrected thyroid problems or optimized thyroid function for some of my coaching clients (www.BioHackingSecrets.com/coaching).

The most important area to start with is diet. I recommend eliminating grains, especially gluten-containing grains that are not organic. The same should be said for non-organic soy. Over 90% of soy (including tofu, edamame, soy milk, etc.) is genetically modified. If you do consume soy, make sure it's organic.

Hashimoto's is an autoimmune condition which results in hypothyroidism. Several studies show a strong link between gluten sensitivity and Hashimoto's.

If you suspect suboptimal thyroid function, start by following the nutrition recommendations in this guide. Make sure to be diligent to completely eliminate gluten and non-organic soy. It's important to note that standard lab tests for gluten intolerance and sensitivity are notoriously inaccurate. Do not rely on these tests, as the most reliable indicator is a 28-day elimination-provocation diet.

Supplements and prescriptions for optimizing thyroid function are:

- *Ashwagandha:* An adaptogenic herb which supports production of thyroid hormone T4
- *Guggul:* This helps convert T4 into the active thyroid hormone T3
- *Korean Ginseng:* Reduces reverse T3 (rT3) and supports healthy T3 and T4 levels
- *Iodine:* Exhibit caution when supplementing with iodine as many sources can initiate a negative feedback loop in the body and are not recommended
- *Tyrosine:* Required for thyroid hormone production
- *Vitamin B12:* As methylcobalamin or hydroxocobalamin taken sublingually if you suspect digestive or absorption issues in the gut
- *Vitamin A:* Supports healthy T3 levels
- *Kelp:* A whole food source of iodine, super-saturated by iodine solution (SSKI available by prescription)
- *WP Thyroid:* Natural pork desiccated thyroid containing T2, T3, and T4. The only two inactive ingredients are coconut and artichoke. This is the prescription choice of Dr. Alan Christianson and usually where I recommend clients start. Other natural desiccated thyroid options include Armour and Nature-Throid (http://getrealthyroid.com/).
- *Cytomel (T3):* In some cases, based on lab work, additional T3 may be needed. In such instances, consider talking with your prescribing physician about Cytomel (liothyronine sodium).
- *iThroid:* Contains balance of iodide and free elemental iodine which is highly absorbable and binds with tyrosine to produce thyroid hormones (www.rlclabs.com).

Prescription Thyroid Medications: I use a number of prescription thyroid medications with coaching clients based on the symptoms and lab work results. Dosages and specific medications used are beyond the scope of this guide. If you do suspect suboptimal thyroid function, it is recommended that you work with an expert in this area.

Many clients have come to me with normal lab work but still exhibit all of the symptoms of hypothyroidism or suboptimal thyroid function. They are usually taking the prescription drug Synthroid (levothyroxine). If you are working with a physician who has prescribed Synthroid, and your symptoms persist despite normal lab work, I would encourage you to investigate other options. An equivalent dosage of WP Thyroid would be a prudent starting place.

When ordering blood work to assess your thyroid function, make sure to get your T4, T3, rT3, and thyroid stimulating hormone levels tested. Many physicians only test for thyroid stimulating hormone, and in some cases T4, but this does not provide a complete picture of how your thyroid is functioning. Unfortunately, a lot of the blood tests for assessing thyroid function are still extremely flawed.

Another proxy for your metabolic rate and thyroid health is taking your body temperature before getting out of bed in the morning. I recommend using a mercury thermometer, which can be purchased on eBay, as opposed to the newer electronic thermometer. If you are unable to invest in a mercury thermometer, I recommend the Geratherm, which is the most accurate non-mercury thermometer. Your temperature should be taken under the armpit first thing in the morning, so keep the thermometer next to your bed. A good reading would be 98.2°F or above.

Do this for at least 5-10 days and your temperature is consistently under 98.2°F, that may be an indicator that you are dealing with suboptimal thyroid hormone levels. Other resources that you can refer to for help with this type of problem are:

- *"Hypothyroidism: The Unsuspected Illness"* by Brenda Barnes
- *"The Thyroid"* by Thomas McAvic
- *"Solved: The Riddle of Illness"* by Stephen Langer

I go into some additional details for home diagnostic tests and recommended blood work for assessing thyroid function in the upcoming troubleshooting section "Keeping Track: Self Monitoring."

TROUBLESHOOTING #7:
BLOOD SUGAR & METABOLIC ISSUES

Signs that you are suffering from blood sugar and metabolic issues include:

- Energy boosts after meals
- Craving sweets or carbohydrates, particularly in between meals
- Agitation or irritability when skipping meals
- Use of coffee or sugar for energy
- Feeling lightheaded when meals are skipped
- Needing to eat to overcome fatigue
- Feeling jittery, shaky, or weak
- Feeling anxious, nervous, or emotionally volatile
- Forgetfulness and poor memory
- Blurry vision
- Feeling the need to nap after meals
- Always feeling hungry

- Cravings for sweets and carbs that are not satisfied by eating these foods
- A need for sweets or desserts after meals
- Frequent urination
- Increased thirst
- Increased appetite
- Diet resistant/hard to lose weight
- Body aches that are unrelated to injuries which tend to migrate throughout the body

Please circle "Yes" or "No" for each statement below:

1. I have been diagnosed with high blood sugar or diabetes. *(Yes or No)*
2. I need coffee, caffeine, or stimulants (including prescription drugs like Adderall, Ritalin, Vyvanse, Dexedrine, Provigil, etc.) to get myself started or get through the day. *(Yes or No)*
3. I have had an increased appetite over the past 12 months. *(Yes or No)*

High blood sugar and metabolic issues are some of the most common causes of compromised energy production and decreased mental clarity. In a healthy individual, when sugars, or carbohydrates which convert to sugars in the body, are consumed the body responds by releasing the appropriate dose of insulin. The insulin works by shoveling those sugars (glucose) our cells, primarily in the liver and muscle, to be used to produce energy or stored for future use.

One key to maintaining healthy blood sugar levels, insulin sensitivity, and metabolic health is to balance between sugar and carbohydrate consumption in relation to energy expenditure. Our modern diet is far too high in these foods, especially when taking into account our sedentary lifestyles. Our bodies have a limited storage capacity for glucose in the muscles and liver, but we have an unlimited ability to convert glucose into body fat and store it this way.

When carbohydrate consumption consistently exceeds energy expenditure, we get fat. This imbalance also causes a cascade of hormonal problems which result in fatigue, low mood, and brain fog. High levels of sugar and carbohydrate consumption result in high levels of insulin release. Over time, too much insulin can result in inflammation, and consequently, our cells can become resistant to insulin's effects.

Similar to other forms of hormonal resistance, our body tries to compensate by releasing larger amounts of insulin, and the downward spiral continues. This leads to more inflammation and more body fat. This excess body fat further increases inflammation, by the way. This also leads to less energy, which results in even less physical activity and compromised cognitive function. While it's unfortunate that these issues have become rampant in our modern society, the good news is that they can be easily corrected with the right lifestyle interventions, supplements, and certain guided actions.

From a nutritional perspective, I advise that you follow the recommendation in this guide, paying particular attention to get your carbohydrates from cellular sources (plants). Most of the plants that you consume should be from non-starchy vegetables, and it is vital that your carbohydrate consumption is in line with your physical activity levels. This is a very individualized calculation, however, as a general rule of thumb, I recommend that most men consume between 65 and 100 grams of carbohydrates per day. Most women should only consume between 50 and 75 grams of carbohydrates per day. Again, these carbohydrates should come from cellular sources.

One of the most effective dietary interventions I've used with clients (www.BioHackingSecrets.com/coaching) suffering from insulin insensitivity is the ketogenic diet. A number of studies have shown that the ketogenic diet is effective in the treatment of diabetes and diabetic complications. Additionally, insulin sensitivity and glucose tolerance are improved when I switch my clients to a ketogenic diet, and blood sugar reductions are also observed.

Some clients also experience an improvement in blood sugar and insulin sensitivity by incorporating strategic intermittent fasting. Having said that, I've also seen an equal amount of clients who are unable to tolerate intermittent fasting protocols until their blood sugars are normalized. It's important that you listen to your body and the signals that it's giving you. Those will be your most accurate barometer for whether a particular strategy is beneficial of detrimental. Other recommendations for correcting blood sugar and metabolic issues include:

- Eating a breakfast that includes high-quality protein, fats, and green vegetables
- Keeping blood sugar low and stable by eating every 2-3 hours, and including small amounts of protein in the form of wild-caught fish or a vegan protein powder with every meal
- Finding your carbohydrate tolerance and keeping your carbohydrate consumption in line with your energy expenditure.
- Avoid high carbohydrate foods (focus on non-starchy green vegetables and 1/2 to 1 cup organic berries maximum per day).
- Utilizing dry saunas. One animal study found that 30 minutes in a sauna, three times a week for three months, resulted in a 31% decrease in insulin levels and a substantial reduction in blood sugar. Dry saunas have tremendous promise in the management of chronic diseases like Type 2 diabetes, metabolic syndrome, cardiovascular disease, as well as many others.

Nutritional supplements and prescription medications that can be beneficial in blood sugar and metabolic issues include:

- Metformin / Glucophage (500 mg 1-2x daily)
- Berberine HCL (500 mg up to 3x daily with meals)
- Exogenous ketones
- Inositol
- Carnitine
- Ubiquinol
- CoQ10
- Cinnamon
- Chromium picolinate
- Magnesium glycinate
- Alpha Lipoic acid
- Lipoic acid
- Pterostilbene
- Vitamin E (tocopherols)
- Glucomannan
- Gymnema Sylvestre
- Biotine
- Niacin
- Bovine adrenal glandulars from grass-fed or pastured cows, bovine liver glandulars from grass-fed or pastured cows, bovine pancreas glandulars from grass-fed or pastured cows

Section Notes: Studies have observed a decrease in blood sugar following the consumption of exogenous ketones. It has been suggested that this may be a result of ketones activating pyruvate dehydrogenase (PDH) which enhances glucose uptake. Alzheimer's disease almost always involves compromised PDH activity. Learn more about exogenous ketones at http://biohacks.pruvitnow.com.

A number of studies have found blueberry consumption, and particularly pterostilbene ingestion, to stabilize blood glucose levels. In one 12-week study, participants supplementing with pterostilbene exhibited 32 mg/dl decrease in fasting glucose and almost 70% of participants were able to bring their blood glucose levels under control.

TROUBLESHOOTING #8:
NEUROTRANSMITTER IMBALANCES

Serotonin:

Signs that you are suffering from serotonin-related issues include:

- Feelings of unhappiness, apathy, frustration, or anger
- Feelings of depression
- A loss in pleasure from things you used to enjoy
- Difficulty staying positive of experiencing joy
- Low mood when it is cloudy or there is a lack of sunlight
- Not enjoying your favorite foods and beverages
- Less socializing
- Isolating oneself or not enjoying relationships and friendships
- Difficulty falling asleep, staying asleep, and waking up refreshed

Please circle "Yes" or "No" for each statement below:

1. I find it difficult to stay asleep at night. *(Yes or No)*
2. Despite not feeling very hungry, I still have a tendency to eat more than I should. *(Yes or No)*
3. I have lost interest in activities that I used to enjoy. *(Yes or No)*
4. I used to be more adventurous. *(Yes or No)*

5. I take a long time when faced with different choices and find it difficult to make decisions. *(Yes or No)*
6. I find myself caught in negative thought loops or thinking about the same things over and over again. *(Yes or No)*
7. I feel like I am surviving but not truly living and thriving. *(Yes or No)*
8. I do not do well resolving conflicts or in times of crisis. *(Yes or No)*
9. I turn small problems into big deals and dwell on them. *(Yes or No)*
10. I've thought about suicide more than once. *(Yes or No)*
11. As a teenager or young adult, I was told that I was moody or hard to get along with. *(Yes or No)*

Dopamine:

Signs that you are suffering from dopamine-related issues include:

- Difficulty getting motivated
- Difficulties starting and finishing tasks
- Low self-esteem or feelings of worthlessness
- Feelings of hopelessness or dread
- Losing one's temper due to minor setbacks
- Difficulty managing stress
- Feeling angry or aggressive when stressed
- Tendency to isolate oneself
- Apathy or lack of concern for family or friends

Please circle "Yes" or "No" for each statement below:

1. Since I was 20 years old, I've gained more than 20 pounds. *(Yes or No)*
2. I smoke cigarettes. *(Yes or No)*

3. I know that I should exercise, but I lack the energy. *(Yes or No)*
4. When I am stressed out, I eat. *(Yes or No)*
5. I have difficulty concentrating or staying focused at home or at work. *(Yes or No)*
6. I find it difficult to get enough sleep or feel refreshed. *(Yes or No)*
7. I need coffee or stimulants to jumpstart me in the morning. *(Yes or No)*
8. I have a low, or no, sex drive. *(Yes or No)*
9. I have been diagnosed with or have experienced the symptoms of heart disease, poor circulation, or cardiovascular issues. *(Yes or No)*
10. I drink 3 or more alcoholic beverages at least two days a week, or I drink more than 6 alcoholic beverages a week. *(Yes or No)*

GABA:

Signs that you are suffering from GABA-related issues include:

- Unexplained feelings of stress, anxiousness, or panic
- Feelings of dread or impending doom
- A tendency to expect the worst in people and situations
- Feelings of inner tension, uneasiness, or excitability
- Unexplained feelings of being overwhelmed
- A racing, restless mind
- Difficulty turning off thoughts when you're trying to relax
- Scattered attention and trouble focusing on one task
- Worrying about situations or things that seem unlikely to occur in reality or that you have not thought of before.
- Feeling uneasy, on-edge, or restless
- Becoming easily tired or fatigued
- Losing your train of thought or having your mind go blank

- Volatile mood or irritability
- Muscle tension or tightness
- Rapid or uneven heartbeat
- Difficulty breathing or shortness of breath
- Sweaty palms
- Cold hands and feet
- Easily scared or startled
- Excessive worry
- Headaches
- Sleeping problems
- Out-of-body feelings
- Obsessive compulsive traits

Acetylcholine:

Signs that you are suffering from Acetylcholine-related issues include:

- Poor memory, or loss of visual, photographic, and/or verbal memory
- Loss of creativity
- Lowered comprehension and word recall
- Difficulty doing mental math
- Difficulty placing people and recognizing faces
- Delayed mental responsiveness
- Difficulty navigating using directions in a car
- Trouble with special orientation or a tendency to be clumsy or bump into things

Please circle "Yes" or "No" for each statement below:

1. People have told me that I am becoming absent minded.
   (Yes or No)

2. I have noticed hair loss. *(Yes or No)*
3. I find it difficult to remember faces. *(Yes or No)*
4. I feel like I need to write everything down (to do lists, directions, groceries, or instructions). *(Yes or No)*
5. I find it difficult to remember phone numbers and addresses. *(Yes or No)*
6. My memory has gotten worse. *(Yes or No)*
7. My management skills have gotten worse. *(Yes or No)*
8. I don't feel like my brain is working the way that it used to. *(Yes or No)*
9. Alzheimer's and/or dementia run in my family. *(Yes or No)*
10. I can be forgetful and lose important things like my car or house keys. *(Yes or No)*
11. I sometimes forget whether I have taken my pills or prescription medications. *(Yes or No)*

Neurotransmitter Imbalances (in general):

Please circle "Yes" or "No" for each statement below:

1. I have been diagnosed with anxiety or depression. *(Yes or No)*
2. Cognitive disorders like Alzheimer's, dementia, or Parkinson's disease run in my family. *(Yes or No)*
3. Depression and/or anxiety run in my family. *(Yes or No)*
4. I'm often stressed or anxious. *(Yes or No)*
5. Anxiety keeps me from doing things like socializing or leaving my apartment as much as I would like. *(Yes or No)*
6. I often experience excessive sweating, rapid heartbeat or heart palpitations, or feelings of anxiousness. *(Yes or No)*
7. Worry and anxiousness affect my ability to sleep. *(Yes or No)*
8. I'm easily frustrated and feel angry in traffic. *(Yes or No)*

9. I often worry about disasters, crises, and illnesses beyond my control. *(Yes or No)*

10. I imagine worst case scenarios and then obsess about them, even if I know they have little basis in reality. *(Yes or No)*

11. I put a lot of stock in, and worry about, what others think about me. *(Yes or No)*

12. I have a low sense of self-worth. *(Yes or No)*

13. It's difficult for me to remember the last time I was happy. *(Yes or No)*

14. I frequently forget words or names that I should know. *(Yes or No)*

15. I often misplace my keys or can't remember where I put things. *(Yes or No)*

16. At times I feel unusually confident, like I can take on the world. *(Yes or No)*

17. I find it difficult to follow the storyline in books and movies. *(Yes or No)*

18. I easily lose my train of thought. *(Yes or No)*

19. I have trouble focusing or concentrating. *(Yes or No)*

20. I can be easily distracted. *(Yes or No)*

21. I experience mental fatigue after working, studying, driving, or other activities that require my focus. *(Yes or No)*

Neurotransmitters are chemicals that facilitate communication between neurons. A neuron will release neurotransmitters and they cross the synapse, which is a gap between neurons. They can then be accepted at receptor sites of another neuron. Neurotransmitters either produce an excitatory or an inhibitory response. An excitatory response (or depolarization) makes it more likely that an electrical signal will be sent. An inhibitory response (or hyper-polarization) makes it less likely that an electrical signal will be sent.

There are many chemicals which act as neurotransmitters in the body. The four that are focused on within this section are: Serotonin, Dopamine, GABA, and Acetylcholine. Healthy neurotransmitter levels play an important role in:

- Energy production
- Cognitive function
- Mood
- Sleep
- Sense of well-being
- Sex drive
- Resistance to stress
- Physical pain
- Many other physiological functions

Factors which contribute to suboptimal neurotransmitter levels include:

- Lack of sleep or poor sleep quality
- Hypothyroidism
- Heavy metal toxicity
- Adrenal fatigue
- Chronic infections
- Chronic inflammation
- Gut dysfunction (80-90% of the body's serotonin is produced in the gut)
- Hormonal imbalances (e.g. low testosterone and low human growth hormone)
- Nutrient deficiencies (esp. B-vitamins, iron, magnesium, zinc, vitamin C, vitamin D)
- Genetic mutations which affect neurotransmitter receptor sites

Neurotransmitter production relies on a delicate balance between homeostasis in the body, amino acid precursors, and enzymes, which make the production, reuptake, and reception of these chemicals possible. Rarely do neurotransmitter imbalances occur in isolation and rarely is there a single underlying cause. So it's important to identify which neurotransmitter imbalances exist, and on top of that, which behavioral and lifestyle factors, or nutrient deficiencies, are exacerbating the problem.

Even if we know exactly which neurotransmitters are being affected and why, implementing the changes necessary to correct these imbalances long-term can be problematic. Here's an example. Let's say that you are a physician who is working with a businessman who travels five days a week and has a bad knee from his college football days. You can't really expect him to not eat out at restaurants, and it's doubtful that he'll put in the 20 minutes of cardiovascular exercise he needs every morning. All of that is just not very feasible.

While it is true that our body possesses the ability to heal itself when provided with the right ingredients, many times we do not fully understand all of the contributing elements. Therefore, we lack an effective game plan (the specific interventions that will produce the desired results), and our ability to implement the required changes is compromised by career obligations, lifestyle preferences, or both. Because of this, the fastest course to correcting neurotransmitter imbalances is often the use of supplements, neutraceuticals, and/or prescription drugs.

How to Increase Serotonin with Supplements, Hormones, and Prescriptions:

– HGH
– Bioidentical testosterone replacement therapy

- Pregnenolone
- Melatonin
- 5-HTP
- Tryptophan
- Vitamin B6 (as Pyridoxal Phosphate)
- Fish oils
- Magnesium Glycinate
- Vitamin B3 (as niacin)
- St. John's Wort
- Passionflower
- Prozac (fluoxetine hydrogen): A number of studies have found long-term Prozac use to upregulate neurogenesis, the birth of neurons in the brain. Additionally, Prozac was found to increase brain plasticity and has exhibited potential to reverse signs of aging in the brain.

How to Increase Dopamine with Supplements, Hormones, and Prescriptions:

- Mucuna Dopa
- Tyrosine
- L-phenylalanine
- Rhodiola rosea
- Methylfolate
- Ginkgo
- Guarana
- Wild green oat extract
- Ritalin (methylphenidate)
- Adderall (amphetamine and dextroamphetamine)
- Wellbutrin (bupropion)
- Selegiline (deprenyl)

- Rasagiline (azilect)
- Modafinil (provigil)
- Gerovital H3 (procaine hydrochloride)
- Anavar (oxandrolone)
- DHEA
- HGH
- Thyroid hormones T4 and T3 (preferably from a natural thyroid glandular)
- Bio-identical testostcronc (as testosterone incipiente or testosterone enanthate)
- Cabergoline (Warning: Use of Cabergoline may result in heart valve complications.)

A company named Nervana recently created headphones that may stimulate the release of dopamine while you listen to music by sending a low-power electrical signal through your ear canal to stimulate the Vagus nerve.

Wild green oat extract operates along the same pathways as the prescription drug Deprenyl, which inhibits the dopamine degrading enzyme MAO-B. In human studies, using wild green oat extract showed improved memory, cognitive function, and was found to have decreased MAO-B levels by 50%.

One of the most effective treatment modalities to combat dopamine is the prescription drug Selegiline (Deprenyl). This MAO-B inhibitor has been shown to increase lifespan in animal studies by 34%. It has also been shown to restore sex drive and sexual activity in 64 of the 66 aging rats. In numerous studies Selegiline has been known to decrease MAO-B activity by 85%.

In another Deprenyl study involving dogs, researchers began administering the treatment of this drug around mid-life. By the end

There's an Adderall doping scandal in the world of professional gaming

Ben Gilbert ⚐🖤
🕘 Jul. 23, 2015, 1:49 PM ⚑ 7,004

Performance-enhancing drugs aren't just for regular sports anymore.

In the world of eSports, however, it's not about bulking up physically. In the world of eSports, performance is about mental acuity and concentration.

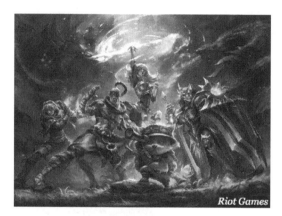

Riot Games

The drug of choice is Adderall, an amphetamine that requires a doctor's prescription. It's used to treat ADHD. Adderall is also common in colleges, where students use it as a study aid. It's a stimulant that enables long periods of concentration, or, as Business Insider science editor Kevin Loria put it: "It's basically speed."

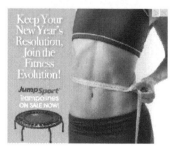

And that's why it's been so easily adopted by the competitive eSports world.

"We were all on Adderall," Kory "SEMPHIS" Friesen, a professional eSports competitor, said in an interview with Launders on YouTube on July 12.

of the study, which lasted just over two years, 39% of the untreated dogs were alive, compared to 80% of the canines who had been given Deprenyl. Given my genetic predisposition to Parkinson's, I take 5 mg of Deprenyl intermittently with frequent drug holidays. During that time off, I take a wild green oat extract, and occasionally, Gerovital H3 (procaine hydrochloride) injections as additional MAO-B inhibitors.

How to Increase GABA with Supplements, Hormones, and Prescriptions:

- Pregnenolone
- DHEA
- GABA
- Phenibut
- Inositol
- Kava
- Niacin
- Branched-chain amino acids (BCAAs)
- Taurine
- Glycine (as bone broth from grass-fed cows or free-range chickens)
- Magnesium glycinate
- Suntheanine
- Tryptophan
- L-phenylalanine
- St. John's Wort
- Melatonin
- Valerian root
- Passionflower
- GABApentin (neurontin): A prescription drug similar to GABA and inositol.
- Growth hormone releasing hormone (GHRH)

How to Increase Acetylcholine with Supplements, Hormones, and Prescriptions

- Alpha-GPC (Alpha-glycerylphosphorylcholine)
- Citicoline (AKA: Cytidine diphosphate-choline or CDP-choline)
- Sunflower lecithin
- Huperzine A
- Acetyl L-carnitine arginate
- Phosphatidylserine
- Alpha Lipoic acid
- R lipoic acid
- Fish oil
- Ginkgo biloba
- Piracetam
- DMAE (dimethylaminoethanol)
- Conjugated linoleic acid (CLA)
- Vinpocetine
- Bacopa Monnieri
- Gotu kola
- Korean ginseng
- Phosphatidylcholine
- Galantamine (ravenel)
- HGH
- DHEA

Other Biohacks for Optimizing Neurotransmitter Balance Include:

- Daily meditation
- Binaural beats
- Brain Sync by Kelly Howell
- Dr. Jeffrey Thompson's neuroacoustics CDs

- Holosync by Centerpoint
- Transcranial direct current stimulation (tDCS)
- DAVID Delight Pro
- David Smart
- Fisher Wallace Stimulator
- NuCalm System
- Marijuana can also be an effective tool for improving neurotransmitter balance, specifically, when it comes to serotonin and dopamine.
- Active CBD oil - Gold 25%
- Active CBD oil capsules 750mg CBD/bottle

For many individuals, the effects of meditation can be enhanced by using the integration of binaural beats. Our brainwaves respond to sound frequencies, beats, notes, and music, and there is a direct correlation between the amplification of these brainwaves and neurotransmitter production.

Transcranial direct current stimulation has been around since the early 1800s. The Fisher Wallace Stimulator is FDA approved and has been prescribed by over 6,000 physicians, including 2,000 board certified doctors. Also, tDCS has been tested in the U.S. Air Force to boost performance. I have a number of these devices, including the David Delight Pro by MindAlive.

Marijuana acts on our own body's cannabinoid receptors. We each have our own endogenous cannabinoid system, and our bodies make our own cannabinoids, which are very similar to the ones found in marijuana. These endogenous cannabinoids signal electrical communication between nerves, similar to our body's neurotransmitters. Our endocannabinoid system helps to regulate many physiological processes, and it plays a vital role in maintaining balance in the body.

As we age, or experience health challenges, our endocannabinoid production can decrease. By supplementing with exogenous cannabinoids through the smoking of marijuana, we may be able to improve and restore:

- Immune health
- Nutrient assimilation and absorption
- Bone regeneration
- Inflammation
- Glycogen uptake and storage
- Physical pain
- Memory and cognitive function
- Emotional stability
- Sleep

I've been fortunate to help many clients overcome anxiety and depression. While this is a very individual process, here are a few strategies that may help elevate your general mood:

- Meditate 5-30 minutes each morning, followed by 20-30 minutes of steady state cardiovascular exercise.
- Ideally, you should jog outdoors, in your target heart rate zone, and verify this with a heart rate monitor like the Garmin Forerunner 220.
- Complete three minute cold thermogenesis (in an ice bath or cold lake) or cryotherapy 3-7 days per week.
- Avoid dairy, grains, alcohol, and processed foods.
- Take the following supplements:
  - 800-1,200 mg of SAMe (S-adenosylmethionine) daily, on an empty stomach.
  - 1,800 mg of DHA daily, through a high-quality fish oil supplement, with food

- A high-dose B vitamin supplement, including the bioactive forms of B2, B6, B12, trimethylglycine, 1,000 mg sublingual methyl B12 lozenge daily, or B12 intramuscular shot (1 CC per week).
- 1,000 mg of magnesium glycinate daily, with food
- One full dropper of Wise Woman Herbals Mood Enhancer up to three times daily
- 100-200 mg of 5-HTP at night before bed, on an empty stomach

– Drink 70% of your body weight in ounces of water each day, filtered using a reverse osmosis water filter to remove water, fluoride, and chlorine chemicals as well as prescription drugs. Add back minerals and electrolytes. Or you can drink natural spring water.

– Expose your eyes to natural sunlight for 5-30+ minutes per day. Look towards the sun about 15-20 degrees off from direct line of sight. The retina lack pain receptors so give yourself a 15-20 degree cushion to prevent damage to the retina and optic nerve.

– Get at least 20 minutes of direct sunlight to exposed skin daily, the safest and most effective way to produce vitamin D. Insufficient vitamin D is linked to virtually every age-related disorder including cancer, vascular disease, and chronic inflammation.

– Use a SunTouch Plus Blue Light or a Sperti Fiji Sun Lamp in the wintertime and during periods when you have less exposure to sunshine. This should only be used as a supplement, not a substitute for exposure to natural sunlight. Emerging evidence suggests that exposure to blue light without the opposing red light to balance it's effects (they naturally occur this way in sunlight) can have detrimental effects long term. It all comes back to getting as much natural sunlight as you can, safely and without burning.

– Use The Five Minute Journal

TROUBLESHOOTING #9: CHRONIC INFECTIONS

Signs that you may be suffering from a chronic infection include:

- Joint pain
- Muscle aches and pain, tightness, or stiffness
- Rashes or redness
- Acne, psoriasis, eczema
- Rosacea
- Low energy or fatigue
- Depression, anxiety, or stress
- Bloating, swelling, or stiffness
- Headaches or migraines
- Stiff neck
- Dizziness
- Changes in heart rate or heart palpitations
- Unexplained hair loss
- Twitching of facial muscles or eyelids
- Muscle cramping
- Tingling in the nose or tongue
- Jaw pain or stiffness
- Sore throat, hoarseness, or easily losing one's voice
- Stuffy nose, runny nose, or difficulty breathing through nostrils
- Blurred vision, difficulty seeing at night
- Floaters in the eyes
- Sensitivity to light and sound
- Decreased hearing in one or both ears
- Buzzing, ringing, or tinnitus in the ears
- Diarrhea, constipation, irritable bowels

- Upset stomach, gas, bloating, or discomfort after eating certain foods
- Symptoms of chronic fatigue or fibromyalgia, including being diagnosed with either condition
- Decreased cardiovascular endurance
- Rapid onset of lactic acid buildup
- Muscle burn during physical activity, especially in the feet or calves
- Decreased circulation
- Cold hands and feet
  Numbness and tingling in the hands, feet, arms, or legs (peripheral neuropathy)
- Poor balance
- Dizziness
- Decreased motor function
- Lightheadedness or wooziness
- Difficulty falling asleep or staying asleep, panic attacks, anxiety
- Feeling as though you are losing your mind or like you are aging at an accelerated rate
- Mood swings, irritability, bipolar disorder, schizophrenia
- Confusion, brain fog, or difficulty concentrating
- Forgetting names, faces, phone numbers, or how to perform simple tasks
- Long-term and short-term memory loss
- Swollen glands or lymph nodes
- Decreased sense of smell
- Allergies or chemical sensitivities
- Low body temperature
- Increased effect from alcohol and worsened hangovers
- Continual infections (sinus, pinkeye, flu, fever, colds)
- Abdominal pain
- Carbohydrate or sugar cravings

- Vaginal or yeast infections
- Impotence
- Infertility
- Rectal itch
- Urinary tract infections
- Athlete's foot
- Dry skin
- Attention deficit disorder or attention deficit hyperactivity disorder
- Nausea, loss of appetite, frequent burping or passing gas
- Unintentional weight gain or weight loss
- Passing a worm in your stool
- Living in or traveling to an area known to have parasites, including most international travel

In his landmark book, *"Plague Time: The New Germ Theory of Disease,"* evolutionary biologist Paul Ewald explores an eye-opening and revolutionary understanding of disease. Newsweek says that this "could change medicine as profoundly during the 21st century as germ theory did in the 20th." In his book, Ewald challenges the conventional wisdom that our genes and lifestyles are the primary causes of the most deadly and debilitating diseases of our time.

Paul Ewald is the Director of Evolutionary Medicine at the University of Louisville. His book offers the following arguments:

- Germs appear to be the root of heart disease, Alzheimer's disease, schizophrenia, many forms of cancer, and other chronic diseases.
- The greatest threats to our health come not from sensational killers such as Ebola, West Nile virus, and super virulent strains of influenza, but from agents that are already here, causing long-term infections which eventually lead to debilitation and death.

- The medical establishment has largely ignored the evidence that implicates these germs to the detriment of our public health.
- New evolutionary theories are available which explain how germs function and offer opportunities for controlling these modern plagues, if we are willing to listen to them.

Many of us see bacteria, viruses, and other microorganisms as our enemies. This perspective was popularized by the germ theory of disease in the 19th century. The truth is that humans and microbes depend on each other for survival. As mentioned earlier, humans have ten times more bacterial cells than human cells in their body.

In the US, over 80% of oral antibiotics are used on livestock to combat the inhumane conditions in which these animals are raised. These factory farms, which produce all of the meats in restaurants and grocery stores (not specified as "organic," "grass-fed," "pastured," "free-range," and/or "wild-caught"), use unnatural practices to produce meat. This includes the overuse of antibiotics. All of this has resulted in a meteoric rise in antibiotic resistant "superbugs." As of 2015, more than 23,000 Americans die every year as a direct result of antibiotic resistant infections. This number is expected to climb each year, unless dramatic changes are made to the way we produce our meat.

It's not just our meat that is posing a threat to our health. While analyzing potential allergens in GMO (genetically modified organisms) crops, the European Food Safety Authority (EFSA) found a viral gene fragment had been encoded in the vast majority of these plants. There are clear indications that this viral gene (called Gene VI) may not be safe for human consumption. Not only that, but this could result in unfavorable gene expression and make us susceptible to a wide variety of infections.

Of the 86 genetically modified crops that have been approved to date, 54 of them contained portions of Gene VI, which is from the cauliflower mosaic virus. Among those 54 engineered plants affected by this virus, are some of the most widely consumed GMOs, including Roundup Ready soybeans and two strains of Monsanto corn (one of which is a strain that has been reported to cause tumors and premature death in laboratory rats).

These are just two out of many examples of how the unnatural alterations we've made to our environment are threatening our health. In these cases, they are doing so by exposing us to pathogens and illnesses that did not exist just a couple of decades ago. In the past four years alone, I've been experiencing more and more clients (www. BioHackingSecrets.com/coaching) coming to me for help with chronic diseases like:

- Fibromyalgia
- Arthritis
- Parkinson's
- Lyme disease
- GI disorders
- Multiple sclerosis
- Chronic fatigue
- Autism spectrum disorders
- Diabetes
- Cardiovascular problems

One of my recent clients, Sara, had been to many of the top Lyme-literate doctors in the Midwest. Despite doing many things right, and following protocols from some of the biggest thought leaders in the field, she was getting worse instead of better.

After we spoke, Sara and her husband Chris asked to be a part of the program. I was straightforward that it could take 12-18 months for these types of situations to resolve themselves. They understood. We got to work.

A few days before we started her program, Sara walked around downtown Chicago for 30 minutes doing errands. Afterwards, she was incapacitated. Literally bedridden and exhausted.

I did an in depth diagnostic assessment and built her a customized program to restore her body's natural ability to heal itself. After three weeks, Sara messaged me that she'd just finished a 30-minute run at 6.0 mph on the treadmill. She said she felt great and there was no crash afterwards. At first, I was not happy she'd pushed herself beyond my recommendations, but that frustration turned to excitement at how quickly she was progressing.

There is a growing body of evidence suggesting that many modern health issues may have ties to infectious causation.

Having gone through my own personal battle with chronic Lyme disease, and its accompanying co-infections, this is an area that I understand all too well.

Left untreated, infections from bacteria, viruses, mold exposure, yeasts, fungi, and parasites can steal our energy, destroy cognitive function, erode our sex drive, and in some cases, lead to early death. Here are some of the chronic infections that can interfere with health, energy, and focus:

- Lyme (borrelia)
- Bartonella/Mycoplasma
- Parasites
- Candida
- H. pylori

- Clostridium
- Molds
- HHV-6 (human herpesvirus six)
- HIV
- Chlamydia
- Clostridium difficile
- Small intestinal bacterial overgrowth (SIBO)
- E coli
- Mycobacterium
- Epstein-Barr virus (EBV)
- Rubella
- Parvovirus B19
- Cytomegalovirus
- Staphylococcus aureus
- Rickettsiaceae
- HSV-1 (herpes simplex)
- Babesia Microti
- Ehrlichia

Many challenges exist in identifying and treating these chronic infections. Simply put, we lack the depth of testing methods necessary to detect many of these pathogens, and the ones that do exist are notoriously inaccurate. These tests produce both false negatives and false positives.

One of the functional medicine practitioners I have worked closely with over the past few years, told me that he no longer orders Lyme tests from one particular laboratory. Why? Because this lab, despite being considered by many to be the gold standard for identifying Borrelia bacteria, is yet to return a single negative test. Interestingly, this was the same laboratory that identified my Lyme disease back in 2011.

Beyond being difficult to identify, these infections are also incredibly difficult to treat. They communicate and interact with one another. For instance, viruses insert their DNA into bacteria. Epstein-Barr and HHV-6 often reactivate in Lyme patients. Furthermore, many clinicians now believe that there is a strong connection between chronic fatigue syndrome, multiple sclerosis, Alzheimer's, and Lyme disease. These are just a few of many, many examples.

It's also been shown that these bacteria have developed sophisticated mechanisms for evading our immune system. They produce biofilms or protective matrices that prevent our body's immune cells from accessing the bacteria and doing their job. Some of the symptoms you may have with a chronic infection include:

- Diarrhea
- Constipation
- Weakened immune system
- Aches, pains, tightness, and/or stiffness
- Stomach distention
- Burning sensations/discomfort in the stomach
- Gas/bloating
- Itching
- Trouble sleeping
- Brain fog/memory and concentration issues
- Hives and rashes
- Fevers
- Allergies/food sensitivities
- Fatigue/low energy
- Cough
- IBS/Mucus in the stool
- Grinding teeth

There are a great deal of lifestyle interventions, supplements, prescription medications, and biohacks that I've used with clients when chronic infections are a concern. A number of them are listed below:

– *Propolair Propolis Vaporizer:* The L3 Propolis Vaporizer eliminates mold spores and unwanted microbes in the environment to improve air quality. Ideal for patients with asthma, bronchitis and as a therapeutic solution for those suffering from autoimmune diseases. With the natural disinfecting properties of propolis, it not only purifies the air and its immediate environment, but also allows one to inhale the healing, protective properties of propolis in a non-invasive manner – just as one absorbs oxygen. The Model L3 also comes with an integrated negative ionizer to further enhance the effects of propolis. Recommended for people with asthma, bronchitis and other respiratory ailments, and those suffering from autoimmune diseases. (www.BioHackingSecrets.com/propolair).

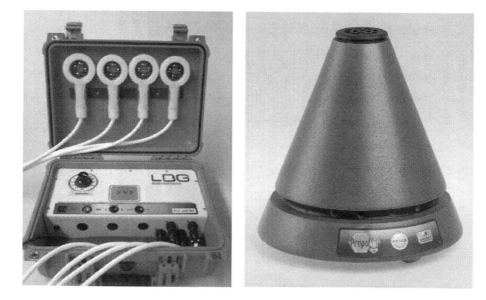

- Biotics Research FC-Cidal
- Biotics Research Dysbiocide
- Metagenics Candibactin AR
- Metagenics Candibactin BR
- Biotics Research ADP
- LBG by ELF Labs Tech (www.elflabstech.com)
- ST-8 by ELF Labs Tech (www.elflabstech.com)
- Oil of oregano
- Byociden's gut cleanse formulas (comprehensive cleansing)
- Garlic, including formulas standardized for high-allicin content
- Oregano
- Berberine
- Oregon grape
- Cinnamon
- Digestive, systemic, and proteolytic enzymes
- Artemisinin
- Liposomal artemisinin
- Olive leaf extract
- Probiotics
- Samento
- Cumanda
- Banderol
- Transfer Factor
- Resveratrol
- Coconut activated charcoal
- Zeolite
- Bentonite clay
- Organic chlorella
- Serrapeptase
- Liposomal vitamin C

- The ketogenic diet and/or fasting-induced ketosis
- Intravascular light therapy system (UVLRX)
- Ultraviolet light therapy devices
- Hyperbaric oxygen chambers
- Doxycycline
- Minocycline
- Vitamin C
- Vitamin E
- Vielight 810 Intranasal blood irradiation device
- The Vielight Neuro
- Curcumin
- Boluoke Lumbrokinase
- Bromelain
- Oral DMPS
- Oral and rectal MMS
- Cistus incanus tea
- Transfer Point Beta 1,3D Glucan
- Apple Cider Vinegar Enemas
- Bentonite Enemas (up to 1x per week)
- Coffee enemas (up to 5x per day)
- Cat's claw
- L-lysine
- Eleuthero
- Astragalus
- Ashwagandha
- Lomatium
- St. John's Wort
- Echinacea
- Burbur

- Pinella
- Pterostilbene
- EGCG (from green tea)
- Magnesium glycinate
- Extra virgin cod liver oil
- Lauricidin
- Rhodiola
- Astaxanthin
- Pure Caprylic acid (C-8 MCT oil as Bulletproof Brain Octane or Parrillo CapTri)
- Valtrex (antiviral; 1,000 mg three times per day for 4-6 weeks)
- Valcyte 450 mg (antiviral; 2 tablespoons twice per day for 3 weeks, then 1 tablespoon twice per day for the remainder of 6 months)
- Albendazole (antiparasite)
- Alinia (antiparasite)
- Ivermectin (antiparasite)
- Metronidazole (antiparasite)
- Tinidazole (antiparasite)
- Xifaxan (Small Intestinal Bacterial Overgrowth)
- Neomycin (Small Intestinal Bacterial Overgrowth)
- Nystatin (Candida)
- Diflucan (Candida)
- Theralumen Immune Laser - www.millenialhealthsystems.com
- *Sota Silver Pulser:* The Silver Pulser by SOTA (www.sota.com) delivers gentle microcurrents of electricity that may kill bacteria, virus, fungi, and molds in the blood and tissues. The microcurrent stimulation helps the body's natural electricity for more energy and improved health. It can also be used to make colloidal silver, a natural antibiotic.

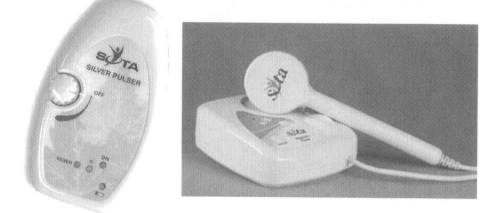

Individuals with underlying health issues should start at just 5 minutes and gradually work up to the recommended 2 hours a day. Minimum treatment duration is 4-12 weeks. Detox (Herxheimer Reaction) reactions are not infrequent. I have used this therapeutic intervention with clients dealing with Fibromyalgia, cancer, Lyme disease, and other conditions with suspected infectious causation. For more information on how to use these devices to improve immune response and neutralize pathogens visit www.bobbeck.com.

- UVLrx Ultraviolet Blood Irradiation Machine
- *Ion Foot Bath Detox System from IonCleanse:* (www.amajordifference.com)

Section Notes:

Therapeutic ketosis can be healthy in repairing mitochondria, which might have been damaged by antibiotic use. It's also useful in treating bacterial and viral infections because bacteria and viruses do not have mitochondria. A ketogenic diet starves them of glucose, their preferred fuel source. If symptoms do not improve on a ketogenic diet, try a low fat diet with a focus mostly on green vegetables with some wild-caught fish, small amounts of organic berries, and fats coming from plant sources, such as olive oil, coconut oil, and C-8 MCT oil (pure caprylic acid).

Hyperbaric oxygen chambers have been found to sensitize spirochetes.

TROUBLESHOOTING #10: BRAIN INFLAMMATION (NEUROINFLAMMATION)

Signs that you are suffering from brain inflammation include:

– Brain fog
– Difficulty thinking or concentrating
– Brain fatigue, particularly after working, reading, driving, or activities that require concentration
– Delayed or slowed mental processing
– Loss of brain function after trauma, particularly head trauma
– Sleepiness, brain fatigue, or poor mental focus after meals
– Fatigue or headaches brought about by chemicals, scents, and cosmetics
– Low mood, depression, or mental disorders

There's a strong correlation between gut health and cognitive functioning, memory, anxiety, depression, and symptoms of other suboptimal performance. The gut-brain axis is one of the most often overlooked factors in energy production and mental clarity. The two systems are inextricably tied, and any imbalance in one will result in an imbalance in the other.

Even the highest performing of my clients, including business leaders, executives, and entrepreneurs, often express concerns about

Cas Lek Cesk. 1996 Jan 31;135(3):74-8.

[Postmenopausal osteoporosis. Treatment with calcitonin and a diet rich in collagen proteins].

[Article in Czech]
Adam M[1], Spacek P, Hulejová H, Galiánová A, Blahos J.
|
CONCLUSIONS:

a) administration of 100 u. calcitonin twice a week for 24 weeks led to a decline of excretion indicators of bone collagen breakdown products, b) the effect of treatment must be monitored using these indicators, c) oral administration of collagen proteins enhanced and prolonged the effect of calcitonin.

unchecked stress, anxiety, low mood, depression, and/or inconsistent cognitive function. When we customize and implement a game plan to optimize the gut-brain axis, they rapidly observe improvements in energy and mental clarity beyond what they previously thought possible.

I believe that one of the most pernicious, and overlooked, culprits of neuroinflammation is the fluoride, chlorine, pesticides, and chemicals in our water supply. Even the most popular water filters are unable to remove fluoride, which has been linked to:

– Hyperthyroidism
– Unfavorable gene expression
– Arthritis
– Joint pain
– Compromised collagen synthesis
– Cancer
– Dementia
– Alzheimer's
– Dementia
– Parkinson's
– Autoimmunity
– Chronic fatigue

- Infertility and damaged sperm
- Heavy metal toxicity
- A number of other biological and physiological health risks

Interesting enough, most developed countries do not fluorinate their water, and according to the World Health Organization (WHO), countries that do fluorinate their water have no less tooth decay than countries who do not. The only effective method for removing fluoride from our water is by installing and using a reverse osmosis water filter. Even bottled water contains fluoride. I recommend using a reverse osmosis water filter to all of my coaching clients (www. BioHackingSecrets.com/coaching), especially those who show signs of toxic overload, and I tell them that this should be their only source for drinking water.

Other mechanisms that increase the risk of brain inflammation include:

- Diets high in carbohydrates, particularly those high in sugar and processed foods
- Lack of exercise
- Chronic stress
- Poor circulation
- Head injuries and trauma
- Environmental toxins
- Systemic inflammation
- GI disorders (including IBS)
- Compromised gut-brain barrier
- Poor antioxidant status (a common consequence of insufficient consumption of organic vegetables and berries)
- Consumption of grains, gluten, alcohol, and other immunogenic and allergenic foods

Once you've installed a reverse osmosis water filter and are using that for drinking water, follow the recommendations outlined in the "Immune Dysregulation" section of this guide. Particularly, you should follow the strategies for restoring intestinal integrity. These will assist in the restoration of the blood-brain barrier and decrease neuroinflammation.

Here are some lifestyle, supplements, prescriptions, and biohacks that are likely to help in the treatment of brain inflammation:

- Consuming large amounts of organic green vegetables and organic berries
- Be sure to include plant-based fats like extra virgin olive oil, MCT oil, avocado, Udo's Choice Oil Blend, flax oil, and raw, organic, unprocessed, extra virgin coconut oil.
- Reduce your use of non-steroidal anti-inflammatory drugs (NSAIDs): Aspirin, Advil, and Ibuprofen.
- Pterostilbene
- Baicalin
- Resveratrol
- Curcumin/turmeric
- Rutin
- Stinging nettle
- Fish oil from extra virgin cod liver oil and a high quality fish oil supplement rich in DHA

DHA is one of the most abundant fats in the brain. It helps to form cellular membranes and protect nerves. It also turns on genes that are involved in the production of brain-derived neurotrophic factor (BDNF). This increases our brain neurons' resistance to free radicals and injury. The National Institute of Health and the Alzheimer's Disease Neuroimaging Initiative (ADNI) have also found that long-term use of high quality fish oil supplements was linked to improved cognitive function and a reduction in brain shrinkage at the end of a three-year study.

Curcumin has been shown to lower inflammation and reduce beta amyloid plaque. This is the compound which is at least partly responsible for Alzheimer's disease by 50%. An observational human study also found that people who frequently ate curry had higher scores on tests of cognitive functioning than those who did not.

If you're in substantial amounts of physical pain, don't freak out about having a couple ibuprofen every once in a while. You don't want to take it daily because it can cause damage to the stomach lining and increase risk of heart attack and stroke. But small amounts of ibuprofen are probably not something you need to be concerned about. And a number of recent studies have linked NSAIDS (non-steroidal anti-inflammatory drugs) to increased longevity across a number of species.

Section Notes:

- A 2009 clinical review in the Cardiovascular, Psychiatry, and Neurology Journal showed a degradation in the blood-brain barrier was found in a vast majority of patients who had been diagnosed with psychiatric disorders including schizophrenia and depression.
- A 2001 study in the Medical Hypothesis Journal found increases in the permeability of the blood-brain barrier to be associated with the symptoms of chronic fatigue syndrome.
- A 2014 study found that patients with dementia, Alzheimer's, and Parkinson's disease also exhibited symptoms of dysfunction in the blood-brain barrier.
- A review published in the year 2000, in the Neurological Focus Journal, found that severe, unexpected headaches and migraines

are an indicator of increased permeability in the blood-brain barrier. These symptoms were found to worsen later in the day.

– It's important to note that NSAIDs have been shown in more than 20 studies to help prevent Alzheimer's, but they also come with a number of GI and cardiovascular complications. So, I recommend starting with nutrition and natural supplements first.

TROUBLESHOOTING #11: IMMUNE DYSREGULATION (INFLAMMATORY IMBALANCE)

Signs that you are suffering from immune dysregulation (inflammatory imbalance) include:

– Muscle weakness
– Fatigue
– Poor cognitive function
– Dizziness
– Numbness, tingling, or burning in the hands and feet
– Brain and neurological symptoms
– Family history of autoimmune diseases

Please circle "Yes" or "No" for each statement below:

1. I have a family history of autoimmune conditions. *(Yes or No)*
2. I have a family history of gluten sensitivity. *(Yes or No)*
3. It takes me a long time to heal from cuts and bruises. *(Yes or No)*
4. I often have a nagging cough that's difficult to get rid of. *(Yes or No)*

5. I get frequent ear or sinus infections. *(Yes or No)*

6. I've seen blood in my pee. *(Yes or No)*

7. I've had pain in my hips, back, knees, neck, or ribs. *(Yes or No)*

8. It's sometimes difficult for me to go to the bathroom. *(Yes or No)*

9. It is not uncommon for more than 24 hours to pass between my bowel movements. *(Yes or No)*

10. I have distention, bloating, or fullness in my stomach that is not related to food. *(Yes or No)*

11. My lab tests show a low T-cell count. *(Yes or No)*

12. I have noticed an increase in warts or cysts (lumps that are slightly painful to the touch - often found around armpits or breasts) on my body. *(Yes or No)*

13. I have asthma or eczema. *(Yes or No)*

14. I'm excessively tired. *(Yes or No)*

15. My muscles and/or joints are often achey or painful. *(Yes or No)*

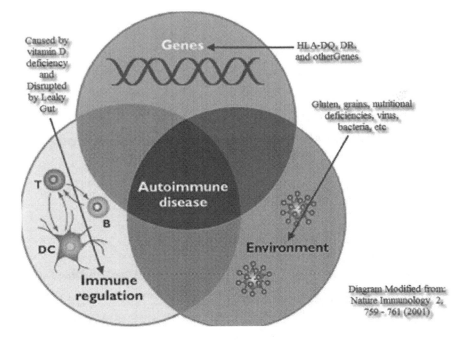

16. I've been diagnosed with or question whether I have chronic fatigue syndrome or arthritis. *(Yes or No)*

17. I've had infections like measles, hepatitis, E. coli, rubella, Epstein-Barr, etc. *(Yes or No)*

18. I have digestive problems. *(Yes or No)*

19. I have food sensitivities. *(Yes or No)*

20. I'm exposed to chemicals where I work or at home. *(Yes or No)*

21. I have elevated c-reactive protein (CPR) and/or Interleukin 6 levels (blood markers of inflammation). *(Yes or No)*

The human immune system is a miraculous set of tools for resisting the onslaught of pathogenic microorganisms like viruses, bacteria, and parasites. When functioning as intended, our immune system keeps us healthy, energized, resistant to stress, and pain free. However, environmental and genetic factors, including our diet, chronic infections, leaky gut, biotoxin illness, can trigger a misdirected immune response where we begin to attack our own cells as foreign invaders. This is one of the most common causes of low energy, brain fog, chronic pain (back pain, joint pain), and poor circulation.

I see these problems occurring every day with my clients. Eventually, when these immunogenic reactions persist, a condition known as immune dysregulation sets in. This condition is responsible for a wide variety of chronic and degenerative diseases, including:

- Multiple sclerosis
- Lupus
- Psoriasis
- IBS
- Rheumatoid arthritis
- Celiac disease

- Type 1 diabetes
- Reactive arthritis (chronic inflammation that is often accompanied by back and joint pain)
- Sjögren syndrome (a condition in which the glands responsible for producing tears and saliva are destroyed, resulting in dry mouth and dry eyes. This can also have adverse effects on the kidneys and lungs)
- Addison's disease (an often overlooked cause of adrenal fatigue and cortisol dysregulation)
- Scleroderma (a connective tissue disease that affects the skin, blood vessels, muscles, and internal organs)
- Pernicious anemia (a decrease in red blood cells due to the stomach's inability to absorb vitamin B12)
- Hashimoto's (a form of hypothyroidism where our immune system attacks the thyroid gland)
- Chronic fatigue
- Neuroinflammation (a.k.a. "brain fog")

Without question, the most common trigger for these autoimmune reactions are the foods we eat every day. Unfortunately, many people fail to make this connection on their own. Here are some of the most problematic, immunogenic, and allergenic foods to avoid if you, or someone you care about, suspects immune dysregulation:

- All gluten containing foods, including: Wheat, Barley, Rye, Breads, Baked goods, and Oats (unless specifically labeled gluten free)
- All processed foods
- All malt products
- All Dairy products, including: Whey protein, Baked goods, Cheeses, Milk, Yogurt (even Greek yogurt), Cream, Ice cream, etc.

- Genetically modified foods, including: Non-organic corn, soy, and canola oil
- Alcohol
- Eggs (including organic and free-range)
- Processed meats, including: Deli meats, Hot dogs, etc.
- Oils and fats other than extra virgin olive oil, or raw, organic, unrefined, extra virgin coconut oil, Udo's Oil 369 blend, flax oil, pure Caprylic acid, and C-8 MCT oil. Some individuals are able to include organic gee or butter from grass-fed cows, but I recommend holding off on these sources of fat until you are able to do a 28-day elimination/provocation diet.
- All sweetened foods, including: Sugar, Artificial sweeteners, and High fructose corn syrup
- All foods containing MSG
- Pay particular attention when consuming Asian cuisine
- Some individuals should remove all grains, beans, peanuts, nuts, nut butters, and soy (including organic soy) from their diets until they are able to reestablish a balanced immune response.

Earlier in this book, I recommended a 28-day elimination/provocation diet. I highly recommend that you follow my instructions to implement this in order to determine whether or not an individual sensitivity exists. When you do this, it is imperative that you eliminate these foods without exception for 28 days. Then you can reintroduce them one at a time in small amounts and observe any changes in energy levels, cognition, mood, and pain. This will help you to determine whether or not your body may have a sensitivity to any particular food. Most people with autoimmune conditions do best staying away from these foods the vast majority of the time.

As you've seen throughout this guide, the gut also plays an important role in the regulation of our body's immune response. In fact, 70% of our body's immune system is located in the gut. Bacterial, viral, fungal, and parasitic gut pathogens interfere with the delicate balance of our gut microbiome, negatively affecting our immune response. They also release toxins which cause intestinal permeability (AKA leaky gut), further amplifying these problems. So, it's vital that you take steps to eliminate unwanted inhabitants of the gut and reestablish the integrity of your intestinal lining.

After you have removed the triggers which are responsible for a leaky gut (I often see SIBO, parasites, candida, H. pylori, and a number of other such conditions affecting my clients). The following can be helpful in healing your intestinal lining:

- Bone broth from grass-fed cows (can be found online at GrasslandBeef.com, AZGrassRaisedBeef.com, BoneBroths.com) Bone broth is rich in gelatin, which contains the amino acids glycine, glutamine, and proline. These amino acids help restore healthy gut integrity. Glutamine also plays an important part in glutathione synthesis, energy production, and the reduction of oxidative stress.

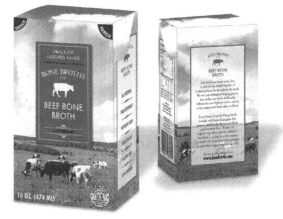

FEBS J. 2011 Sep;278(17):3152-63. doi: 10.1111/j.1742-4658.2011.08241.x. Epub 2011 Aug 8.

Glutamine and α-ketoglutarate as glutamate sources for glutathione synthesis in human erythrocytes.

Whillier S[1], Garcia B, Chapman BE, Kuchel PW, Raftos JE.

⊕ Author information

Abstract

Glutathione (GSH) is an intracellular antioxidant synthesized from glutamate, cysteine and glycine. The human erythrocyte (red blood cell, RBC) requires a continuous supply of glutamate to prevent the limitation of GSH synthesis in the presence of sufficient cysteine, but the RBC membrane is almost impermeable to glutamate. As optimal GSH synthesis is important in diseases associated with oxidative stress, we compared the rate of synthesis using two potential glutamate substrates, α-ketoglutarate and glutamine. Both substrates traverse the RBC membrane rapidly relative to many other metabolites. In whole RBCs partially depleted of intracellular GSH and glutamate, 10 mm extracellular α-ketoglutarate, but not 10 mm glutamine, significantly increased the rate of GSH synthesis (0.85 ± 0.09 and 0.61 ± 0.18 μmol·(L RBC)(-1) ·min(-1), respectively) compared with 0.52 ± 0.09 μmol·(L RBC)(-1) ·min(-1) for RBCs without an external glutamate source. Mathematical modelling of the situation with 0.8 mm extracellular glutamine returned a rate of glutamate production of 0.36 μmol·(L RBC)(-1) ·min(-1), while the initial rate for 0.8 mM α-ketoglutarate was 0.97 μmol·(L RBC)(-1) ·min(-1). However, with normal plasma concentrations, the calculated rate of GSH synthesis was higher with glutamine than with α-ketoglutarate (0.31 and 0.25 μmol·(L RBC)(-1) ·min(-1), respectively), due to the substantially higher plasma concentration of glutamine. Thus, a potential protocol to maximize the rate of GSH synthesis would be to administer a cysteine precursor plus a source of α-ketoglutarate and/or glutamine.

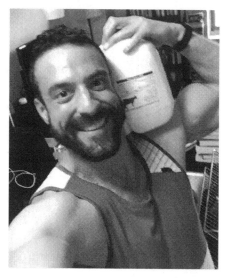

- L-Glutamine
- Designs4Health GI Revive
- GI Renew (available at Store.ChrisKresser.com)
- Aloe Vera (whole leaf juice and extract)
- Slippery Elm
- Marshmallow (althaea officinalis)
- Cat's claw (uncaria tomentosa)
- Quercetin
- MSM (methylsulfonylmethane)
- Deglycyrrhizinated licorice (DGL)

Signs and symptoms of leaky gut include:

- Muscle pain, aches, tightness, stiffness
- Arthritis or other joint conditions
- Allergies
- Migraines
- Asthma

- Diet resistant/hard to lose weight
- IBS
- Chronic fatigue/low energy
- Food intolerances and sensitivities
- Rashes, eczema, rosacea, acne
- Anxiety
- Depression
- Brain fog
  Gas, bloating, burping
- Constipation
- Diarrhea
- Etc.

Cyrex Labs offers a number of tests for autoimmune patients which test for both IgG and IgA antibodies. These tests are able to detect intolerances to a broad array of foods. I occasionally utilize Cyrex Labs' Array 10 and Array 4 with my autoimmune clients.

Other beneficial lifestyle interventions, supplements, prescriptions, and biohacks I've used to help (www.BioHackingSecrets.com/coaching) with immune dysregulation include:

- Cold Thermogenesis (CT):
  - Cryotherapy
  - Cold showers
  - *Ice Baths:* The protocol for an ice bath is to fill your bathtub with cold water and then add 2-3 bags of ice from your local grocery store or convenience store. Allow that ice to melt about 80% of the way. This should bring the water to around 40°F or 50°F. After the water reaches this sort of temperature, get in and hangout for 8-12 minutes while breathing deeply. After

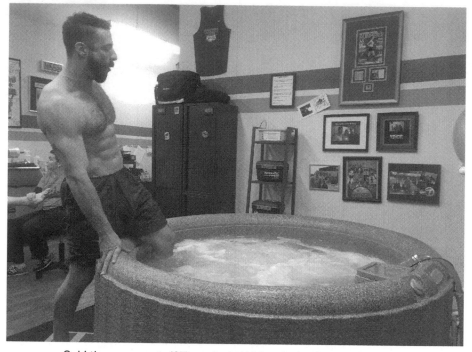

Cold thermogenesis (CT) can be helpful with immune dysregulation.

some practice with this method, I recommend integrating the breathing strategies outlined in the "Wim Hof Method" section of this book. For more information about this strategy of breathing, you can visit WimHofMethod.com.

- *The Quantlet:* Physical performance is deeply tied to your body's temperature. When you get hot, your performance suffers. This is because key respiratory proteins and cellular enzymes change shape and may even malfunction if they overheat, which impacts certain metabolic processes. Keeping the body cool during exercise or exertion can therefore help you perform better. But that's not all! Cold Thermogenesis (CT), as it is known scientifically, is an exciting new area of research which has recently shown positive effects on thyroid function,

TROUBLESHOOTING

fat loss, exercise efficiency and inflammation reduction. This is because recent studies have found that adults have more brown adipose tissue (BAT) than was previously believed, which can significantly increase energy expenditure in response to cold exposure. (www.thequantlet.com/biohacks)

- Cold plunges (lakes, rivers, oceans, streams)

I am lucky enough to live in Chicago, which has a number of recovery facilities where you can access ice baths and cryotherapy. If you live close to the Chicago area, I have done work with Liz at the Chicago Recovery Room and do cryotherapy occasionally at Chicago Cryospa. Occasionally I'll take clients to Red Square or the Chicago Sweatlodge, which have dry saunas and cold plunge pools. All of these facilities make it convenient to integrate these strategies into your weekly routine.

The best form of CT will always be cold plunges in a natural body of water like a cold lake, river, or ocean. Just make sure you have someone there with you so you don't black out and drown. In the wintertime, I'll also do cold plunges in Lake Michigan and spend anywhere from 3-7 minutes in a seated position freezing my ass off. You can do the same if you have a lake that gets cold enough nearby your residence. This does take some getting used to, but the benefits are worth it. Other helpful biohacks are:

- Hyperoxygenation
- Vibrant breathing
- Wim Hof Method
- Ozonated Water
- Structured water via vortexing or a wine aerator
- PEMF Therapy
- Sota Silver Pulser (www.sota.com): Use for 30 minutes every other day for week one. Then 30 minutes every day for week two. One hour a day week three. And sleep with it running week four.

457

- Book: *"Healing is Voltage"* by Jerry Tennant, MD
- Kangen water
- Structured water
- Essiac tea
- Liposomal glutathione
- IV glutathione (Dr. Jack Kruse suspects IV and IM glutathione require photonic light for assimilation and may be dangerous when administered exogenously)
- Intramuscular glutathione (see above)
- Liposomal vitamin C
- Curcumin/turmeric
- AHCC
- Transfer Point Beta 1, 3-D Glucan
- Resveratrol
- Fungi perfecti host defense
- Colloidal Silver
- High quality probiotics
- Low dose naltrexone
- Echinacea
- Prebiotics (to feed the good bacteria in the gut)
- NAC (N-acetylcysteine)
- Sublingual vitamin D3 (5,000-10,000 IU daily)
- Book: *"The Body Electric"* by Robert Becker, M.D.
- Vitamin C injections (Make sure the vitamin C is not derived from GMO corn)

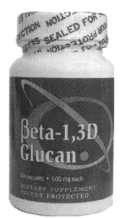

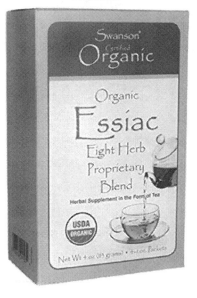

When taking vitamin D, always be sure to keep a diet rich in vitamin A to prevent vitamin D toxicity. As an added measure, I recommend including supplemental extra virgin cod liver oil.

Essiac tea originated in the 1920's when a Canadian nurse, Rene Caisse (essiac is her last name spelled backwards), got the formula from a patient who had gotten the recipe from an Ojibwa medicine man. She went on to use the essiac tea formula with cancer patients and individuals dealing with autoimmune conditions for many years with positive results. Some of the clients I have who are dealing with cancer have included essiac tea in their regimen, and some have even experienced full remission after being in Stage 4 and given a poor prognosis for survival.

Curcumin is a supplement that can be incredibly effective or provide very little benefit, depending on the type used and the dosage. There are only two forms of curcumin I use with my clients (www.BioHackingSecrets.com/coaching) because many do not produce the desired physiological results.

The same is true of probiotics, the brand, dosage, and bacterial strains included are of paramount importance.

In the 1980s, New York physician, Dr. Bernard Bihari, discovered the beneficial effects of low dose naltrexone on the immune system at dosages between 3 and 4.5 mg. Low dose naltrexone has a broad range of benefits, including healing autoimmunity, improving sleep, increasing intestinal motility, and elevating mood by releasing endorphins and increasing circulating opioids.

Low dose naltrexone has also been shown to promote T-regulatory cell function (Tregs). This lowers inflammation and provides many therapeutic benefits. Because of this, naltrexone has many applications in treating chronic inflammation, fatigue, sleeplessness, cognitive problems, anxiety, depression, and mood disorders.

A number of studies have shown low dose naltrexone to be beneficial in treating conditions like:

- Alzheimer's
- Parkinson's
- Chronic fatigue
- Psoriasis
- Lupus
- Hashimoto's
- Grave's disease
- Rheumatoid arthritis
- Multiple Sclerosis

I've used low dose naltrexone myself and recommend it to many of my executive coaching clients. I recommend starting with 2 mg at night before bed the first month, 3 mg at night before bed the second month, and 4 mg at night before bed the fourth month and beyond.

I also often recommend treatment with echinacea, which is widely used in Europe and North America for colds and flu. It has been shown in a number of studies to decrease the severity and duration of acute illness. A 2007 study found that echinacea decreased the probability of contracting the common cold by 58% and reduced the duration of colds by 1.4 days.

TROUBLESHOOTING #12: IMPAIRED METHYLATION (AND GENETIC POLYMORPHISMS)

Signs that you are suffering from problems related to impaired methylation include:

- Depression, anxiety, and stress
- Premature graying of the hair
- Asthma, allergies, arthritis, joint pain
- Cognitive problems
- Obsessive compulsive disorder or perfectionism
- Panic attacks
- Addictions
- Infertility
- Hair loss
- Anemia
- Ringing in the ears (Tinnitus)
- Difficulty sleeping
- Headaches
- Slow metabolism
- Hypothyroidism
- Poor memory
- High blood pressure
- High blood sugar
- Addictive behavior

Many individuals who exhibit energy fluctuations, suboptimal cognitive function, and symptoms of chronic illness, more often than not have genetic mutations contributing to these conditions. Three of the more common genetic mutations I see in my clients are:

MTHFR: This is a gene responsible for producing the methylenetetrahydrofolate reductase enzyme, which is an enzyme that plays an important role in energy production, brain function, detoxification, and the body's ability to maintain healthy homocysteine levels. Mutations in the MTHFR gene can result in toxic overload, low mood, fatigue, brain fog, cardiovascular disease, hypertension, glaucoma, mood disorders, psychiatric disorders, and various cancers.

HLA (Human Leukocyte Antigen): HLA mutations also make it difficult to detoxify and remove pathogens, particularly those related to mold, Lyme, and coinfections. Genes associated with gluten sensitivity and celiac disease also overlap with HLA genotype. So, finding out your HLA type is an important indicator of understanding your predisposition for these conditions.

A number of individuals who seek help because they exhibit the symptoms and characteristics of Lyme disease may actually be dealing with problems from other causes like mold, coinfections, GI disorders, etc. They get hung up trying to identify a culprit using various Lyme tests, all of which are notoriously inaccurate.

APOE (apolipoprotein E): The APOE gene is responsible for encoding a protein which combines with lipids (fats) to form cholesterol transporting lipoproteins. Certain APOE polymorphisms (mutations) increase the risk of Parkinson's, Alzheimer's, dementia, endothelial problems, and cardiovascular diseases, including heart attack and stroke.

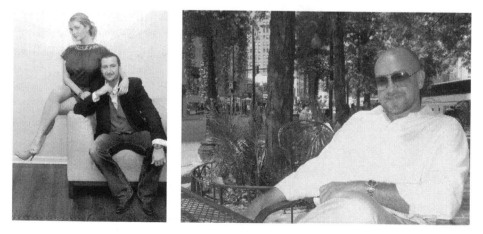

TROUBLESHOOTING

There are three slightly different versions of the APOE gene ranging from e2, e3, and e4. The most common allele is e3, which is found in about half of the general population. People who are at the highest risk for Alzheimer's have the e4 allele from both parents. By the way, everyone carries two copies of the APOE gene, one from each parent. The combination of the two determine your APOE "genotype": e2/e2, e2/e3, e2/e4, e3/e3, e3/e4, or e4/e4.

Individuals with an e4/e4 APOE genotype are roughly 15 times more likely to develop Alzheimer's disease. These statistics seem to be more relevant for women and not all individuals with this APOE genotype end up developing Alzheimer's. Lifestyle factors do contribute more than genetic predisposition in almost all cases. My APOE genotype is e4/e4.

Other genetic mutations associated with cognitive decline and Parkinson's including PINK1, PARK7, SNCA, and LRRK2. For more information about genetics and genetics testing visit The National Human Genome Research Institute website at www.genome.gov.

Impaired methylation is perhaps the most significant side effect of genetic mutations pertaining to energy and focus. Methylation is a vital

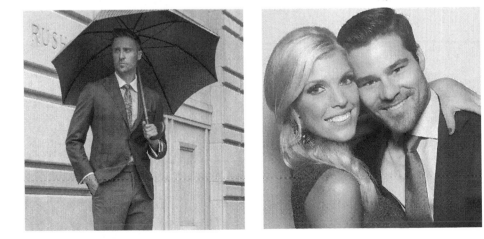

THE BIOHACKER'S GUIDE: TO UPGRADED ENERGY & FOCUS

Exact Means And Methods to Eliminate Infectious Viruses, Bacteria and Other Pathogens to Help Maintain or Regain Health

Copyright © 1998 Robert C. Beck, D.Sc. March, 1999
Revised by Sharing Health from the Heart Inc. August 2000

The complete process is described here in detail to allow anyone to successfully achieve recoveries and insure that the currently proven methods will never again be "lost" or suppressed.

What You Do

1) Blood electrification for a minimum of 2 hours per day for a minimum of four to twelve weeks. Apply salt–water moistened electrodes over Ulnar and Radial arteries on opposite insides of same wrist. A Velcro® and elastic strap holds electrodes in place. You must electrify blood for two hours every day for at least four to twelve weeks. This should not interfere with other activities. As your blood circulates normally, enough will be flowing along this path in the forearm until most blood in your body is eventually treated by the 50 to 100 microampere current flowing internally. About 3 to 5 milliampere is necessary at the skin to overcome resistive losses through tissue before current reaches blood.

2) Drink 3 to 5 ppm self–made Ionic Silver Colloid daily. Costing under 1¢ per gallon, colloids are shown to easily control opportunistic infections. This helps your immune system.

3) Apply your magnetic pulse generator for a minimum of 20 minutes daily by positioning and pulsing coil over lymph nodes and internal organs. Pulse each time it recharges at several second intervals. Pulses of high intensity time–varying magnetic flux generate a measurable back-e.m.f. in adjacent tissue thus neutralizing any residual germinating and incubating pathogens. Without this step, sufferers have been known to sometimes re–infect themselves. Conventional *permanent* magnets cannot be substituted for this purpose.

4) Drink as much ozonated water as you can comfortably ingest daily. You must generate fresh ozone yourself each time and drink immediately since O_3 has a half-life of only a few minutes. All known pathogens and cancers are anaerobic. O_3 aids their elimination by oxidation and speeds your detoxification and recovery with no discomfort. Consuming O_3 water flushes pathogens, wastes and toxins from your system.

THESE FOUR STEPS WORK SYNERGISTICALLY AND SHOULD BE USED TOGETHER.

How to Do This & Why - A Technical Explanation

1) *The blood electrifier* and ionic silver colloid maker are usually combined in one small plastic box typically 3¾ x 2¼ x 1 inch (pack of cards size) containing one outlet for wrist electrodes and a second for colloid making. A single 9V transistor radio battery drives a voltage tripler, and a single-IC-chip switches the 27–33V from negative to positive 3.92 times each second. A biphasic square wave with sharp rise-time output is fed to a 3.5 mm jack connecting to two 3/32" stainless steel or gold–plated electrodes 1" long each covered with two layers of 100% cotton flannel saturated with diluted salt water. A potentiometer allows users to adjust output until comfortable. Red and green LED's show polarity reversal (essential for safe blood electrification) and overall system functioning. A grain-of-wheat lamp indicates current flow when making ionic colloid. Precise electrode locations are determined by carefully feeling arterial pulse points on opposite insides of same wrist and positioning saturated electrodes precisely along the paths where arteries come closest to surface. Locations are critical, since the objective is to supply maximal current into blood and not waste it in surrounding flesh. Typical impedance measured from electrode–to–electrode may be as low as 2000 Ohms. Adjust output for strongest comfortable level. Schematics, parts lists and instructions for a three 9 V battery design are detailed in this paper. Anyone can build his own system; you need nothing except replacement batteries. However commercially available systems are inexpensive, reliable and are useable immediately.

2) *Ionic silver colloids* of excellent quality and freshness are easily user–made as follows: Pure silver (.999) or better yet, .9999 (4 Nine) 14 gauge (0.064" dia.) electrodes providing anode and cathode about 8" long, are immersed in distilled water. Some prefer "golden" colloids, easily made by heating 2 cups of distilled water to the boil in a non–metal container. Immerse silver wires and activate the 27–33 Volt DC output for ~15–20 minutes to produce 3 to 5 ppm.

464

metabolic process that occurs in every cell of our body, more than a billion times every second. It's a fairly simple biochemical process that involves passing a methyl group from one molecule to another in order to produce hormones, enzymes, and other compounds like CoQ10, melatonin, creatine, carnitine, and phosphatidylcholine. This is one of the reasons why these compounds are awfully deficient in individuals with impaired methylation.

People with MTHFR polymorphisms usually show high blood levels of folic acid, which is the synthetic form of folate. That's because our bodies are unable to process this form of the B vitamin. While there are laboratory tests whether you possess the MTHFR, HLA, or APOE single nucleotide polymorphisms (genetic mutations), the simplest approach is often providing your body with nutrients to support these biochemical processes and observing whether you experience an improvement in energy, cognitive function, and mood.

I recommend that you begin with a high quality B vitamin complex which contains riboflavin-5-phosphate sodium, vitamin B6 as pyridoxal 5-phosphate, folate as l-5-methyltetrahydrofolate (L-5-MTHF), B12 as methylcobalamin, and betaine anhydrous (trimethylglycine).

Other nutritional recommendations, lifestyle changes, supplements, and biohacks to support methylation include:

- *Eating more dark leafy greens:* Bok choy, Escarole, Charred kale, Spinach, Dandelion, Collard greens, Mustard greens, Beet greens.
- *Getting more B vitamins in your diet from healthy sources:* Wild-caught fish, Free-range or pastured organic eggs, Sunflower seeds, Organically-sprouted legumes, Walnuts, Asparagus, Dark, leafy green vegetables, Almonds, Organic gluten-free grains, Liver from grass-fed cows.

- *Reduce your consumption of the following:* Meat, Sugar, Saturated fat, Animal protein, Alcohol (no more than 3 drinks per week), Cigarette smoking/exposure to secondhand smoke.
- *Maintain a healthy gut microbiome by taking:* Probiotics supplements, Prescript Assist, VSL3 (double strength available by prescription), Advanced Orthomolecular Research Probiotic-3, Gut Pro Powder, and a few others I use depending on the client's symptomatology.
- *Whole food prebiotics:* Kimchi, Fermented vegetables, Water kefir, Coconut kefir, Bubbie's Pickles (brand), etc.
- *Improve digestion using digestive enzymes:* Digestive Enzymes, Betaine HCL, Digestive bitters, Ox Bile (if gallbladder has been removed or client has difficulty digesting fats).
- *Take supplements that support methylation and prevent damage from high levels of homocysteine, including:* The B vitamins mentioned above, Magnesium glycinate, Zinc, SAMe (S-Adenosylmethionine), Vitamin B6 as P-5-P, Sublingual or intramuscular B12 as methylcobalamin or hydroxocobalamin. Animal protein increases homocysteine levels in the body, and processing saturated fats and sugars can lower levels of vital nutrients in the body.

Here are some specialized tests that can detect genetic abnormalities and SNPs, like MTHFR:

- *Genova Diagnostics NeuroGenomic:* This test evaluates single nucleotide polymorphisms (SNPs) in genes that modulate methylation, glutathione conjugation, oxidative protection and the potential to evaluate vascular oxidation.
- SpectraCell MTHFR genotyping test
- Vitamin Diagnostics Methylation Pathways Panel Troubleshooting

TROUBLESHOOTING #13: MITOCHONDRIAL DYSFUNCTION

Signs that you are suffering from problems related to impaired methylation include:

- Low energy, fatigue, or malaise
- Muscle weakness or loss of coordination
- Hearing and/or visual problems
- Digestive disorders, particularly if they have a propensity towards constipation
- High blood sugar or diabetes
- Hypothyroidism or slow metabolism
- Adrenal fatigue
- Confusion or disorientation
- Memory loss
- Exercise intolerance (excessive fatigue after intense exercise, may include a decrease in sex drive)
- Seizures
- Heart, kidney, or liver disease
- Dizziness or lightheadedness when standing up
- Excessive sweating
- Low appetite, bloating, and/or difficulty swallowing
- Difficulty ejaculating or keeping an erection

Mitochondria are the tiny, bacteria-like energy production centers of our cells. They take in nutrients and then convert those nutrients into ATP (adenosine triphosphate), the fundamental energy unit of the body. There are many forms of mitochondrial disease, and this can stem from both genetic and environmental factors.

467

We are just now starting to recognize the prevalence of mitochondrial dysfunction and the various ways that it affects everything from energy, to cognition, to mood, and even the prevention of chronic degenerative diseases. Factors which increase the risk of mitochondrial dysfunction include:

- Poor diet
- Genetic mutations
- Antibiotics in our meat
- Prescription drugs
- Impaired methylation
- Exposure to dietary and environmental toxins
- A number of other causes

A 2013 study showed, "Bactericidal antibiotics induce mitochondrial dysfunction and oxidative damage in mammalian cells." Symptoms of mitochondrial dysfunction include:

- Slowed reaction time
- Low energy
- Chronic fatigue
- Impaired coordination
- Muscular weakness
- Multiple sclerosis
- Parkinson's
- Alzheimer's
- Dementia
- Heart disease
- Liver disease
- Learning disabilities

- Delayed development in children
- Visual and hearing problems
- Autism and autism spectrum disorders
- GI disorders, including gas, bloating, constipation, diarrhea
- Diabetes
- Chronic infections
- Thyroid and adrenal problems
- Memory problems
- Confusion and disorientation

Diseases linked to mitochondrial dysfunction include:
- Type 2 diabetes
- Parkinson's
- Heart disease
- Stroke
- Alzheimer's
- Multiple sclerosis
- Chronic fatigue syndrome
- Fibromyalgia
- Various forms of cancer

Nutritional interventions, lifestyle changes, supplements, and biohacks for improving mitochondrial function include:

- Therapeutic ketosis via the ketogenic diet and intermittent fasting
- Caloric restriction (reduce calories by 20-30%)
- Avoid eating within 3 hours of bedtime (has been shown to improve mitochondrial health)
- Supplemental beta hydroxyl butyrate (increases ATP production)
- Exogenous ketone bodies (you can check out the exogenous ketones I'm taking at www.Biohacks.PruvItNow.com)

- Organic, raw, unprocessed extra virgin coconut oil
- MCT oil
- C-8 pure caprylic acid MCT oil (Bulletproof Brain Octane, Parrillo CapTri)
- Creatine HCL
- Creapure pharmaceutical grade creatine monohydrate
- Pterostilbene, resveratrol, and curcumin (all upregulate mitochondrial function and support the electron transport chain, turn on longevity genes, and lower inflammation)
- D-ribose
- Ubiquinol CoQ10
- PQQ (pyrroloquinoline quinone)
- NAC (N-acetyl cysteine)
- Organic coffee
- Nicotinamide riboside
- Sublingual NADH (Nicotinamide adenine dinucleotide)
- Baking soda
- Cold exposure (cryotherapy, cold plunge, ice baths, and cold showers)

You should also dramatically reduce or eliminate alcohol consumption as alcohol lowers the coenzyme NAD+ (nicotinamide adenine dinucleotide). NAD+ is an essential enzyme needed for the production of testosterone and energy. NADH is the same as NAD+ except that it includes hydrogen. This is shown to improve alertness, concentration, mental clarity, energy production in addition to being a beneficial treatment for Alzheimer's disease, chronic fatigue, and athletic performance. People have also found NADH to be helpful with cholesterol, jet lag, depression, Parkinson's, and high blood pressure.

A number of studies have shown oral ingestion of baking soda to increase exercise performance, buffer lactic acid, and increase cerebral blood flow. It has also been known to improve the mitochondrial builder protein Â (PGC)-1Î±Â in a dose-dependant manner. I've not personally taken oral baking soda but may consider this as a possibility in the future after I have done more research.

Section Notes:

- The detrimental effects of antibiotics were reversed in mice through the administration of the antioxidant N-acetyl cysteine.
- Coffee is one of the highest sprayed crops in terms of pesticide content, so always go organic.
- Nicotinamide riboside is a newcomer to the scene but provides much promise for upregulating mitochondrial function. Due to its cost, most people don't take effective dosages, and therefore, have unfavorable experiences with the compound.

TROUBLESHOOTING #14: CIRCULATION & OXYGEN DELIVERABILITY

Signs that you are suffering from problems related to circulation and oxygen deliverability include:

- Poor focus and concentration
- Mental fatigue
- Reliance on coffee or exercise to "wake the brain up"
- Nail issues or fungal growth on toes
- Cold tip of nose, hands, and feet

- Nail beds are white instead of bright pink
- Swollen legs or ankles

Please circle "Yes" or "No" for each statement below:

1. I often experience swelling of the legs or ankles (edema). *(Yes or No)*
2. I get short of breath when I exercise. *(Yes or No)*
3. I often feel lightheaded. *(Yes or No)*
4. Sometimes I find it difficult to breathe when I'm lying down. *(Yes or No)*
5. I'm often tired during the day. *(Yes or No)*
6. I have a persistent cough. *(Yes or No)*
7. I have felt heaviness or pressure in my chest. *(Yes or No)*
8. Sometimes my lips are a bluish color. *(Yes or No)*
9. I experience pain in my feet, especially during exercise. *(Yes or No)*
10. During exercise I experience a burning sensation in my muscles (lactic acid buildup) frequently. *(Yes or No)*
11. I have a family history of heart disease. *(Yes or No)*
12. I've had a heart attack. *(Yes or No)*
13. I'm a smoker. *(Yes or No)*
14. I do not like fish, and I rarely eat cold water fatty fish. *(Yes or No)*
15. I do not perform steady state cardiovascular exercise like jogging or swimming. *(Yes or No)*
16. I do not get 30 minutes of physical activity every day. *(Yes or No)*
17. I sit most of the day. *(Yes or No)*
18. I have another autoimmune condition. *(Yes or No)*
19. I have had herpes or hepatitis. *(Yes or No)*
20. I eat processed foods that come in a box, a bag, a can, a tube, a jar, or a wrapper. *(Yes or No)*

21. I have high blood pressure. *(Yes or No)*
22. I am overweight or obese. *(Yes or No)*
23. I have high blood sugar, insulin resistance, or diabetes. *(Yes or No)*
24. I have high triglycerides. *(Yes or No)*
25. I have a hard time managing stress. *(Yes or No)*
26. I have low HDL (good) cholesterol. *(Yes or No)*

As we get older, we lose the ability to utilize oxygen. A number of internal and external factors contribute to the rise of circulation and oxygen deliverability issues including, but not limited to:

– Anemia
– Nutrient deficiencies
– Mitochondrial dysfunction
– Chronic infections
– Chronic inflammation
– Methylation problems
– GI disorders
– Environmental toxins, especially air pollution
– Lack of exercise
– Poor diet
– Coronation of drinking water (which removes oxygen)
– Consumption of meat from grocery stores and restaurants (due to it's high antibiotic content)
– Overcooking our foods
– Lack of adequate raw, organic vegetables and berries in one's diet
– Poor antioxidant status
– Inadequate consumption of healthy, unsaturated fatty acids and omega-3s, among others

Air normally contains about 20% oxygen. However, in many of our polluted cities, these levels have dropped to around half that (10%). Oxygen is an important precursor in the production of ATP. It strengthens our immune system, improves brain function, boosts mood, and kills pathogens in our blood and tissues. For many of us, these oxygen needs are not being met, and we see this exhibited by increased cases of:

- Asthma
- Allergies
- GI disorders
- Intestinal parasites
- Cancers
- Chronic fatigue
- Depression
- Anxiety
- Mood disorders
- Bacterial and viral diseases
- Platelet aggregation, blood viscosity, blood "stickiness" (can be due to genetic or environmental factors)

Many nutritional supplements used to treat these conditions function by increasing cellular oxygenation. A few examples are:

- Ubiquinol CoQ10
- Niacin
- Vitamin E
- L-Citrulline
- Arginine
- Pycnogenol

TROUBLESHOOTING

When addressing circulation and oxygen deliverability issues, I recommend starting with nutrition. Focus on a plant-based diet with 80% of your nutritions coming from organic, living plants. Most of those plants should be vegetables, and most of those vegetables being green, and to a much lesser degree, organic berries. Focus on healthy, plant-based fats like extra virgin olive oil, MCT oil, coconut oil, Udo's Choice oil blend, avocado, etc. Make wild-caught fish your primary protein source, and reduce or eliminate other forms of meat (we can reintroduce and experiment with these after symptoms have been resolved).

Pay particular attention to avoid the dietary toxins that cause immunogenic and allergenic inflammatory responses in the body. These have already been covered at nauseam throughout this guide. There are a number of studies that have also shown an organic Mediterranean diet to be beneficial for improving cardiovascular health and oxygen deliverability issues. This type of diet may also be helpful in the prevention of many cancers, and it is also one of the highest recommended diets for diabetics and those suffering from metabolic issues. Other strategies for improving circulation and oxygen deliverability include:

- A daily 20-30 minute outdoor, steady state jog in your target heart rate zone, with lots of skin exposure to direct sunlight
- Breathing exercises like the Wim Hof Method and other vibrant breathing techniques
- The ketogenic diet and/or fasting-induced ketosis
- Address anemia and low iron
- The Elevation Training Mask
- The PowerLung
- The Expand-a-Lung
- A Cardio Cap
- Restricted breathing exercises

- The 02 Trainer by Bas Rutten
- Hypoxic training
  - Hypoxico altitude training products (www.Hypoxico.com)
  - Hyperbaric chambers
- Inversion
  - Handstands
  - Headstands
  - Inversion tables
  - Inversion boots and pull up bar
- Chew gum
- NormaTec PULSE Recovery System
- Hot and cold contrast
  - Three cycles of 20 minutes in the sauna followed by a 2 minute cold shower
  - 2-12 minute cold plunge in an ice bath or lake, followed by the sauna
  - 3 minutes in a cryotherapy chamber, followed by a sauna or hot shower
- Exercise with Oxygen Therapy (EWOT)

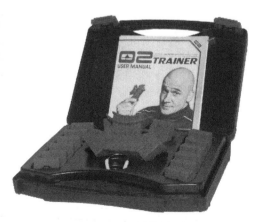 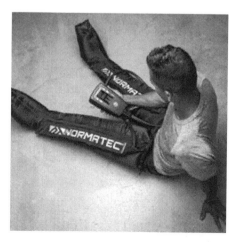

- Drink Ozonated Water and Hydrogen-Rich Water:
  - Sota Water Ozonator (www.sota.com)
  - Dr. Hayashi's Hydrogen-Rich Water Stick
- Pulsed Electromagnetic Fields (PEMF) Therapy (www. BiohackingSecrets.com/PEMF)
  - Ondamed (in less than a week doing daily 40-60 minute sessions with the Ondamed I felt a quantifiable improvement in circulation and flexibility)
  - MAS Special Multi+ -
  - Parmeds Super (one of the best full body PEMF machines I've used)
  - EarthPulse (great for enhancing sleep quality and reducing time to onset)
  - PEMF-120 (best device for back pain)
  - FlexPulse portable PEMF device (device I use the most due to it's versatility and portability)
  - MicroPulse portable PEMF (good entry level device based on NASA research)

Exercise boosts nitric oxide (similar to the amino acid L-Arginine, which is used for erectile dysfunction and by bodybuilders to increase vascularity). Studies have shown that regular exercise increases eNOS expression and nitric oxide production while decreasing free radical generation in humans. This has beneficial effects on the vascular and antioxidant systems of the body, and subsequently, may reduce the risk of hypertension, diabetes, and heart disease.

EWOT is also known as oxygen multi-step therapy. This involves exercising while breathing oxygen in high conversation (as close to 100% as possible). Exercising with oxygen has been shown to improve endothelial health, slow down the aging process in our capillaries and improve blood and tissue oxygenation. Other benefits of EWOT include:

- Recovery from stress-related illnesses
- Prevention of cancers
- Increase of energy
- A slowing down/reversing of the aging process
- Improvement in the diameter of the blood vessels
- Increased oxygenation of the tissues and cells
- Strengthened immune response
- Easier/Faster Weight Loss
- Amplified memory

At home oxygen concentrators can be purchased. A good concentrator can deliver about 90% oxygen at a rate of around 10 liters per minute. This is the bare minimum for EWOT. For exercise, most people need 15 liters per minute. This requires the use of oxygen tanks or two concentrators. Oxygen concentrators and ozone generators can be purchased through Longevity Resources (www.ozonegenerator.com).

Here are some supplements that are helpful in treating circulation and oxygen deliverability:

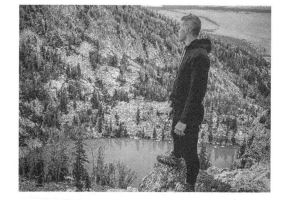

- Butcher's broom
- Piracetam
- Cordyceps
- Chia seeds
- Vinpocetine
- Ginkgo
- Huperzine
- Alpha GPC

- N-acetyl l-carnitine
- Cayenne
- Malic acid
- Pycnogenol
- Grape seed extract
- Resveratrol
- Pterostilbene
- *Vitamin K2:* Vitamin K2 plays a vital role in blood coagulation and vascular health. It may also help to prevent coronary artery disease, blood clots, heart attacks, and stroke. In addition, it is an essential nutrient in that it helps bone to absorb calcium and preventing this calcium from adhering to arterial walls. This is known as vascular calcification. I recommend supplementing with vitamin K to many of my clients (K1, MK4, and MK-7) along with vitamin D not only to improve circulation and oxygen deliverability, but also to prevent cardiovascular complications.

Section Notes:

- Studies and animal models show that the ketogenic diet helps mitochondria to more efficiently utilize oxygen and produce more energy per oxygen molecule.
- Early signs of low iron can include hair loss, fatigue, and muscle cramps.
- The Cardio Cap is a device used by swimmers, which can be affixed to the end of your snorkel.
- Neuroscience researchers have found chewing gum to increase cognition, attention, and memory. It may also improve blood flow to the brain and upregulate nutrient delivery. Just make sure to choose a brand that is free of artificial sweeteners, chemicals, artificial colors, etc. I use B-Fresh spearmint and cinnamon gum.

- The NormaTec PULSE Recovery System utilizes compressed air to massage your limbs, detoxify the lymphatic system, mobilize fluid, and speed up recovery. This is very similar to the kneading and stroking that takes place during a massage. It is used by many athletes to accelerate recovery.
- The recommended protocol for ice baths and ice tubs is 8-12 minutes at 52-53°F.
- Researchers have found that people with fibromyalgia have muscle hypoxia (low levels of oxygen in their muscles). Evidence suggests that magnesium glycinate and malic acid may help ease pain and discomfort caused by low muscle oxygenation. They may also help the body to produced more ATP. Furthermore, malic acid increases cardiovascular and muscular endurance.

TROUBLESHOOTING #15: MOVEMENT PATTERNS & BIOMECHANICS

Please circle "Yes" or "No" for each statement below:

1. I have poor posture. *(Yes or No)*
2. I find it difficult to jog. *(Yes or No)*
3. When playing sports, I am frequently injured. *(Yes or No)*
4. I experience pains, aches, tightness, or stiffness in my back, joints, neck, or muscles. *(Yes or No)*
5. I am not flexible. *(Yes or No)*
6. I have hurt my back more than once doing heavy squats, dead lifts, weight training, cross-fit, or high-intensity workouts. *(Yes or No)*

Use it or lose it. That's the way it goes with the human body. If you look at a professional dancer, you'll see someone who is overflowing with energy. Their appearance is youthful, and their body is supple from hours of daily use. I have been fortunate to have had the chance to work with a number of professional dancers, and without exception, they all look 10 to 15 years younger than their biological age. Their statuesque bodies are strong, yet flexible and pliable. Their posture is immaculate.

Professional and high-level dancers train from 8-12 hours a day. Their posture, mobility, movement patterns, and over all biomechanics reflect this training. Now, let's contrast the lifestyle of a dancer to that of your average American. Statistically, most modern Americans sit an average of 13 hours each day. Average men and women of other countries at least walk an average of 10,000 steps a day. Americans only average about half of that.

Not surprisingly, my clients (www.BioHackingSecrets.com/coaching) with the biggest health challenges are those who walk less than 2,000 steps per day. That's basically the steps that you would take going from your bed, to your car, to your office, and then doing all these things in reverse. There may also be tiny pockets of movement in between, like going to the bathroom or getting something to eat, but that's about it. On the other hand, many of my healthiest clients take an average of around 20,000-30,000 steps per day. One even sent me a screenshot where he nearly hit 45,000 steps in a single day.

Here's the truth. The more energy you expend, the more energy you will have. Movement and deep breathing oxygenate and alkalis the body. Most people only utilize about 20% of their lung capacity, but when we move, we increase our heart rate and our body's oxygen demands, we breathe deeper and fill ourselves with oxygen. This not only upregulates cellular ATP energy production, it also expels greater amounts of CO_2, which is the most significant source of acidity in the body.

When we don't move our bodies daily, the way they are intended to be used, and when we don't appreciate the gift of this movement and our physical body, these luxuries are taken from us. Our muscles and joints turn stiff and tight. We become rigid and inflexible. We hunch forward from our backs and our knees begin to ache. Over time, we lose the ability to perform even the simplest movements, like jogging, without experiencing pain or discomfort.

Next time you have the opportunity to watch a child play, notice how effortlessly he runs and jumps without worry or concern, without even a second thought. This is our natural state. Tony Robbins famously teaches that motion creates emotion, and the fastest way to change your emotional state and energy is to change your physiology (the way you move and use your body).

Try this exercise. First, imagine someone who is depressed. They are exhausted and unhappy. Picture what this person would look like. Now, stand up and walk, assuming the posture and movement patterns of this individual. Walk around the room the same way that they would. Mirror their pace, their gaze, and everything else you can imagine about them, and pay particular attention to how you feel as you are doing so.

Do this for a minute or so, and then imagine someone who is overflowing with positive energy. How is their posture different? Where are their eyes in relation to the floor, the ceiling, and other people? When they walk, do they walk fast or slow? Take a quick second to adopt the posture, head position, and movement patterns of this person, and walk around the room mirroring their physiology. Think about how this person would breathe. Would their breathing be deep or shallow? Think about which of the two personas you would rather take on.

In order to change your emotional state, your energy levels and your mental clarity, you'll need to start by correcting your posture, breathing, and the speed at which you walk. We all know that good posture is important. At least, we've been told this our entire life, but why is it so critical? Not only does this help your appearance, it makes your body healthier.

Psychol Sci. 2010 Oct;21(10):1363-8. doi: 10.1177/0956797610383437. Epub 2010 Sep 20.

Power posing: brief nonverbal displays affect neuroendocrine levels and risk tolerance.

Carney DR[1], Cuddy AJ, Yap AJ.

⊕ Author information

Abstract

Humans and other animals express power through open, expansive postures, and they express powerlessness through closed, contractive postures. But can these postures actually cause power? The results of this study confirmed our prediction that posing in high-power nonverbal displays (as opposed to low-power nonverbal displays) would cause neuroendocrine and behavioral changes for both male and female participants: High-power posers experienced elevations in testosterone, decreases in cortisol, and increased feelings of power and tolerance for risk; low-power posers exhibited the opposite pattern. In short, posing in displays of power caused advantaged and adaptive psychological, physiological, and behavioral changes, and these findings suggest that embodiment extends beyond mere thinking and feeling, to physiology and subsequent behavioral choices. That a person can, by assuming two simple 1-min poses, embody power and instantly become more powerful has real-world, actionable implications.

A study titled "Power Posing: Brief Nonverbal Displays Neuroendocrine Levels and Risk Tolerance" was conducted back in 2010. In this study, it was found that in as little as one minute, high power postures elevations in testosterone, decreases in cortisol, increased feelings of authority and increased risk tolerance. Individuals assuming low power postures exhibited the opposite patterns. More specifically, two sessions consisting of one minute of power postures each brought about a 33% increase in risk tolerance, a 20% increase in testosterone, and a 25% decrease in cortisol.

These findings are echoed in professor Amy Cuddy's own findings, which show that people with high power poses have increased feelings of dominance, risk taking, and power, as well as reduced anxiety. The benefits don't stop there, however. The Cleveland Clinic found that people who suffer from back pain experience positive changes simply by consciously improving their posture.

We now know just how biochemically important oxygen is in the production of energy. Well, when we slouch, our body takes in 30% less oxygen than when we exhibit upright posture and proper breathing patterns. A number of studies carried out by Erik Peper found that participants who are upright and dynamic felt more energetic, happier, and more positive, whereas people who slouched reported feeling sad, lonely, and isolated. Other studies have found that just adopting an upright posture when you're stressed can reduce negative mood and elevate self esteem.

Furthermore, one study at Indiana University found that sitting upright allows our central nervous system (brain and spinal column) to function more efficiently. It also improves our memory and learning. If you implement just two simple changes that will dramatically impact your energy and focus, you should:

- Consciously correct your posture
- Walk with energy and purpose

Admittedly, this is much easier said than done. You'll find yourself, at first, having to correct your posture what feels like 100 times a day, and you will have a tendency to slip back into old movement patterns. However, I am absolutely sure that if you set your mind to this task, correcting the way you stand, sit, and move, you will permanently change your energy, emotions, and mental sharpness. Here are some biohacks, supplements, and strategies that will also help increase your mobility, movement patters, and restore healthy biomechanics:

- Hanging
- Inversions
  - Teeter Hang Ups
  - Inversion table
  - Headstands
  - Handstands
- Whole body vibration training
- Soft tissue work and myofascial release
  - Lacrosse ball
  - TriggerPoint roller

- RumbleRoller
- Joe DeFranco's "Limber 11" video (available on YouTube)
- The Stick (a device used to roll out muscles, can be found on Amazon)
- Cranial Sacral therapy (Try Dr. Berg's Back & Neck Massage Tool)
- Body Back BuddySelf-Massage Tool
- Theracane
- The Foot Rubz Massage Ball
- Acupuncture
- Deep tissue massage
- Active release technique (ART)
- Functional range conditioning (FRC)
- Voodoo floss bands
- YogaToes
- MarcPro Plus (save $47 on the MarcPro Plus at www.BiohackingSecrets.com/marcpro with discount code "biohacks").
- Budokon Yoga DVDs (My favorite is the "Flow and Flexibility" workout)
- Rolfing (think massage meets chiropractic work - on steroids)
- MAT (Muscle Activation Techniques)

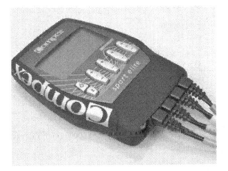

  - Advanced muscle integration therapy
  - Graston technique
  - Trigger Point Therapy
  - Compex Sport Elite Muscle Stimulator

Deep tissue massage can also be extraordinarily helpful to correcting and realigning biomechanics. I try to get a 30-60 minute deep tissue massage once a week or every other week. Unfortunately, it doesn't always happen. But energy, flexibility, stress, and movement are discernibly improved when I do.

I also try to hang each morning from my pull up bar, after I do a few pull ups. This has many benefits, including decompressing the spine, enhancing grip strength, and stretching abdominal muscles. Headstands and handstands can be done on parallettes or using a wall to assist. When it comes to the whole body vibration training, I use the Power Plat Pro machine. A 2014 study found that long term whole body vibration training improved posture and stability in young men, so this is something I highly advise that you try while you are working on correcting your posture. Recommended supplements for pain, stiffness, flexibility, and mobility are:

- Astaxanthin
- Proteolytic enzymes/Systemic enzymes
- Serrapeptase
- Boluoke
- Bromelain
- AHCC fermented medicinal mushroom mycelia (roots)
- Curcumin/Turmeric
- Ecklonia Cava (brown seaweed extract)
- Cat's claw
- Betaine HCL
- Glucosamine
- Chondroitin
- Collagen Generators (i.e. BioSil, Neocell Collagen Type 1 & 3, CellFood Silica, bone broth from grass-fed cows, Great Lakes Gelatin)

- MSM (methylsulfonylmethane)
- Hyaluronic acid
- Liposomal vitamin C
- High dose natural vitamin C or Quali-C
- Liposomal Curcumin
- PhytOriginal live phytoplankton
- Nattokinase
- Papain
- Protease (bacterial and fungal)
- Pancreatin
- Trypsin
- Rutin
- Fish oil
- Magnesium glycinate
- Malic acid
- D-ribose
- Carnitine
- Boswellia
- Cayenne
- Cherry fruit extract
- DMSO (dimethyl sulfoxide)
- Valerian root
- Minocycline (typical dosage 100 mg 2x daily, taken at meal time. This can interact with other drugs, including iron pills, blood thinners, and antacids)

Other strategies, treatments, and biohacks are:

- Stem cell therapy (heal injuries, accelerate recovery, and regrow cartilage)

- Hyperthermic conditioning
  - Ultra baths
  - Dry saunas
  - Jacuzzi or hot tub
- Posture/body alignment
- Pilates
- Yoga
- Chiropractic work
- Airrosti
- BioMat
- Medicinal marijuana
- PEMF therapy
- The Alexander Technique
- "Foundation Training" DVD by Dr. Eric Goodman
- *Becoming a Supple Leopard* by Dr. Kelly Starrett
- *Ready to Run* by Dr. Kelly Starrett
- *Unbreakable Runner* by TJ Murphy and Brian Mackenzie (founder of CrossFit Endurance)
- *The Trigger Point Therapy Workbook* by Clair Davies
- *The New Arthritis Breakthrough: The Only Medical Therapy Clinically Proven to Induce Long Term Improvement and Remission* by Henry Scammell

Sometimes taking Lyrica combined with Cymbalta (both prescription drugs) may be an effective treatment for pain. Typically, recommended dosages would be 125 mg of Lyrica at bedtime for three days, then 50 mg at bedtime for four days a week. Then, for the second week, you would take 25 mg in the morning and 50 mg at bedtime for three days. Finally, you would take 50 mg in the morning and 50 mg at bedtime for four days. From then on, you would take 50 mg in the morning and 50 mg at bedtime.

When it comes to Cymbalta, you would want to take 20 mg daily in the morning Week 1 and 2, and Week 3 and 4, you would take 30 mg in the morning. Then, Week 5 and 6 take 40 mg in the morning, and thereafter take 60 mg in the morning. For a more in-depth explanation, I recommend checking out *"The Fatigue and Fibromyalgia Solution"* by Dr.Jacob Teitelbaum, MD.

Marijuana has also proven itself to be effective in this area. In 2010, a review of 14 clinical studies on the use of marijuana for pain revealed that marijuana not only controls pain, but in many cases, does so better than pharmaceutical alternatives. When compared to prescription painkillers, it was found that marijuana is much safer. For example, the prescription painkiller Vioxx killed over 60,000 people before being pulled from the market. In 2010 alone, prescription painkillers were responsible for almost 17,000 deaths. Marijuana has still not been shown to kill a single individual in all it's centuries of use.

Section Notes:
- Many cities offer community acupuncture clinics, which make getting acupuncture much more affordable. The one that I've gone to in Chicago provides a full hour of acupuncture and a full diagnostic assessment.
- The Combat Sport Relief Muscle Stimulator is one of my new favorite tools to use. It offers nine different training programs which focus on endurance, resistance, strength, explosive strength, potentiation, active recovery, warm up, and massage.
- An ultra bath would consist of 2 cups Epsom salt or magnesium chloride, 1 cup baking soda, 12-15 drops lavender oil and an optional 1 cup 35% food grade hydrogen peroxide added to a tub of water.

- The book by Henry Scammell (listed above) discusses the use of minocycline antibiotic therapy in the treatment of arthritic conditions.

TROUBLESHOOTING #16: ESTROGEN DOMINANCE, ELEVATED ANDROGENS, AND PCOS (IN WOMEN)

Symptoms of estrogen dominance:

- Accelerated aging
- Stuffy nose, sinuses, and allergies
- Autoimmune disorders such as lupus erythematosis, thyroiditis, and Sjoegren's
- Breast cancer
- Breast tenderness (including cysts in breasts and armpits)
- Cervical dysplasia a.k.a. cervical intraepithelial neoplasia (CIN)
- Cold hands and feet as a symptom of thyroid dysfunction
- Decreased sex drive
- Depression with anxiety or agitation
- Dry eyes
- Early onset of menstruation
- Endometrial (uterine) cancer
- Fat gain, especially around the abdomen, hips and thighs
- Fatigue
- Brain fog
- Gallbladder issues
- Loss of hair
- Headaches

- Hypoglycemia (low blood sugar)
- Increased blood clotting (increasing risk of strokes)
- Infertility
- Irregular menstrual cycles
- Moodiness (irritability)
- Insomnia
- Magnesium deficiency
- Memory issues
- Osteoporosis
- Polycystic ovaries
- Premenopausal bone loss
- Slow metabolism
- Thyroid dysfunction mimicking hypothyroidism
- Uterine cancer
- Uterine fibroids
- Water retention & bloating (edema)

Conditions linked to estrogen dominance:

- Endometriosis
- Blood Clots
- Elevated Blood Pressure
- Fibroid Breasts
- Infertility
- Irregular Menstrual Flow
- Uterine Fibroids
- Breast Tenderness
- Mood Swings
- Uterine Cancer
- Hair Loss

- Depression
- Weight Gain
- Migraine Headaches
- Spotting
- Breast Cancer Risk
- Insomnia
- Inflammation
- Abnormal Pap Smears
- Fluid Retention
- Cramping
- Vaginal Dryness
- Thyroid Imbalances
- Decrease in Memory
- Low or No Sex Drive

Elevated Androgens and PCOS (Polycystic Ovarian Syndrome): Around 10% of menstruating women in the U.S. have polycystic ovarian syndrome (PCOS), which effects reproductive health and can cause frustrating physical and emotional changes. Women with PCOS are prone to:

- weight gain
- excess hair on the face, chest, stomach, thumbs, or toes (including male-pattern hair growth)
- decrease in breast size
- deeper voice
- thin hair
- acnes and skin issues
- water retention (include edema)
- anxiety and stress

- depression or low mood
- pelvic pain
- irregular periods
- ovarian cysts
- diabetes, high blood sugar, or insulin insensitivity
- circulatory problems

These hormonal imbalances can be complicated which makes it difficult to give generic recommendations. I see them often with my female clients and usually have to do in depth analysis of their situation before moving forward with a protocol.

Here are a few of the tools I have used to help with estrogen dominance, elevated androgens, and PCOS in female clients:

- Reduce toxic burden by switching to a plant-based, organic diet. 80% of food should come from a wide variety of vegetables, most of those vegetables being green. At least half of plants consumed should be raw.
- Ketogenic diet
- Intermittent fasting (when appropriate)
- Limit foods that spike insulin and blood sugar. For fruit, I usually start out by keeping clients to no more than one cup of organic blueberries, raspberries, or blackberries daily. Insulin spikes upregulate an enzyme called 1720-liase which further elevates testosterone. This can be beneficial at times if you're a man looking to build muscle. But not in this particular instance.
- Metformin (500 mg twice per day with meals)
- Berberine HCL
- Tons of cruciferous vegetables
- Dry saunas

- Infrared saunas
- Cold Thermogenesis (cold showers, ice baths, cold plunges, cryotherapy)
- Bioidentical hormone replacement therapy
- Systemic/proteolytic enzymes
- Iodine (form organic kelp and bladderwrack)
- Organic green tea and EGCG supplements
- DIM
- Calcium D-Glucarate
- Vital Berry
- Magnesium Glycinate
- CoQ10 (ubiquinol form)
- Bioactive B-Vitamin Complex (if MTHFR genetic mutation present)
- Milk Thistle
- Artichoke
- Curcumin/Turmeric
- Broccoli extracts (sulforaphane glucosinolate) - increases Phase 2 detoxification enzymes and protects DNA.
- Organic chlorophyll
- Chlorophyllin
- Easily absorbed, non-constipating iron supplement (when anemia may be a compounding factor)

BONUS: BOOST BRAIN POWER
WITH NUTRACEUTICALS, SUPPLEMENTS, & PHARMACEUTICALS

Here are some of the biohacks that may boost memory and cognition:

Caffeine:
- Prolab Advanced Caffeine
- Yerba Mate
- Guayusa tea
- Pu-erh tea
- Green tea
- Organic coffee with C8 Pure Caprylic acid MCT oil

Supplements:
- Jarrow Brain Boost
- Nicotine gum (2 mg)
- Huperzine A
- Piracetam
- Aniracetam

- AgmaSet brand Agmatine (for nerve health)
- Pregnenolone
- Gastrodin
- Vinpocetine
- Phosphatidylserine
- Alpha-GPC
- Ginkgo biloba
- Bacopa
- Pterostilbene
- Tyrosine
- Phenylalanine
- L-DOPA
- Rhodiola rosea
- Ashwagandha
- Gotu Kola
- DHA (docosahexaenoic acid)
- Acetyl L-carnitine arginate
- Bioactive B complex (see "Impaired Methylation" section in Troubleshooting)
- Ubiquinol
- CoQ10
- PQQ (pyrroloquinoline quinone)
- Magnesium L-Threonate
- Phosphatidylcholine from sunflower lecithin: Lipids make up 60-80% of the central nervous system and a deficiency in them can expose us to the energy-sapping toxic heavy metals like mercury (esp. from dental amalgams). By replenishing lipids like phosphatidylcholine and phosphatidylserine many clients report increased energy, elevated mood, and enhanced cognitive function. It's also why I use or create liposomal forms of many vitamins and nutrients to enhance absorption and uptake.

- HGH
- Bioidentical hormones
- DHEA
- Green tea
- Pre-formulated nootropics
  - LifeExtension Cognitex
  - Onnit Alpha Brain
  - De Novo Nutrition Utopia(n)
  - TruBrain
  - Jarrow Neuro-optimizer
  - HerbWorks
- Taurine
- Aniracetam
- Citicoline (CDP-choline)
- Centrophenoxine
- DMAE
- Galantamine
- GABA (gamma-aminobutyric acid)
- Phenibut
- Picamilon
- Tryptophan
- 5-HTP
- Sulbutiamine
- DL-phenylalanine
- Mucuna pruriens
- Suntheanine
- Alpha-lipoic acid
- Creatine (as pure creatine monohydrate)
- Creatine HCL
- Vitamin D6 as pyridoxal 5-phosphate

- Vitamin B8 as inositol
- Vitamin B12 as methylcobalamin
- Iodine
- SAMe (s-adenosylmethionine)
- Uridine
- Lion's mane
- Lemon balm
- Marijuana
- Wild green oat extract
- Resveratrol
- Saint John's Wort
- Melatonin

Prescription Drugs:

- Prozac

Prozac May Be Involved in Creating New Brain Cells

By Rick Nauert PhD
~ Less than a minute read

A new study reports the antidepressant fluoxetine, commonly called Prozac, Sarafem, or Fontex, is associated with the development of new nerve cells in the adult brain.

Researchers had previously determined that progeny nerve cells exist at the surface of the adult cortex and that a lack of blood, or ischemia, enhances the generation of new inhibitory neurons from these neural progenitor cells.

These cells were accordingly named "Layer 1 Inhibitory Neuron Progenitor cells" (L1-INP).

However, until now it was not known whether L1-INP-related neurogenesis could be induced in the normal adult cortex.

Researchers used fluoxetine, a selective serotonin reuptake inhibitor and one of the most widely used antidepressants, to stimulate the production of new neurons from L1-INP cells.

Investigators determined a large percentage of these newly generated neurons were inhibitory GABAergic interneurons, and their generation coincided with a reduction in cell death following ischemia.

Researchers believe the finding shows that fluoxetine has a neuroprotective response and that the purposeful creation of new nerve cells in the brain is prevention/treatment option for neurodegenerative diseases and psychiatric disorders.

The study is published online in the journal *Neuropsychopharmacology*.

Source: National Institute for Physiological Sciences

Simvastatin as an Anti-Inflammatory and Neuroprotective Agent in Parkinson's Disease

Groundbreaking research suggests that the cholesterol lowering drug **simvastatin** may provide powerful neuroprotection in Parkinson's disease. A little known fact among the public is that statin drugs do more than simply lower cholesterol, they are also anti-inflammatory agents. In fact, many researchers believe that some of the cardiovascular benefits are due to their anti-inflammatory properties (Quist-Paulsen 2010).

Simvastatin is efficient at crossing the blood-brain barrier, and it has been shown to exert potent anti-inflammatory and neuroprotective action in the dopaminergic tract (Roy 2011; Yan 2011).

In animal models, simvastatin was shown to attenuate the neurotoxicity of MPTP. In fact, simvastatin accumulated in the nigra and suppressed microglial activation, leading to reduced expression of inflammatory cytokines and increased dopaminergic neuroprotection (Ghosh 2009). Another animal experiment found that simvastatin was able to completely reverse the decline in dopamine receptors associate with exposure to the neurotoxin 6-hydroxydopamine (Wang 2005).

In a large human clinical study involving over 700,000 subjects, use of simvastatin was associated with a 49% reduction in the likelihood of onset of Parkinon's symptoms, as well as a 54% reduction in the risk of dementia, suggesting a substantial neuroprotective effect (Wolozin 2007).

Due to the emergence of strong evidence that simvastatin may have anti-inflammatory and neuroprotective actions, **Life Extension** encourages those Parkinson's disease patients taking a cholesterol-lowering medication to talk with their doctor about switching to **simvastatin**. Even those whose cholesterol is not significantly elevated may benefit from low-dose simvastatin – those not taking cholesterol-lowering medication should discuss this with their doctor.

Importantly, those taking any statin drug should be aware that statins deplete coenzyme Q10 (CoQ10) levels. If taking statins, supplement with CoQ10 and ensure maintenance of healthy CoQ10 blood levels by periodically having a CoQ10 blood test.

- Simvastatin (low dose, supplement with ubiquinol form CoQ10 100-300 mg per day)
- Hydergine (ergoloid)
- Deprenyl (selegiline)
- Rasagiline
- Modafinil (provigil)
- Amphetamines & Stimulants
  - Adderall (D-amphetamine salt)
  - Vyvanse (lisdexamfetamine dimesylate)
  - Dex (dextroamphetamine)
  - Methylphenidate (Ritalin)

Paul Erdös, who was on of the most prolific mathematicians to ever live, had a habit of working 19-hour days. He's published more peer review papers than any other mathematician in history and was notorious for heavy amphetamine use.

Science writer Paul Hoffman said: "Like all of Erdös' friends, fellow mathematician Ronal Graham was concerned about his drug taking. In 1979, Graham bet Erdös $500 that he couldn't stop taking amphetamines for a month. Erdös accepted the challenge and went cold turkey for 30 days. After Graham paid up - and wrote the $500 off as a business expense - Erdös said, 'You showed me that I'm not an addict, but I didn't get any work done. I'd get up in the morning and stare at a blank piece of paper. I had no ideas, just like an ordinary person. You've set mathematics back a month.'"

Section Notes:

- Research also suggests nicotine may be helpful in the prevention of Parkinson's disease.
- New research has found that Taurine increases growth of brain cells by activating sleeping stem cells. It also increases the survival of neurons, and it has unique biochemical properties that promote new brain cell formation.

BONUS: KEEPING TRACK
(SELF-MONITORING)

We live in an incredible time with access to tools and testing methods that provide real time feedback on the most important biomarkers of health. To a great degree, many of the biggest threats to our energy and mental clarity can be prevented through consistent monitoring. Without question, the best treatment for fatigue and brain fog is prevention.

There are many diseases and imbalances that can contribute to suboptimal energy and focus. One of the reasons why these imbalances are able to get a foothold is because they often fly under the radar until they reach such a point that their deleterious effects cannot be ignored. The two most important practices you can adopt in order to optimize energy and focus as well as ensure a high quality of life are:

1. A full blood panel every six months (tracking the biomarkers suggested within this section, not just the standard tests issued by your physician).
2. Tracking basic biomarkers of health using simple, at-home monitoring tools.

Another reason why so many people suffer from poor circulation, high blood sugar, high blood pressure, heart disease, cancer, and stroke is poor surveillance. We are simply not aggressive enough when it comes to monitoring and taking responsibility for our own health. Your health, energy, mental clarity, and quality of life is not your doctor's responsibility. That's on you.

AT-HOME MONITORING AND LAB TESTS

Quite frankly, doctors treat symptoms and diseases - and high performance has little to do with the avoidance of disease and everything to do with the pursuit of optimal health. Here are some of the most important at-home monitoring tools and laboratory tests you can use to track biomarkers of health and maintain high levels of energy and cognitive performance:

Fasting blood sugar (glucose): This test measures the concentration of glucose in the blood after an 8-12 hour fast. It's limitation is that it only tells us how blood sugar behaves in a fasted state. It tells us very little about how your blood sugar and insulin respond to the food you consume.

Marker	Ideal
Fasting blood glucose (mg/dL)	<86*
OGGT / post-meal (mg/dL after 2 hours)	<120
Hemoglobin A1c (%)	<5.3

A study of nearly 2,000 men was conducted over a 22-year period, and it was found that when fasting glucose was over 85 mg/dL, those men had a 40% increased risk of death from cardiovascular disease.

This test can easily be taken at home, using a glucometer and testing strips. One of the products I most highly recommend is the Precision Xtra NFR by Abbot, which can also be used to test blood ketones. You'll need the former when initiating therapeutic ketosis, either through a ketogenic diet or fasting. My clients and I will often use both the True Result glucometer and the True Test Blood Glucose Test Strips. This is a more economical option, but it does not test blood ketone levels.

Optimal fasted blood glucose levels are 70 to 85 mg/dL. If your levels are 86 and 99 mg/dL, measures should be taken to lower your fasted glucose levels. Values greater than 99 mg/dL put you at significant risk for heart attack, cancer, stroke, and vascular disease. Levels such as these require more drastic interventions and perhaps the help of an expert. Also, take note that if you're on a low-carb or ketogenic diet, slightly elevated blood sugar levels that are in the 90s or even low 100s may not be an issue provided that your post prandial (after meals) blood glucose levels and hemoglobin A1C are within a healthy range.

Glucose tolerance test: This test gives you the ability to measure your body's insulin response to glucose. The process involves consuming 75 grams of dissolved glucose in a fasted state. Your blood sugar is then tested one or two hours afterwards. There are many studies illustrating the harmful effects of elevated post prandial blood sugar levels. These data points are indicative of your body's insulin sensitivity and elevated levels put you at risk for cardiovascular disease, diabetes, and atherosclerosis.

If you experience "food comas" after eating a meal which contains higher amounts of sugar and carbohydrates, this is often a sign of high post-meal blood sugar and insulin levels. This will affect your energy production, and it may also lead to other health problems involving inflammation and your circulatory health. Ideally, for oral glucose tolerance testing, you'll want your fasting glucose levels to be less than 86 mg/dL. One hour after consuming a 75 gram glucose load, you'll want your blood sugar level to be less than 140 mg/dL. Two hours after the 75 gram glucose load, your levels should be lower than 120 mg/dL, and after three hours, your blood sugar levels should be back to the baseline.

Peak blood sugar levels usually occur 45 minutes after eating, and then for healthy individuals, it should drop back to around 100 mg/dL around the 2-hour mark. If your values are above these metrics, interventions should be made. If your blood sugar is greater than 140 mg/dL after you have consumed a 75 gram glucose load, immediate action should be taken, and you should probably begin working with an expert in order to get your body functioning optimally once more.

Ketones: For individuals implementing therapeutic ketosis through a ketogenic diet, intermittent fasting, or both, the only accurate way to ensure that you are in a state of ketosis is by measuring the ketone levels in your body. To do this most accurately, you'll need to measure the levels of beta-hydroxybutyrate in your blood. This can be done at home

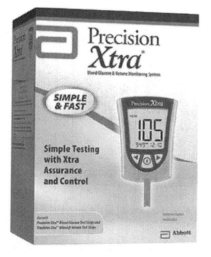

using the Precision Xtra blood glucose monitoring system, which measures both ketone and blood glucose levels with a finger prick approach.

The Precision Xtra blood ketone test strips can get expensive, but it really is worth the investment. Most benefits are derived once ketone levels exceed 1.0 mM, and the recommended range is between 0.5 and 3.0 mM. For many people, there's little need to go above 2.0 mM.

Another ketone testing methods is testing levels of acetoacetate in the urine. This is the easiest way to get started but also may not accurately reflect blood ketone levels once you become fat adapted. In other words, once you start to mobilize ketones routinely in your blood, these tests may no longer work for you. For testing your ketone levels this way, you can use Ketostix test strips, but again, blood testing is recommended.

You could also test for acetone ketones in your breath. Research has shown that there is a correlation between breath acetone levels and blood ketone levels of beta-hydroxybutyrate. One tool that you can use for this is the Ketonics Ketone Breath Monitor. It estimates your beta-hydroxybutyrate in the blood based on the acetone levels in your breath.

Blood Pressure: Hypertension affects one in three people and is a major risk factor for cardiovascular disease and stroke. It's also a useful metric for observing the effects of adrenaline in people who have hypothyroidism, as this condition is one of the major causes of secondary hypertension. The same way that someone does not go from having normal blood glucose levels to being diabetic overnight, there's a gradual progression from healthy blood pressure levels to hypertension. This is great because consistent monitoring allows us to intervene and make the adjustments needed to keep these types of problems from getting out of hand.

Normal blood pressure levels should be less than 120/80 mm Hg. Prehypertension is defined as systolic pressure (the top number which indicates the pressure in the arteries when the heart beats) of 120 to 139 or a diastolic pressure (the bottom number) indicates the pressure in our arteries between heartbeats) between 80 to 89. Hypertension is defined as blood pressure readings of 140/90 or above.

A manual blood pressure reading performed by a trained medical professional is the most accurate way to have your blood pressure

SYSTOLIC CHANGE	POSSIBLE FINDING
Increases 6-10 mm/Hg	Healthy adrenal function
Does not change	Fair adrenal function
Drops 1-10 mm/Hg	Poor adrenal function
Drops more than 10 mm/Hg	Adrenal exhaustion

tested. However, there are a number of digital, at-home blood pressure monitors like the Omron 3 Series Wrist Blood Pressure Monitor. Other recommended at-home monitoring devices are the Omron 10 Series Wireless Upper Arm Blood Pressure Monitor and the Omron 7 Series Ultrasilent Wrist Blood Pressure Monitor.

It is very important that you take your at-home digital blood pressure monitor in to your next doctor's appointment with you. That way, you can have your blood pressure taken by a member of the medical staff using the manual cuff, and then immediately after that, you should measure your blood pressure using your digital at-home device in order to compare the differences between your systolic and diastolic pressures. This process is important in determining the inaccuracy of your digital at-home device, as they all have them.

Personally, I try to keep my blood pressure around 110/75, and I'm usually fairly close. If you have slightly elevated blood pressure levels, I recommend consuming more living, organic plants and gluten-free grains, in addition to getting most of your healthy fats from plant sources like extra virgin olive oil, coconut oil, MCT oil, Udo's Oil 369 blend, flax seed oil, chia seeds, avocados, etc.

You should also discipline yourself so that you are getting 20-30 minutes of cardiovascular exercise each morning, ideally outdoors with lots of skin exposed to direct sunlight. While you do so, you should use

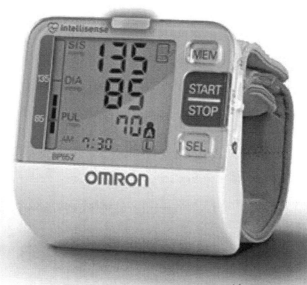

Omron 3 Series Wrist Blood Pressure Monitor

a heart rate monitor to ensure that you are within your target heart rate zone. Furthermore, you should continually work on optimizing your health by following the recommendations within this guide and/or work with an expert to help optimize your health.

Blood Pressure Tests for Adrenal Function: There's a simple adrenal test that you can perform using a blood pressure monitor. It's called the orthostatic hypotension test. Here are the steps to this test:

Step 1: Lay down for five minutes, and then take your blood pressure and make note of the systolic pressure (the top number)
Step 2: Stand up and take your blood pressure again
Step 3: Assess your adrenal functioning

If your systolic pressure drops more than 10 mm Hg, this may be indicative of adrenal fatigue.

If your systolic pressure drops between 1 and 10 mm Hg, this may be indicative of poor adrenal function.

If your systolic pressure does not change, that may be indicative of fair adrenal function.

If your systolic pressure increases 6-10 mm Hg, this may be indicative of healthy adrenal function.

Body Temperature & Your Health: Body temperature can be used to assess thyroid function. Adults with healthy thyroid hormone levels and metabolic health have temperatures around 98.6°F or 37°C in the mid-afternoon (around 3:00 pm, if you wake up between 5-9 am). If you take your mid-afternoon temperature and find that it's in the lower 98°F or even 97°F, this may be a sign that you have suboptimal thyroid function or hypothyroidism.

Another test that I use with clients (www.BioHackingSecrets.com/coaching) who exhibit symptoms of compromised thyroid function is a morning basal temperature reading before getting out of bed. Use a traditional mercury thermometer (which can be purchased on eBay) or a Geratherm thermometer if you're unable to get a traditional

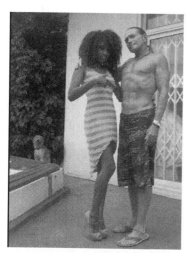

thermometer, and keep it next to your bed so that you can take your temperature first thing in the morning. Again, you'll want to do this before you get out of bed. Take note that using a mercury thermometer will take about ten minutes, but it will give you the most accurate reading. A healthy basil temperature should be between 97.8°F and 98.2°F. If your temperature is lower than 97.8°F it may be a sign of hypothyroidism.

You can also use your body temperature to gauge your adrenal function. A simple test is to take your temperature 3 times a day. The first time, you should take it 3 hours after you wake up, then 3 hours after that, and then again 3 hours later. Total these 3 readings up, and then divide this total by 3 to get an average for the day. This is your daily average temperature. Repeat this process for five consecutive days. If one or more of those daily average temperatures are more than 1.2°F off from one another (or 1.1°C off from one another) this could be a sign that you have cortisol dysregulation or adrenal fatigue.

Static Breath Hold: Prior to his passing, fitness model and industry icon Greg Plitt, had a pool workout that combined resistance training with high intensity sprints and steady state cardio. I did a lot of pool work and yoga on my road to recovery from Lyme Disease. This workout made frequent appearances in the rotation.

At the end of the workout, Plitt had you take a few deep breaths then do an underwater swim to see how far you could go. High level swimmers have done this for decades to strengthen lung capacity, oxygen utilization, and cardiovascular endurance.

Recently static breath holds reemerged in my life when I was introduced to The Wim Hof Method (www.wimhofmethod.com). I now try to incorporate them a couple times a week.

What's most important with static breath holds are not the nuances of how you do it, so much as you do it the same way each time. Reason being you want to compare apples to apples.

Here's how I do my static breath holds, modeling Wim's approach:

- Take 30-35 deep breathes in through the mouth, inhaling deep into the belly until you cannot take in any more air. Let each breath go, but don't force the air out. Imagine letting go the same way air escapes from a deflating air mattress when you first pull the plug.

- After 30-35 breaths, let your last breath go.
- Now, start your stopwatch, and hold your breath as long as you can.
- When you can't physically go any longer, take a deep breath in and hold it for 15 seconds. This trains your body to more efficiently utilize and partition oxygen in a deficit.

Keep in mind the first round is usually unimpressive. Look at it like a warmup. You get better, and more oxygenated, with each full round. Most times, I only do two rounds.

I've been having some conversations with fellow biohacker, and the man behind the EarthPulse PEMF machine, Paul Becker. Here's Paul at age 58, still in amazing shape and looking at least 15 years younger than his chronological age.

Well, one of the cool things about PEMF therapy is it increases mitochondria in the cells, ATP production, and oxygen efficiency. Knowing I've been sleeping on the EarthPulse for a while now, Paul has been eager to see where my static hold time is at. The truth is, I've been putting it off because my sleep schedule has been erratic and my nutrition lacking, at least compared to where it's usually at when I'm not finishing a book.

After a few days of consistent harassment on Skype, I gave in to Paul's request. I always do my static breath holds after exhaling. Some people do them with their lungs filled with air. That obviously affords for longer hold times. It's really whatever you prefer. My best time was right around 2 minutes and 30 seconds.

Just now I did two full rounds of 35 breaths followed by a static hold. The second round I did for time. Despite suboptimal sleep, fewer workouts, and dietary conditions inferior to my norm going in, I held for 3 minutes and 7 seconds after the exhalation. I crushed my previous best time in spite of the circumstances I was up against. You can imagine the results professional athletes see when we combine advanced strategies with optimal nutrition and lifestyle conditions.

Other Important Tests: More important than the results of any test on the planet is paying attention to how your body feels when you first wake up in the morning and throughout the day. Also pay attention to any physical changes that have taken and are taking place. For example, you may have noticed a significant reduction in your sex drive lately, and this could be an indicator that negative changes in your body are taking place. If you have a good night's rest but find yourself tired again just a couple of hours after you wake up, you may need to seek help for whatever is causing that problem. These are obviously just a few examples of many different things that your body is trying to tell you day to day, but paying attention to these sorts of things is the most important test to use for optimizing your overall health.

You can't always just rely on the tests that your doctor recommends. A good example of this is the clients (www.BioHackingSecrets.com/coaching) that I have with thyroid problems. Their tests were not indicating that there was a problem, yet they didn't feel well and knew that something had to be wrong.

If you don't feel as though your are performing optimally as you go about your day, pay attention to what signals your body is sending you and then take action to identify and correct whatever the root cause of those symptoms may be. That being said, here are some tests that will help you monitor what's going on with your body and optimize your health, energy, and focus:

- *Full Blood Panel* (sex hormones, thyroid panel including TSH T4 T3 Reverse T3, blood sugar, lipids, comprehensive metabolic panel, nutrients like B12, magnesium, vitamin D, inflammatory markers like C-reactive protein and homocysteine, GGT, alkaline phosphatase, lactate dehydrogenase, and a CBC complete blood count with basic immune markers, serum iron, ferritin, iron saturation, iron binding capacity). Some companies I have used with clients or had recommended include Life Extension Foundation (they have an annual blood super sale where you can get 50% off labs), WellnessFX, DirectLabs.com, Inside Tracker (www.insidetracker.com), Theranos, and Optimal Wellness Labs MAP Test.
- *Gut Testing:*
  - Doctors Data Comprehensive Stool Analysis with 3 samples
  - MALDTOF method
  - BioHealth 401 (culture-based stool method)
  - SIBO breath testing (Genova)
  - Urinary organic acids profile (Genova Comprehensive Organic Acids Profile)
  - Organic Acids from Great Plains Lab (Genova's is superior)
- *Hormone Testing:*
  - BioHealth 201 (cortisol rhythm, DHEA, total cortisol)
  - 24 hour urine hormone testing (cortisol, tetrahydracortisol, tetrahydracortisone, DHEA) by Genova
  - Adrenal hormone profile (Pharmasan Labs)
- *Methylation Testing:*
  - Functional Methylation Profile by Health Diagnostics and Research Institute
  - Neurotransmitter profile (Pharmasan Labs)

- *Immunological Testing:*
  - Array 3 by Cyrex Labs
  - Array 4 by Cyrex Labs
  - Array 5 by Cyrex Labs
  - Array 7 by Cyrex Labs
  - Array 11 by Cyrex Labs
- *Nutrient Status & Toxic Overload Testing:*
  - Genova NutrEval (or Metametrix One)
  - Urine Amino Acids through Genova or Doctors Data
  - Quicksilver Scientific Heavy Metals test
  - Serum 25-hydroxy vitamin D test (should be > 50 ng/ml)
  - Biological Monitoring test from Pacific Toxicology Laboratories in Los Angeles which look for exposure to environmental contaminants (www.Pactox.com)
  - Food sensitivity profile with separate gluten sensitivity testing (Food Sensitivity Elimination/Reintroduction Eating Program recommended within this guide)
  - Dark Field Microscopy (Live Blood Analysis) - Can reveal and pin-point many underlying issues which are contributing to a current health challenge. Although not diagnostic in itself, Blood Analysis will highlight the factors compromising the ability to achieve balance and health.

Section Notes:

If you have sub-optimal energy and don't know how your adrenals are functioning, it's an excellent idea to do a salivary adrenal panel which will measure your cortisol output over four different intervals during the day. This is different from having your cortisol level tested at the doctor's office, as this is a one-time test and doesn't give you a complete picture of what the adrenals are doing the whole day. In some states, you can order your own test kit from DirectLabs.com. Otherwise, you'll have to have your healthcare practitioner order one for you.

CLOSING

That's everything I have. You now have every piece of biohacking knowledge I can give you. All of my tips, tricks, techniques, tools, and tactics. You're most likely asking, "Okay...what do I do now?"

That's easy. Go back to the foundational program. Twenty-Eight days eating a diet consiting of 80% plant based, mostly vegetables and leafy greens, and 20% animal proteins. Get your fats from plant based source, like extra vigin olive oil, MCT oil, coconut oil, etc.

Remove dairy, alcohol, GMO's, and gluten/grains from your diet. There's a whole list of additional things you should cut out, but at least start with those four.

During the 28 days, go back through the guide and use it to make a plan. Then follow that plan and test and tweak based on how you feel and the home measurements we just discussed.

Look, there is no right or wrong. It's all about making small changes and sticking to them. The smallest change that sticks is better than the largest change that last a week.

Don't be tough on yourself, if you mess up... *start over.*

This is a journey about being the best you you can be. There is no competition, no time limit, and no way for you to be wrong.

Decide which day you're going to start the 28 days foundational diet.

In the meantime start something today. Start small...make a leafy green smoothie. Stop drinking cream in your coffee, and wake up a few minutes earlier so you can make yourself a healthy breakfast rather than eating through a window on your way to work.

If you're already past that stage, start meditating.

Whatever you need to do to take the next step... do it. There's no journey too long that it can't be made, unless you refuse to start.

I'M LOOKING FOR A FEW MORE OF MY
Dream Clients...

"If That's You... I Will PERSONALLY Work With You One-On-One To Create A Custom, Rapid Fat-Loss And Optimal Performance Program For Your Genetic Blueprint And Health Status!"

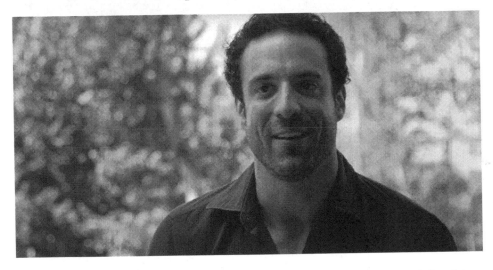

I'm opening an incredible opportunity for you to see *why* Biohacking Secrets Inner Circle is known as *"the place"* where entrepreneurs and executives seeking *fast and dramatic* fat-loss and greater energy, focus, and health come together.

Just for applying, I'll send you a free copy of the lost chapter, "Psychedelics & Controlled Substances" that was so controversial, my lawyers wouldn't allow me to put it in this book. In it, you'll learn:

- How micro-dosing certain psychedelics can expand our consciousness and allow us to *tap into the potential of our subconscious mind.*

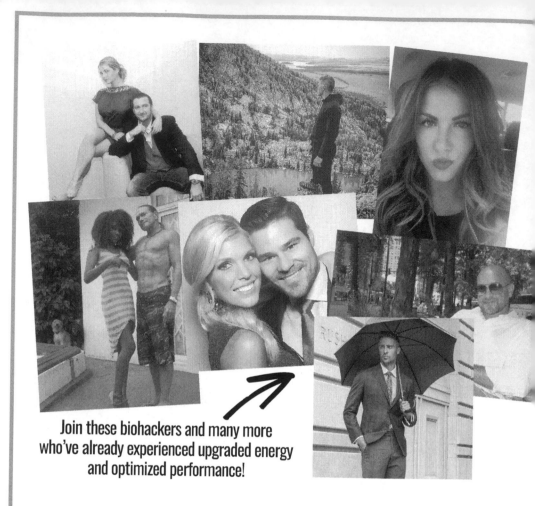

Join these biohackers and many more who've already experienced upgraded energy and optimized performance!

- How micro-dosing specific hallucinogens can be used to *reduce anxiety and stress,* alleviate the symptoms of obsessive-compulsive disorder, and *decrease the frequency and severity of migraines.*
- *How these substances have been used for centuries* by some of history's most prominent leaders and wealthy businessmen, including Barack Obama, Steve Jobs, the Beatles, Richard Branson, Bill Gates, Thomas Edison, and many others.
- The hallucinogen that has been shown to have *therapeutic potential in alcohol addiction.*
- How this natural compound can be used to *enhance recall, improve recollection of memories, and upgrade cognition and memory.*
- Safe and natural ways to therapeutically *overcome depression and*

- *anxiety* without potentially dangerous prescription drugs.
- Plus *much, much more.*

I also want to *give you* $613.91 worth of free Biohacking information including two months as an "Elite" Gold Member of our VIP Training area, where you will receive a steady stream of cutting edge information to make you feel superhuman and optimize your physical and mental performance including:

- ***The 7 Day Weight Loss Kickstart:*** How to lose up to 20 lbs in 7 days without exercise... and keep it off for good!

- ***The Excercise Blueprint:*** Discover the tiniest changes that yeild the biggest returns!

- ***A Digital copy*** of *"The Biohacker's Guide to Upgraded Energy & Focus: An Uncommon System to Rapidly Optimize Physical and Mental Performance"*

And to help you put it all to work, my team and I will give you a ***free health assessment*** to start building the *perfect* program to optimize performance in every area of your life, customized for *your* body type...

We Can Only Work With 8 Clients At A Time, So Apply Now At:
www.BiohackingSecrets.com/apply
or send a text message to 847-989-3743
To Schedule Your Free Health Assessment!

Made in the USA
San Bernardino, CA
04 September 2016